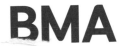
Oxford Case Histories
in Anaesthesia

D1435126

Oxford Case Histories

Series Editors:

Sarah Pendlebury and Peter Rothwell

Published:

Neurological Case Histories (Sarah Pendlebury, Philip Anslow, and Peter Rothwell)

Oxford Case Histories in Cardiology (Rajkumar Rajendram, Javed Ehtisham, and Colin Forfar)

Oxford Case Histories in Gastroenterology and Hepatology (Alissa Walsh, Otto Buchel, Jane Collier, and Simon Travis)

Oxford Case Histories in Respiratory Medicine (John Stradling, Andrew Stanton, Najib Rahman, Annabel Nickol, and Helen Davies)

Oxford Case Histories in Rheumatology (Joel David, Anne Miller, Anushka Soni, and Lyn Williamson)

Oxford Case Histories in TIA and Stroke (Sarah Pendlebury, Ursula Schulz, Aneil Malhotra, and Peter Rothwell)

Oxford Case Histories in Neurosurgery (Harutomo Hasegawa, Matthew Crocker, and Pawan Singh Minhas)

Oxford Case Histories in Oncology (Thankamma Ajithkumar, Adrian Harnett, and Tom Roques)

Oxford Case Histories in Anaesthesia

Edited by

Jon McCormack
Consultant Anaesthetist,
Royal Hospital for Sick Children,
Edinburgh, Scotland, UK

Keith Kelly
Consultant Anaesthetist,
Royal Hospital for Sick Children,
Edinburgh, Scotland, UK

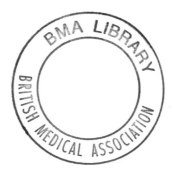

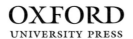

OXFORD
UNIVERSITY PRESS

OXFORD
UNIVERSITY PRESS

Great Clarendon Street, Oxford, OX2 6DP,
United Kingdom

Oxford University Press is a department of the University of Oxford.
It furthers the University's objective of excellence in research, scholarship,
and education by publishing worldwide. Oxford is a registered trade mark of
Oxford University Press in the UK and in certain other countries

Published in the United States of America by Oxford University Press
198 Madison Avenue, New York, NY 10016, United States of America

British Library Cataloguing in Publication Data
Data available

Library of Congress Control Number: 2014936673

ISBN 978–0–19–870486–7

Printed and bound by
CPI Group (UK) Ltd, Croydon, CR0 4YY

Oxford University Press makes no representation, express or implied, that the
drug dosages in this book are correct. Readers must therefore always check
the product information and clinical procedures with the most up-to-date
published product information and data sheets provided by the manufacturers
and the most recent codes of conduct and safety regulations. The authors and
the publishers do not accept responsibility or legal liability for any errors in the
text or for the misuse or misapplication of material in this work. Except where
otherwise stated, drug dosages and recommendations are for the non-pregnant
adult who is not breast-feeding

Links to third party websites are provided by Oxford in good faith and
for information only. Oxford disclaims any responsibility for the materials
contained in any third party website referenced in this work.

A note from the series editors

Case histories have always had an important role in medical education, but most published material has been directed at undergraduates or residents. The Oxford Case Histories series aims to provide more complex case-based learning for clinicians in specialist training and consultants, with a view to aiding preparation for entry- and exit-level specialty examinations or revalidation.

Each case book follows the same format with approximately 50 cases, each comprising a brief clinical history and investigations, followed by questions on differential diagnosis and management, and detailed answers with discussion.

At the end of each book, cases are listed by mode of presentation, aetiology, and diagnosis. We are grateful to our colleagues in the various medical specialties for their enthusiasm and hard work in making the series possible.

Sarah Pendlebury and Peter Rothwell

From reviews of other books in the series:

Neurological Case Histories
'. . . contains 51 cases that cover the spectrum of acute neurology and the neurology of general medicine—this breadth makes the volume unique and provides a formidable challenge . . . it is a heavy-duty diagnostic series of cases, and readers have to work hard, to recognise the diagnosis and answer the questions that are posed for each case . . . I recommend this excellent volume highly . . . '

Lancet Neurology

'This short and well-written text is . . . designed to enhance the reader's diagnostic ability and clinical understanding . . . A well-documented and practical book.'

European Journal of Neurology

Oxford Case Histories in Gastroenterology and Hepatology
'. . . a fascinating insight into clinical gastroenterology, an excellent and enjoyable read and an education for all levels of gastroenterologist from ST1 to consultant.'

Gut

Preface

This textbook is the latest in the *Oxford University Press Case Histories* series. It has tried to stay true to the basic form of the earlier works, i.e. the case histories are largely based on (anonymous) real cases, and a small amount of information is given, followed by a question posed as to how the patient should be managed. The reader should thus try to formulate a management plan in their own mind at each stage before reading further. However, the authors recognize that a book on anaesthetic management is subtly different from other specialties.

First, the diagnosis has generally been made, and one is usually asked to provide an anaesthetic intervention for a procedure to treat that diagnosis. That said, one should always keep an open mind. Thus, there is a break from the pattern in other books of history–investigation–diagnosis–treatment. Each chapter in this book has a brief introduction with some learning outcomes for the following cases. As some of the chapters could warrant a book in their own right, we have not attempted to give a comprehensive overview of all possible cases within one area. Rather, we have attempted to report important cases which illustrate learning outcomes within this field.

Second, there is often a lack of what would arguably be called the gold standard of treatment in medicine (an adequately powered randomized controlled trial in humans) in the practice of anaesthesia. The decision as to which anaesthetic technique is used will be determined by such factors as the condition and comorbidities of that patient, the experience of the individual anaesthetist, and, in some circumstances, the equipment available. There is thus generally a discussion of the advantages and disadvantages of the techniques used.

There are also some concepts in anaesthesia that do not fit easily into a case-based discussion yet are still important to the practice of anaesthesia as a whole. This is best exemplified in Chapter 1, which touches on the efficient running of an anaesthetic list and department, as well as the discussion of anaesthetic risk.

Whilst every care has been taken to ensure that the book is free from factual errors, it is left to the reader to ensure the correct dosage of any drug regimen mentioned.

We hope this textbook will be of use to not only anaesthetic colleagues in training, particularly those preparing for professional examinations, but also to the established anaesthetist in terms of their continuing education.

We acknowledge that there is some overlap between cases. However this merely emphasizes the multi-faceted way that similar problems may present to colleagues regardless of which subspecialty of anaesthesia they practice.

We would like to thank all the colleagues who contributed to this book. Most of all, we would like to thank our respective families for their tolerance and unstinting support during the preparation of this work.

JG McCormack, KP Kelly
Edinburgh, July 2014

Contents

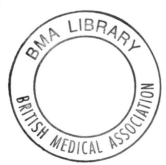

Symbols and abbreviations

<	less than
>	more than
≥	equal to or greater than
≤	equal to or less than
=	equal to
±	plus or minus
°C	degree Celsius
®	registered trademark
™	trademark
α	alpha
β	beta
γ	gamma
AAA	abdominal aortic aneurysm
AAGBI	Association of Anaesthetists of Great Britain and Ireland
ABG	arterial blood gas
AC	alternative current
ACE	angiotensin-converting enzyme
ACOM	anterior communicating artery
ACoT	acute coagulopathy of trauma
ACT	activated clotting time
ADH	antidiuretic hormone
ADHD	attention deficit hyperactivity disorder
A&E	accident and emergency
AECC	American-European Consensus Conference
AF	atrial fibrillation
AFOI	awake fibreoptic intubation
Alb	albumin
ALF	acute liver failure
ALI	acute lung injury
ALP	alkaline phosphatase
ALT	alanine transaminase
a.m.	before noon (*ante meridiem*)
ANH	acute normovolaemic haemodilution
AP	anteroposterior
APACHE	Acute Physiology and Chronic Health Evaluation
APLS	advanced paediatric life support
APTT	activated partial thromboplastin time
ARDS	acute respiratory distress syndrome
ASA	American Society of Anaesthetists
ASDH	acute subdural haematoma
AT	anaerobic threshold
ATLS	advanced trauma life support
atm	atmosphere
ATP	adenosine triphosphate
AVR	aortic valve replacement
bd	twice daily
BE	base excess
Bil	bilirubin
BIS	bispectral index
BMI	body mass index (kg/m^2)
BNP	brain natriuretic peptide
BP	blood pressure
bpm	beat per minute
BSA	body surface area
BTS	blood transfusion service
BURP	backward, upward, and rightward pressure
CABG	coronary artery bypass grafting
CAP	community-acquired pneumonia
CAT	Combat Application Tourniquet
CBG	capillary blood gas
CCU	coronary care unit
CEA	carotid endarterectomy; continuous epidural analgesia

CEMACH	Confidential Enquiry into Maternal and Child Health
CEPOD	Confidential Enquiry into Perioperative Deaths
CGA	corrected gestational age
CICV	'can't intubate, can't ventilate'
Cl^-	chloride
cm	centimetre
CMACE	Centre for Maternal and Child Enquiries
$CMRO_2$	cerebral metabolic rate of oxygen
CNS	central nervous system
CO	carbon monoxide
COHb	carboxyhaemoglobin
COPD	chronic obstructive pulmonary disease
CPAP	continuous positive airway pressure
CPB	cardiopulmonary bypass
CPET	cardiopulmonary exercise testing
CPM	central pontine myelinolysis
CPP	cerebral perfusion pressure
CPSP	chronic post-surgical pain
Cr	creatinine
CRP	C-reactive protein
CRPS	complex regional pain syndrome
CRT	capillary refill time
C&S	culture and sensitivity
CSE	combined spinal and epidural
CSF	cerebrospinal fluid
CT	computed tomography
CTG	cardiotocography
CVC	central venous catheter
CVP	central venous pressure
CVVH	continuous veno-venous haemofiltration
CXR	chest X-ray
DHS	dynamic hip screw
DIC	dissseminated intravascular coagulation
DIND	delayed ischaemic neurological deficit

dL	decilitre
DLT	double-lumen tube
DMSO	dimethyl sulfoxide
DNIC	diffuse noxious inhibitory control
DVT	deep vein thrombosis
ECF	extracellular fluid
ECG	electrocardiogram
ECMO	extracorporeal membrane oxygenation
ED	emergency department
EEG	electroencephalogram
eGFR	estimated glomerular filtration rate
EMG	electromyography
ENT	ear, nose, and throat
ERAS	enhanced recovery after surgery
ERCP	endoscopic retrograde cholangiopancreatography
$ETCO_2$	end-tidal carbon dioxide
ETT	endotracheal tube
EuroSCORE	European System for Cardiac Operative Risk Evaluation
EVD	external ventricular drain
FAST	focussed assessment sonography in trauma
FBC	full blood count
FEV_1	forced expiratory volume in 1 second
FFP	fresh frozen plasma
FiO_2	fraction of inspired oxygen concentration
FRC	functional residual capacity
ft	foot/feet
FVC	forced vital capacity
g	gram
GAS	Group A β-haemolytic *Streptococcus*
GCS	Glasgow coma score
GI	gastrointestinal
GP	general practitioner
γGT	gamma glutamyl transferase
GTN	glyceryl trinitrate
H^+	hydrogen ion

HAI	hospital-acquired infection	LRTI	lower respiratory tract infection
Hb	haemoglobin		
HCC	hepatocellular carcinoma	LV	left ventricle/ventricular
HCO$_3^-$	bicarbonate	Lymph	lymphocyte
HDU	high dependency unit	m	metre
HELLP	haemolysis, elevated liver enzymes, and low platelet	mA	milli ampere
		MAC	minimum alveolar concentration
HiB	*Haemophilus influenzae* B (vaccine)	MACE	major adverse cardiovascular events
HIV	human immunodeficiency virus	MAP	mean arterial pressure
HLS	helicopter landing site	MCA	middle cerebral artery
HR	heart rate	MCF	maximum clot firmness
hsCRP	high-sensitivity C-reactive protein	MELD	Model for End-stage Liver Disease
IABP	intra-aortic balloon pump	MET	metabolic equivalent
IASP	International Association for the Study of Pain	mg	milligram
		MI	myocardial infarction
IBS	irritable bowel syndrome	MILS	manual in-line stabilization
IC	ileal conduit	min	minute
ICF	intracellular fluid	ml	millilitre
ICP	intracranial pressure	mm	millimetre
ICU	intensive care unit	MMF	mycophenolate mofetil
ID	internal diameter	mmHg	millimetre of mercury
IFR	instrument flight rules	mmol	millimole
IM	intramuscular	MODS	multiorgan dysfunction syndrome
INR	international normalized ratio	mol	mole
IPPV	intermittent positive pressure ventilation	mph	mile per hour
		MPS	mucopolysaccharidoses
IR	interventional radiology	MRI	magnetic resonance imaging
IU	international unit	MRSA	methicillin-resistant *Staphylococcus aureus*
IUGR	intrauterine growth restriction		
IV	intravenous	mV	millivolt
JVP	jugular venous pressure	MV	minute ventilation
K$^+$	potassium	Na$^+$	sodium
KCC	King's College criteria	NAC	N-acetylcysteine
km	kilometre	NaCl	sodium chloride
kPa	kilopascal	NAP4	National Audit Project 4 (RCoA audit of airway complications)
L	litre		
LBW	low birthweight		
LFT	liver function test	NBM	nil by mouth
LMA	laryngeal mask airway	Neutr	neutrophil
LMWH	low molecular weight heparin	ng	nanogram

NG	nasogastric
NHS	National Health Service
NHSLA	National Health Service Litigation Authority
NIBP	non-invasive blood pressure
NICE	National Institute for Health and Clinical Excellence
nmol	nanomole
NPSA	National Patient Safety Agency
NSAID	non-steroidal anti-inflammatory drugs
NT-BNP	N-terminal brain natriuretic peptide
od	once daily
OLV	one-lung ventilation
OPCABG	off-pump coronary artery bypass graft
p	probability
$PaCO_2$	partial pressure of carbon dioxide
PACU	post-anaesthetic care unit
PAD	preoperative autologous blood donation
PaO_2	partial pressure of oxygen
PAOP	pulmonary artery occlusion pressure
PCA	patient-controlled analgesia
PCC	prothrombin complex concentrate
PCEA	patient-controlled epidural analgesia
PCI	percutaneous coronary intervention
PE	pulmonary embolus
PEEP	positive end-expiratory pressure
PET	positron emission tomography
PICU	paediatric intensive care unit
PLP	phantom limb pain
Plt	platelet
p.m.	after noon (*post meridiem*)
PNL	percutaneous nephrolithotomy
POCD	post-operative cognitive dysfunction

PONV	post-operative nausea and vomiting
POSSUM	Physiological and Operative Severity Score for Enumeration of Mortality and Morbidity
PPI	proton pump inhibitor
PPV	positive pressure ventilation
PR	per rectum
PRC	packed red cell
PT	prothrombin time
PVR	pulmonary vascular resistance
qds	four times daily
RCC	red cell concentrate
RCOG	Royal College of Obstetricians and Gynaecologists
RCRI	revised cardiac risk index
RCT	randomized controlled trial
RR	respiratory rate
RRT	renal replacement therapy
RSI	rapid sequence induction
RSV	respiratory syncytial virus
s	second
SAPS	Simplified Acute Physiology Score
SCBU	special care baby unit
SDD	selective decontamination of the digestive tract
SGA	supraglottic airway
SIRS	systemic inflammatory response syndrome
SOD	selective oral decontamination
SOMCT	short orientation memory concentration test
SpO_2	peripheral oxygen saturation
SVR	systemic vascular resistance
TACO	transfusion-associated cardiac overload
TAo	transaortic
TAp	transapical
TAP	transversus abdominal plane
TAVI	transcatheter aortic valve implantation
TBW	total body water

TCI	target-controlled infusion
tds	three times daily
TED	thromboembolism deterrent
TEG	thromboelastography
TENS	transcutaneous electrical nerve stimulation
TF	transfemoral
TIA	transient ischaemic attack
TIVA	total intravenous anaesthesia
TOE	transoesophageal echocardiography
TRALI	transfusion-associated acute lung injury
TRiM	Trauma Risk Management
TRIM	transfusion-associated immunomodulation
TURP	transurethral resection of the prostate
U	unit
U&E	urea and electrolytes
UK	United Kingdom
URTI	upper respiratory tract infection
USS	ultrasound scan
UTI	urinary tract infection
V	volt
VALI	ventilator-associated lung injury
VAP	ventilator-associated pneumonia
VAS	visual analogue scale
vHLD	von Hippel–Lindau disease
VILI	ventilator-induced lung injury
VLBW	very low birthweight
VO_2 peak	peak oxygen consumption
V/Q	ventilation/perfusion
VRIII	variable rate intravenous insulin infusion
vs	versus
VTE	venous thromboembolism
WCC	white cell count
WHO	World Health Organization

Contributors

Dr Talat Aziz
Clinical Director & Consultant
Anaesthetist,
Department of Anaesthesia,
Critical Care and Pain Medicine,
Western General Hospital,
Edinburgh, Scotland

Dr Clair Baldie
Consultant Anaesthetist,
Department of Anaesthesia,
Critical Care and Pain Medicine,
Western General Hospital,
Edinburgh, Scotland

Mr Peter Bodkin
Consultant Neurosurgeon and
Honorary Senior Lecturer,
Aberdeen Royal Infirmary, Scotland

Dr Caroline Brookman
Consultant Anaesthetist,
Department of Anaesthesia,
Critical Care and Pain Medicine,
Western General Hospital,
Edinburgh, Scotland

Dr Vicki Clark
Consultant Anaesthetist,
Simpson Centre for Reproductive
Health, Royal Infirmary,
Little France Crescent, Edinburgh

Dr Alistair Gibson
Specialty Trainee,
Department of Anaesthetics,
Critical Care and Pain Medicine,
Royal Infirmary of Edinburgh,
Edinburgh, Scotland

Dr Simon Heaney
Specialist Trainee,
South East of Scotland School
of Anaesthesia

Dr Christopher Hoy
Specialist Registrar in Anaesthesia,
East of Scotland Deanery,
Ninewells Hospital, Dundee,
Scotland

Dr Vanessa Humphrey
Specialist Trainee,
South East of Scotland School
of Anaesthesia

Dr Keith Kelly
Consultant Neuroanaesthetist,
Department of Anaesthesia,
Critical Care and Pain Medicine,
Western General Hospital,
Edinburgh, Scotland

Dr Rosie Macfadyen
Consultant in Critical Care,
Western General Hospital,
Crewe Road, Edinburgh, Scotland

Dr Jon McCormack
Consultant in Paediatric Intensive
Care Retrieval and Emergency
Medical Retrieval,
Royal Hospital for Sick Children,
Edinburgh and City Heliport,
Glasgow, Scotland

Dr Karen McGrath
Consultant in Paediatric Anaesthesia,
Royal Hospital for Sick Children,
Edinburgh, Scotland

Dr Euan McGregor
Specialty Trainee,
South East Scotland School
of Anaesthesia, Scotland

Dr Omair Malik
Consultant in Paediatric
Anaesthesia and Paediatric
Intensive Care Retrieval, Royal
Hospital for Sick Children,
Edinburgh, Scotland

Dr Ivan Marples
Consultant Neuroanaesthetist,
Department of Anaesthesia,
Critical Care and Pain Medicine,
Western General Hospital,
Edinburgh, Scotland

Dr Rory Mayes
Consultant in Critical
Care Medicine and Anaesthesia,
Scottish Liver Transplant Unit,
Royal Infirmary of Edinburgh,
Scotland

Dr Sheena Millar
Consultant, Cardiothoracic
Anaesthesia,
Department of Anaesthetics,
Critical Care and Pain Medicine,
Royal Infirmary of Edinburgh,
Edinburgh, Scotland

Dr Colin Moore
Consultant, Cardiothoracic
Anaesthesia,
Department of Anaesthetics,
Critical Care and Pain Medicine,
Royal Infirmary of Edinburgh,
Scotland

Dr Anil Patel
Consultant Anaesthetist, Royal
National Throat Nose & Ear Hospital
and University College Hospital,
London

Dr Linzi Peacock
Consultant Anaesthetist, Simpson
Centre for Reproductive Health,
Royal Infirmary, Edinburgh, Scotland

Dr Joanna Renée
Specialist Trainee, South East
of Scotland School of Anaesthesia

Dr Mark Ross
Specialist Trainee South East of
Scotland School of Anaesthesia

Dr Matthew T Royds
Consultant Anaesthetist,
Western General Hospital, Crewe
Road South, Edinburgh, Scotland

Dr Prit Singh
Consultant Anaesthetist,
Department of Anaesthesia,
Critical Care and Pain Medicine,
Western General Hospital,
Edinburgh, Scotland

Dr Alastair J Thomson
Consultant Anaesthetist,
Royal Infirmary of Edinburgh,
Edinburgh, Scotland

Dr Alasdair Waite
Consultant Anaesthetist, Department
of Anaesthesia, Critical Care and
Pain Medicine, Western General
Hospital, Edinburgh, Scotland

Dr Jonathan Wedgwood
Consultant Anaesthetist,
Department of Anaesthesia,
Critical Care and Pain Medicine,
Western General Hospital,
Edinburgh, Scotland

Dr Neil H Young
Consultant in Critical Care Medicine
and Anaesthesia, General Intensive
Care Unit, Royal Infirmary of
Edinburgh

Chapter 1

General anaesthesia

Dr Jonathan Wedgwood
Dr Talat Aziz

Waiting times: improving theatre productivity and minimizing expenditure

Background

The aim of all anaesthetic departments ought to be the delivery of a high-quality, safe, and efficient service. Quality and safety in the delivery of health care must not be compromised in our pursuit for increasing efficiency and productivity.

Learning outcomes

1 Understand where system inefficiencies impact on theatre utilization

2 Identify processes for improving utilization within current resources

3 Consider options for additional resources to improve theatre efficiency.

CPD matrix matches

1I02; 1I05

Case history

In order to achieve waiting time targets, your trust has introduced waiting list initiatives and is using the independent sector to help with capacity. Your chief executive feels that the theatre suite is not working as well as it ought to be. You are asked to introduce changes that will increase productivity without incurring additional costs but maintaining safety and quality. Is this possible?

The use of operating theatre sessions and the time within each session are sources of angst for health care providers worldwide. The perfect operating list remains the 'holy grail', and much work has focussed on trying to achieve this. Many a consultancy has developed to help organizations improve their processes in order to help attain this.

Acquiring data to establish our position and how we benchmark against others will provide information on our current status. Successful and sustainable implementation of recommendations for change is more likely if they have been identified by our own staff groups in a 'bottom-up' approach. Data collection is necessary in order to comply with local and national requirements. There often is a disconnect between data collection and its role in introducing change within an organization.

An appropriately scheduled theatre day should ensure maximum productivity. A smooth running day improves staff morale, and this is enhanced further when the day's scheduled activity is completed as predicted. The fiscal benefit is a reduction in overtime benefits. Our patients benefit in having their procedure performed on the identified day, and there is no diversion of resources from our emergency cases.

Scheduling is often performed by non-clinical waiting list managers and is reliant upon the information provided by the referring surgeon. This may include information relating to the anticipated duration of the procedure and the predicted length of hospital stay. This information is used to populate the theatre list, and the durations of procedures are summed up until the total time available for that particular session has been achieved. Inaccuracies in this information will result in either an under- or oversubscribed list. Anecdotally, experienced theatre personnel are often able to predict the likelihood of either outcome.

More accurate theatre lists may be produced by changing from a manual, subjective method to a list populated by historical data. Various software packages exist and require the input of information, in order to establish a 'total' time frame for a specific procedure performed by a named surgeon. The total time is made up of a number of discrete units, e.g. time in the anaesthetic room, time of the actual operation, and time to transfer the patient to the recovery area. This would result in fewer operating lists overrunning that affect staff morale but also in generating fewer overtime payments.

Improving the scheduling of our theatre sessions will also have a positive impact on our patient population: fewer patients cancelled on the day of their surgery or fewer emergency surgery being delayed due to late-running elective theatre lists. Urgent and emergency surgery carried out overnight is associated with a higher incidence of morbidity and mortality. Our staff morale will improve, as their personal lives will be less disrupted because of the need to stay beyond their agreed hours. If undersubscribed sessions were also better populated, we may be able to demonstrate increased productivity by performing more procedures and rely less on expensive alternatives such as waiting list initiatives and engaging with the private sector.

A National Theatres' Project Steering Group was established to investigate how operating theatres could improve patient experience and outcome. A further objective was to treat more patients by using resources more productively and efficiently to deliver best value. The report highlighted the requirement for continuous improvement and a focus on:

- Comparability: development of consistent data collection and performance management for theatre services
- Efficiency: management of limited and expensive theatre resources more efficiently
- Quality: improving patient experience and health outcomes.

In order to benchmark our activity, there has to be agreed theatre definitions, together with a systematic reporting of key performance indicators, including:

- Percentage of sessions used
- Underruns
- Overruns
- Percentage of time used in session
- Theatre utilization: defined as the percentage of actual hours used as a percentage of the planned allocated hours and is a key measure used to identify theatre efficiency.

Using the data

'88% theatre utilization and 99.9% time used—time to celebrate?'

Whilst 88% session utilization appears good, it is important to recognize that 12% of available sessions are not being used. Ninety-nine per cent of the utilization of the available time appears to be excellent, with virtually no available time being unused. However, this may mask a large degree of variation within this figure, with many operating lists either finishing >45 min early (the minimum time required to perform an additional case) or overrunning by 30 min, thereby impacting on our staff.

Suboptimal use of the available time has a number of possible implications:

- Patient experience: theatre lists that are overbooked are more likely to lead to patients being cancelled, due to lack of operating time
- Staff experience and morale: overrunning lists require staff to work beyond their contracted hours. Staff accept that, on occasions, procedures can and do take longer than expected. Accurate scheduling would minimize elective list overruns
- Impact on waiting times: lists that are consistently underrunning could have been used to support additional activity

- Overtime payments: lists which overrun may result in additional costs
- Absenteeism: there is a correlation between areas which regularly overrun and higher levels of sickness absence.

Theatre efficiency and productivity continue to challenge the National Health Service (NHS) and also private and public health care providers globally. There is a great deal of theory published, underpinning the implementation of change, but there is no single solution that resolves all issues, and the 'perfect operating list' remains elusive.

How do we use our time better?

Historically, little regard has been paid to the capacity planning for each specialty. Analysing retrospective data will allow us to make a more accurate prediction of the needs of each service in the forthcoming year. If it transpires that a specialty has consistently used 75% of its available capacity over the last few years, this is highly suggestive of a surplus of supply vs demand. These unused, but funded, sessions ought to be offered to specialties where demand exceeds supply.

There is a need to establish a weekly meeting of all stakeholders, in order to ensure maximal utilization of funded theatre sessions. Communication is the key component for the meetings to be successful, with all surgical leave approved at least 6 weeks in advance. The multidisciplinary team meeting requires representation from all surgical disciplines, anaesthesia, theatre and ward staff, radiographers, and waiting list managers, in order to ensure:

- Theatre resources are used appropriately
- Weekly review of required sessions and list construction
- Changes to average procedure times are agreed.

An example of how these meetings may be used successfully is as follows:

1 Six weeks before the scheduled list: vacant theatre lists can be offered to another surgeon within the same specialty

2 Four weeks before the list: vacant theatre sessions can be offered out to other specialties to use

3 Three weeks before the list: review of lists, patients booked. Agree the order of operating list; identify any equipment, staffing issues. Identify any potential unused capacity (unless time slots are required for urgent patients) or potential overruns

4 One week before the list: finalize the order of list; confirm equipment availability; ensure operating lists are full

5 Forty-eight hours before surgery: booking coordinator to confirm all lists are final

6 Day of surgery: changes to lists on the day of surgery must be regarded as the exception. Any changes required on the day of surgery must be notified through the identified theatre coordinator and the reasons recorded. This needs to be the subject to ongoing monitoring

7 Compliance: monitoring of compliance with agreed standards. Poor or no compliance should be discussed with the clinical management team concerned and corrective actions agreed.

The introduction of such a meeting to an organization can significantly increase theatre utilization, thereby reducing waiting times. Achieving this aim requires a structured programme of ongoing practical education to ensure all staff can work flexibly across more than one specialty.

Three-session days?

The surgical case-mix of certain specialties does not lend itself well to the traditional office hours that we tend to adhere to. A three-session day (1 session = 1 half day) may be adopted in a theatre list which has traditionally overrun. This requires consultation with all key stakeholders; staff ought to be given the opportunity of opting into this new way of working. It may suit some individuals to work a longer day, but no individuals should be coerced into this work pattern. Staff groups may be willing to adapt to the needs of the service, as a predictable longer work day is more preferable than a day that overruns because of an overbooked list.

Any other factors that may reduce efficiency?

In order to ensure these changes result in the expected benefits, a robust pre-assessment process is required to ensure that all patients present for surgery in their optimal state; the first patient arrives in the anaesthetic room at an appropriate time, and the turnaround time between successive patients is minimized.

Summary

Operating theatre productivity can be increased, without increasing costs, by better utilization of the number of funded sessions, together with an improved use of time within each session. This can be achieved by improving communication between specialties and increasing the accuracy of the scheduling process. A process of ongoing education and personal development will allow all theatre team members to be both comfortable and competent, covering specialties other than their core activity, thereby maintaining quality and safety.

Further reading

NHS Institute for Innovation and Improvement. *The productive series.* Available at: <http://www.institute.nhs.uk/quality_and_value/productivity_series/the_productive_series.html>.

Pandit JJ, Abbott T, Pandit M, Kapila A, and Abraham R (2012). Is 'starting on time' useful (or useless) as a surrogate measure for 'surgical theatre efficiency'? *Anaesthesia*, **67**, 823–32.

Pandit JJ and Tavare A (2011). Using mean duration and variation of procedure times to plan a list of surgical operations to fit into the scheduled list time. *European Journal of Anaesthesiology*, **28**, 493–501.

Scottish Executive (2006). *National theatres final project report: national benchmarking project.* Available at: <http://www.scotland.gov.uk/Publications/2006/11/24135440/2>.

University of Iowa, Carver College of Medicine. *Bibliography*. Available at: <http://www.franklindexter.net/bibliography_TOC.htm>.

Case 1.2

Assessing and explaining risk and predicting outcome

Background

'Risk' is the probability or likelihood of loss, injury, or other undesirable event, which, although unintended, occurs as a consequence of a particular course of action. Clinicians often perceive these as death or serious morbidity, but, for the patient, increased dependence, loss of independence, or prolonged recovery and rehabilitation may be as important, particularly in the elderly or near the end of life. 'Risk assessment' is an objective structured investigation to determine and quantify those factors that could cause an adverse outcome. This must be coupled with the formulation and implementation of a management plan to ameliorate those risks. Notwithstanding, risk will remain, and the patient should be aware of this.

Learning outcomes

1 Understanding the need for risk assessment
2 Awareness of different tools available for assessing risk
3 Applying risk assessment to the clinical context.

CPD matrix matches

2A03

Case history

You are asked by a colorectal surgeon for your expert opinion on an 85-year-old woman with a tumour in her sigmoid colon and a single hepatic metastasis. She has controlled hypertension, chronic kidney disease stage 3, ischemic heart disease, and a past history of myocardial infarction (MI). She cares for her 92-year-old husband who is blind and has mild dementia. She would require sigmoid colectomy and segmental hepatic resection. The surgeon is concerned about her fitness for anaesthesia. How do you respond?

Introduction to risk assessment

Make sure that you know what you are being asked. The surgeon may be asking for an objective structured assessment of risk, prior to making decisions on further management. They may already be of the opinion that major surgery is inappropriate or be reluctant to undertake it and asking you to confirm their assessment and reinforce that view with the patient.

If the referral request is not explicit, clarify the request before seeing the patient. When you see the patient, establish from the outset what they have already been told, what they understand, and what they expect of the consultation with you.

Try to gain an impression early on of the patient's appreciation of the potential risks. Some patients who have significant comorbidity or who have had surgery before already have an awareness that significant risks are involved; others have no concept at all or prefer not to think about them.

What is fitness for anaesthesia?

It is a misconception of many patients and other clinicians that anaesthesia poses the major risk and consequently is the primary determinant of outcome, but it is also unhelpful to consider the risks attributable solely to anaesthesia, which are, in fact, very low. The final outcome is dependent on the interactions between the patient, the controlled trauma of surgery, the anaesthetic, the perioperative care, and the system delivering that care. Consequently, one might say all patients are fit for anaesthesia; the real question is what degree of risk is acceptable. However, it should be remembered that knowledge of risk is of little value; it is balanced against the benefits of the proposed treatment.

What is the purpose of risk assessment?

We have an obligation to act in the best interests of our patients and to refrain from doing harm. Knowledge of the risks associated with a particular course of action allows:

1 Informed consent: the patient must be informed of the benefits and risks of a particular treatment or surgical procedure; importantly, this should include the risks and benefits of any alternative treatment, including non-operative interventions. It is difficult for the anaesthetist to have an in-depth understanding of the benefit of a surgical procedure: 5-year survival, disease-free survival, functional outcome, and, equally and importantly, the consequences of undertaking a modified procedure or not performing the procedure at all. This requires close cooperation and communication between the surgeon, the anaesthetist, other clinicians, the patient, and, where appropriate,

the carers and relatives. In the absence of a well-organized multidisciplinary team, this can be difficult to achieve smoothly. Consequently, there may be a degree of uncertainty. At the first meeting with the patient, this should be explained and the opportunity for a further consultation offered

2 Consideration of a modified, less extensive procedure with lower overall risk: clearly, this also alters the potential benefits. This may include non-operative interventions. In this case, segmental, rather than curative, resection, avoidance of hepatic resection, placement of a colonic stent, or no surgical intervention, until there is incipient bowel obstruction (in which case, palliative colostomy could be performed), are all possibilities. Patients often have a misconception that non-surgical treatment means no treatment at all. It is important to reassure them that this is not the case

3 Targeted perioperative care:

   (a) Optimize medical care and control comorbidity preoperatively

   (b) Initiate specific treatments designed to reduce risk: this may include the prescription of beta (β)-blockade or statins in patients at high risk of cardiovascular complications. In this case, the patient is on both of these classes of drug; they should be continued perioperatively

   (c) Choice of anaesthetic technique and intraoperative management strategy, including the use of invasive monitoring

   (d) Planned use of level 2 or level 3 care post-operatively.

What means/tools are available to assess risk?

In attempting to predict outcome, simply identifying characteristics or factors which have been shown to be associated with increased risk is not sufficient. These risk factors must be correlated with outcome in a predictable way. Ideally, there will be a graded relationship between these factors and outcome, allowing stratification of risk. For example, there is an increased risk of renal injury in patients with pre-existing renal impairment, diabetes, congestive cardiac failure, or liver disease, undergoing major surgery, but the risk is not quantifiable.

The key aims of a risk prediction strategy are:

- Objective
- Patient-specific
- Simple
- Easy to use
- Low cost
- Reliable

- Allows gradation or stratification of risk
- Non-interventional.

Scoring systems or risk indices have been developed, using multiple variables weighted for significance and combined to produce an overall score. One of the best known is the American Society of Anaesthetists (ASA) physical status grading system developed in 1941 and revised in 1960. This relies solely on the assessment of the absence or presence and severity of systemic disease and is easy to use and can be applied preoperatively. However, it has been shown to be subject to significant interobserver variability. Importantly, it does not include patient-specific data (e.g. age, gender), information on type or extent of surgery, or surgical pathology. Consequently, although ASA status has been shown to correlate with risk and outcome, it can only give a general impression of the overall risk which is not patient-specific. Despite this, its usefulness for a rapid prospective assessment of risk should not be underestimated.

Increasing the number of variables in the score tends to increase the predictive value, and increasing the amount of patient-specific data should make the score more applicable to that individual; however, this also increases the complexity of the scoring system.

Key elements of a preoperative scoring system

It is useful if the scoring system also identifies factors or variables that can be altered or improved, but only if changing these factors preoperatively ameliorates risk. Factors to consider include:

- Patient demographics
- Fixed characteristics (ischaemic heart disease, renal impairment, diabetes)
- Functional assessment
- Type/extent of surgery
- Surgical pathology.

Scoring systems may be:

1 Organ-specific: designed to predict adverse outcome in one organ system, e.g. Goldman's Cardiac Risk Index and the more recent, simplified Revised Cardiac Risk Index (as described by Lee). This index assigns a score of one point to the presence of each of six variables and grades the risk of a cardiac event according to the total point score. Practically, this approach is limited to cardiovascular risk which can be useful if that can be identified as the predominant risk or if the patient has specific concerns about cardiovascular risk

2 Disease-specific: designed to predict outcome in patients with a specific disease where that has the predominant effect on outcome, e.g. in liver dysfunction:

(a) Child–Turcotte–Pugh score

(b) MELD (Model for End-stage Liver Disease) score.

Whilst both these scores have proved useful, they also highlight some of the problems with scoring systems; the Child–Turcotte–Pugh takes no account of the renal function, a known significant risk factor, and has been criticized for a lack of objectivity caused by the difficulty in assessing the presence and severity of ascites and encephalopathy. Neither score includes any assessment of the cardiopulmonary function.

3 General: designed to predict overall outcome, usually expressed as the likelihood of mortality or serious morbidity:

(a) Charlson comorbidity index

(b) Simplified Acute Physiology Score 2 (SAPS 2)

(c) Acute Physiology and Chronic Health Evaluation 2 (APACHE 2).

All three scoring systems are disease severity scoring systems that have been used to predict outcome in surgical procedures, with varying success, depending on the surgical procedure. This suggests that each needs to be validated for the particular surgical procedure to which it is applied and probably needs to be modified to include in the score data about the surgical procedure and pathological diagnosis.

(d) Physiological and Operative Severity Score for Enumeration of Mortality and Morbidity, colorectal modification (Cr-POSSUM)

(e) Surgical Apgar score.

Both of these scoring systems require intraoperative data. Although POSSUM has been used to predict outcome preoperatively by using a 'best and worst case' entry for intraoperative data, it is not validated for this purpose. They are designed to predict outcome post-operatively to track the performance of surgical units and/or individual surgeons, using observed/expected mortality ratios.

(f) Association of Coloproctology of Great Britain and Ireland Colorectal Cancer Resection Score (ACPGBI-CRC): this is a simple scoring system, developed from a mathematical model, to predict mortality after surgery for colorectal cancer using: age, ASA grade, Dukes stage (surgical pathology severity), urgency of procedure, and whether or not the cancer was excised. It could be used preoperatively by using intention to treat to answer the last question

4 Age: in elderly patients, frailty or functional age, as opposed to chronological age, has been used successfully to predict the likelihood of the need for supported accommodation post-operatively, using a simple five-category assessment, developed from the Canadian Veterans Heart Study. The REASON study demonstrated convincingly that increasing age, higher ASA status, decreasing albumin (Alb) level, and emergency surgery correlated significantly with death and poor outcome

5 Biochemical markers: N-terminal brain natriuretic peptide (NT-BNP) and high-sensitivity C-reactive protein (hsCRP) have been used to predict major cardiovascular events in non-cardiac surgery. Rather than being used in isolation, their utility will be in increasing the predictive power of existing or future risk indices.

Some of these scoring systems listed include an assessment of exercise capacity or cardiopulmonary function. It is intuitive that the current cardiopulmonary function of the patient is important; the problem is how it can be assessed. Patient-reported estimates of physical activity are unreliable, particularly in the elderly, even when supported by structured questioning using activity scales (Duke Activity Status Index Questionnaire) which attempt to correlate activities of daily living with defined metabolic capacity expressed in metabolic equivalents (METs).

Formal assessments of exercise capacity, using the ability to climb two flights of stairs or timed walking (the 'shuttle' test), have been used to address this problem. Over the past 10 years, cardiopulmonary exercise testing (CPET) has been developed. This is an objective test to evaluate the integrated cardiopulmonary function under conditions of submaximal exercise. This allows the assessment of physiological reserve as well as the opportunity to detect occult cardiac failure and myocardial ischaemia. Various physiological variables are assessed to grade the test, of which the details are beyond the scope of this text. Predictive value has been shown for patients undergoing thoracic and major abdominal surgery. CPET needs to be used as part of an overall assessment and not as an isolated tool.

How can we communicate predicted risk effectively?

We have a duty to communicate risk clearly in a way that allows the patient to use the information to make an informed judgement.

Patients vary widely in their perception and appreciation of risk. It is important to gain an understanding of what they perceive the risks to be, if any, before starting on a detailed discussion. For some patients, it is not a matter of probability or percentages; it is an all-or-nothing event—'I will get through or I won't'.

For others who have faced significant risks in their life before, it can be a judgement based on comparison or perceived relative risk. The National Institute for Health and Clinical Excellence (NICE) and the Association of Anaesthetists of Great Britain and Ireland (AAGBI) have published guidance on discussing risks and benefits:

◆ Personalize risks and benefits, as far as possible; as the foregoing discussion has revealed, it is difficult to assign specific risks to an individual; often the best that can be achieved is to place the patient in a particular group that is associated with a given risk

◆ Use natural frequency (10 in 100), rather than a percentage (10%)

◆ Use of positive and negative framing is encouraged: a mortality risk of 10 in 100 and a survival rate of 90 in 100

◆ Be consistent in the use of data. Use the same denominator when comparing risk, e.g. 7 in 100 for one and 20 in 100 for another, rather than 1 in 14 and 1 in 5

◆ If using terms, such as common, uncommon, rare, extremely rare, to describe probabilities, these should framed by using numerical data; it can be useful to support this with comparisons with everyday events that have relevance to the patient's own life: risk of being a pedestrian hit by a car, risk of being struck by lightning. Remember that these risks are often expressed as a lifetime risk, whereas a surgical procedure is a specific event in a short time frame.

All of us have preferences for the way in which we perceive information; for some, it is auditory, for others visual. It is useful to support oral information with written word and to accommodate visual preferences with the use of pictures and diagrams. This has the added benefit of allowing patients to take information away with them. Consider the use of recorded consultations. It has been demonstrated that patients often remember very little of the consultation, once they leave the clinic.

What influences a patient's decisions?

Whilst we may like to think that these decisions resolve simply into chance of cure or extension of life vs risk of death or damage, for the patient, it is often considerably more complex. Patients may view increased dependence, loss of independence, or prolonged recovery and rehabilitation as unacceptable, particularly if this impacts something else of great importance to them, e.g. the ability to care for a loved one or to live independently. Any discussion of risk should examine the wider aspects of the patient's life, in order to understand and address these issues.

We have a duty to present the patient with an objective assessment of the risks and benefits of any treatment, as far as is possible, but not to cajole or force them to accept a particular course of action. In this case study, the likelihood of a curative resection was low, although the perioperative risk was considered moderate by the clinicians involved, namely her modified cardiac risk, frailty, and ASA status. The patient considered that the most important thing to her was her ability to continue to live with, and care for, her husband, faced with what the anaesthetic team perceived to be a moderate perioperative risk but the likelihood of a prolonged recovery and rehabilitation. This patient opted to have a colonic stent.

Summary

Remember it is the patient's risk, not yours. We must respect the patient's autonomy and dignity, and their beliefs and attitudes. Their decision is based in the context of their wider life: hopes, ambitions, expectations, relationships, perceived duties, as well as the information and expectations given by the medical team. The patient has the right to make a decision which may be at odds with what you believe to be in their best interest; this may include refusing treatment.

Further reading

Association of Anaesthetists of Great Britain and Ireland (2005). *Catastrophes in anaesthetic practice—dealing with the aftermath*. Available at: <http://www.aagbi.org/sites/default/files/catastrophes05.pdf>.

Frappell-Cooke W, Gulina M, Green K, Hacker-Hughes J, and Greenberg N (2010). Does trauma risk management reduce psychological distress in deployed troops? *Occupational Medicine*, **60**, 645–50.

Staender SE and Manser T (2012). Taking care of patients, relatives and staff after critical incidents and accidents. *European Journal of Anaesthesiology*, **29**, 303–6.

White SM and Akerele O (2005). Anaesthetists attitudes to intraoperative death. *European Journal of Anaesthesiology*, **22**, 938–41.

Case 1.3

'Did I really do that?' Managing the aftermath of a serious adverse event

Background

The importance of open disclosure of the facts following a serious critical incident or clinical catastrophe has been stressed by many authors and medical regulatory authorities. It is part of the duty of care both to the patient or their relatives and to the process of learning from incidents, in order to prevent recurrence, improve safety, and enhance the delivery of care.

Anaesthetic training teaches how to deal with the technical, and increasingly the non-technical, skills required for the management of a clinical emergency, but less attention is given to managing the aftermath of a serious critical incident, particularly the effects on those involved. There is a need for training in how to:

- Disclose a serious adverse event to an injured, distressed, and possibly aggrieved patient or, as in this case, the patient's relatives
- Understand and assist in managing the potential effects on the members of the medical team involved in the incident
- Recognize the potentially serious effects such an incident may have on you as the clinician directly involved.

Learning outcomes

1 Recognize the important initial steps following an adverse event
2 Acknowledge support processes for patients, relatives, and staff involved.

CPD matrix matches

1B04; 1I01; 2B05

Case history

A 41-week pregnant, multiparous lady with an uneventful pregnancy was admitted to the obstetric ward for induction of labour at 6 p.m. At 10 p.m., 3 hours after the induction pessary, she started complaining of abdominal pain. This was attributed to early labour, and she was kept on the ward, with intermittent monitoring, as per hospital protocol. At about 1.30 a.m., she started seizing and collapsed on the ward. An emergency call-out was sent by the ward staff. Anaesthetic, critical care, and obstetric team members immediately responded, finding the patient in a post-ictal state. with a Glasgow coma score (GCS) of 8, a feeble central pulse, and a dusky colour around the peripheries. No external bleeding was seen, but she had severe fetal bradycardia and a tense abdomen. A major haemorrhage protocol was activated. Immediate resuscitation was commenced, according to Resuscitation Council protocols.

After a rapid sequence induction (RSI), initially, there was difficulty in intubation, but, on the third attempt, it was successful, with no further compromise in the cardiovascular status. Both the obstetric and anaesthetic on-call consultants were called in to the hospital immediately for help and guidance. A decision to do a perimortem Caesarean section was taken. The patient was immediately rushed to theatre, and the baby was delivered at 2 a.m. The patient lost about 3 L of blood with continuing ooze from the uterine bed. Invasive monitoring was commenced, whilst the resuscitation continued. The wound was packed, and all measures were taken by the team to arrest the bleeding. She continued to deteriorate, despite the use of blood products and inotropic agents, and she had multiple episodes of pulseless electrical activity after childbirth, with return of spontaneous circulation intermittently. She was extremely acidotic and hyperkalaemic on serial arterial blood gas (ABG) analyses. She eventually went into asystole at 4 a.m., and, despite all aggressive attempts at resuscitation to treat the reversible causes, she was pronounced dead at 5.30 a.m., after agreement with all involved team members. The post-mortem examination found conclusive evidence of amniotic fluid embolism.

How would you deal with breaking the bad news to the family?

Bad news should always be given face to face. This requires practice, when possible, by direct observation of an experienced colleague, supplemented by simulated communication training. When relatives are not in the hospital, it may be helpful to get a third party to telephone them to come in; this avoids you being drawn into a difficult conversation over the telephone, with potentially devastating consequences for the relative hearing the news at home alone with no support. If you have been directly involved in the event, recognize that you may not be in a fit state to break the news. Remember that the delivery of bad news is about caring for the family, and it is vital that it is done well. This can have a significant effect on their perception of the event and their eventual recovery from it. If necessary, ask a senior, experienced colleague to speak to the family in your presence. It is helpful to have a nursing colleague with you to support the relatives, particularly when the interview is over. Cardinal points include:

- Ensure that you have privacy and that you are not going to be interrupted
- Be aware of, and sensitive to, different cultural perspectives and values
- Use the services of an interpreter, if necessary
- Ensure that you are in possession of all the facts relating to the incident, as far as they are available; discuss only what you know to be true; do not speculate, and, if more information is likely to available later, say so
- Make sure, before beginning, that you know to whom you are speaking
- Establish what they know already
- If the patient is very seriously ill or, as in this case, has died, attempt to set the tone of the interview by giving a warning. For example, 'the condition that X came to hospital with is a very serious one, and I am afraid I have bad news'
- Avoid medical terms or jargon
- Pause, and give space and time for them to deal with the information and their emotions
- Allow time for questions
- If, as in this case, the patient has died, ensure that, before the interview is concluded, you have said so. Do not allow the interview to conclude, having only used euphemisms for death
- Ask the relatives if they would like a religious representative to meet with them
- It is appropriate and desirable to express regret and an apology for what has happened, but do not apportion blame to yourself or anyone else
- It should be standard practice for an investigation to take place after a serious adverse event or perioperative death; relatives should be told this and that, as a consequence, more information may be available later
- Ensure that they have a named point of contact for further questions and support
- Ensure that they are supported if they wish to make contact with additional relatives or friends
- Keep a full, contemporaneous written record of what has been discussed.

Failure to fully disclose what has happened and why it has happened is likely to seriously damage the relationship between the affected individuals and the hospital staff. It can cause the patient or relatives increased distress, dissatisfaction, and anger and increases the likelihood of litigation. It is important to reassure and demonstrate to the patient or relatives that, where appropriate, lessons have been learned from the incident and strategies put in place to prevent recurrence. This applies both where an actual error has been made and, as in this case, where a complex case is appropriately managed but has a bad outcome. All events present an opportunity for learning and improvement that should not be missed.

How would you deal with the management of the team and its members?

It is known that many medical personnel suffer a strong emotional response to the injury or death of a patient. These include concerns for the patient, anger directed at themselves or possibly other members of the medical team, and guilt. The emotional impact may be stronger in junior or less experienced medical staff. This impact is also likely to be higher in the case of an unexpected death, particularly that of a mother and child. It is also seen that the majority of clinicians would wish for support from others in coping with this emotional response. Unfortunately, many do not receive it. Direct and early involvement of a senior colleague is vital, even if the anaesthetist involved is senior, to help with ongoing clinical management and initiate post-incident care for relatives and staff members. It must be recognized that involvement in a serious adverse incident or death may seriously impair the clinician's ability to deal with the ongoing management not only of that patient, but also for a period of time thereafter. Where possible, those members of the team directly involved in an unexpected death should have the opportunity to remove themselves from clinical work, certainly for the remainder of that day. It must be recognized that, in certain situations such as lack of another team or a mass casualty situation, this may not be possible, but all possible practical support should be provided. Rarely, it may be necessary to remove an individual from work, because they are unfit to carry on. This must be recognized and undertaken sensitively.

The opportunity to discuss the event with a trusted, experienced colleague openly and honestly without fear of blame is valuable and effective in coming to terms with the event. This certainly does not replace, but rather complements, the more formal subsequent investigation in root cause analysis and mortality and morbidity meetings. Nor does it mean that accountability can be overlooked; indeed, recognizing and accepting responsibility, where appropriate, is a vital part of learning and development for the clinician involved.

How would you deal with the debriefing and/or morbidity and mortality meetings?

It is suggested that debriefing should happen at a time that suits all those involved; ideally, this should be within a few hours of the event. Many argue that debriefing should be a routine part of daily clinical practice. This makes it a familiar experience, rather than a potentially threatening one after what is clearly an unusual event. The purpose of informal debriefing is to allow those involved to express their perceptions of the event, to gain insight and feedback whilst details are still fresh, to identify any problems that can be rectified immediately, and to allay anxieties, misconceptions, or misunderstandings experienced by any of the team members. It should foster open communication and may help to identify individuals requiring further support. However, it is not meant to be a full and comprehensive investigation of the incident. More formal stress debriefing can be held later, ideally within 72 hours. The United Kingdom (UK) Royal Marines use TRiM (Trauma Risk Management), a support system operating through practitioners embedded within operational units. The aim is to promote the recognition of psychological illness, to provide social support, and to promote further specialist management. Key to this is that the initial support is provided by peers or colleagues. Other approaches have been described in the civilian emergency services; all require a moderator with some formal training.

Further follow-up—how should the anaesthetist in the team be supported in the longer term by the anaesthetic department and the hospital trust, if identified to have psychological distress?

Clinicians, and indeed the organizations for which they work, have a duty to ensure that their colleague's health is not damaged by their experiences in the workplace—this is mandated in law in the UK.

It is therefore incumbent on colleagues, the hospital, and, where possible, the family and society in general to provide practical help and support to the anaesthetist and other team members involved, according to individual needs. This is part of good clinical and corporate governance and risk management. It is important to note that team members who were apparently remote from the incident or seemed to have had little or no responsibility for managing it may be affected. This should be looked for at the initial debriefing. Whilst these individuals may not be the direct responsibility of the anaesthetic staff, they must be looked after. Action should be taken to ensure that this occurs.

Following the initial actions described already, an experienced and sympathetic senior anaesthetic colleague should be assigned to act as mentor and provide support for as long as necessary. The mentor should be known and accepted by the anaesthetist concerned. Members of the department may have to take over the involved anaesthetist's duties, including on-call commitments, for a period of time. It is known from the literature that doctors are reluctant to seek professional help, and some continue to feel traumatized long after the event. Each individual also has a responsibility to ensure they are fit to work. It is important for colleagues and mentors to recognize signs of stress and remind individuals of the psychological resources available to them.

How might you be affected by your involvement in a serious traumatic adverse event?

It is important to recognize how a serious adverse event may affect behaviour and performance at the time of the event and afterwards. When the event occurs, the ability to deal with it depends on knowledge, skills, and experience; if the event is perceived as being within the individual's previous successful experience, then a degree of stress may enhance performance. However, if the complexity or seriousness of the event is perceived to exceed the ability to deal with the event, this may induce an acute stress reaction. This is likely to be exacerbated if the individual perceives themselves as, in some way, responsible for the event, e.g. a failed intubation, total spinal or drug administration error. Clinicians should be aware that this can degrade performance. Calling for help is well recognized as a high priority during a critical incident, which not only provides practical and clinical support, but also emotional support. This should be appreciated by the clinician called to assist as well.

After the event, many clinicians report feelings of guilt, anger, inadequacy, concerns about future performance, concerns for the well-being of the patient or relatives, and worry about the potential consequences for them. Individuals may experience disturbed sleep and recurrent thoughts about the event. Significant numbers report an effect on their personal life.

Good support and pastoral care, as described earlier, can do much to mitigate this, and these responses may be considered normal in the short term; however, if these feelings persist for >2–3 weeks, this should be considered abnormal and specialized help sought.

A minority of clinicians experience problems of such severity that their ability to continue working is undermined. This must be recognized and acted upon by them or those who have a responsibility for them and the safe delivery of patient care.

Indicators of serious ongoing problems described are:

- Dreams, flashbacks, recurrent distressing thoughts
- Persistent attempts to remember and reinterpret the incident

- Avoiding similar situations; this may manifest as absenteeism and sickness
- Disordered sleep
- Irritability or bouts of anger
- Persistent anxiety feelings of being constantly 'on edge' or under threat
- Social withdrawal, either from colleagues or family
- Problems with concentration and/or memory.

In the long term, this can lead to drug or alcohol dependence and, in a small, but significant, minority, self-harm or suicide.

It is also important to appreciate more subtle effects on thinking and performance.

Clinicians unconsciously use rules of thumb or heuristics to problem-solve, particularly during crises. These responses depend on pattern recognition or how closely the current situation resembles those previously experienced. Unfortunately, the ease with which the apparent solution is brought to mind depends not only on how often it has occurred before, but also on how recently it occurred and importantly on the emotional impact it had. Therefore, a previous adverse event may lead one to overestimate the risk of it occurring again when a similar, but not identical, event occurs, potentially leading to another error in management, these being well-recognized characteristics of human performance and behaviour.

What guidelines are available for the medical personnel to deal with consequences of major catastrophes in the workplace?

The AAGBI produced a guideline in 2005 *Catastrophes in anaesthetic practice—dealing with the aftermath*. This publication offers guidance on the wider aspects of dealing with incidents, including the development of departmental protocols for the investigation of incidents and support of staff.

Simulation training dealing with the clinical management of various crises in the perioperative setting and management of resources in cases of simulated catastrophes is gaining rapid popularity, and various courses are available from such centres across the country. The scenarios require complex decision making, interaction with different personnel, and debriefing sessions and have been found to have good evidence base for practice. Whilst great attention is given to human performance and teamwork and non-technical skills are practised and enhanced, less attention is given to self-reflection and understanding how and why one reacts or behaves in a particular way. Understanding one's own behaviour and responses is highly valuable in dealing with critical incidents and their aftermath.

Who should be informed and what steps should be taken by the individuals when dealing with potential complaints in this scenario?

First and foremost, after any serious adverse event, keep accurate and contemporaneous records. They should be legible, timed, dated, and signed. These records, once completed, should not be tampered with at a later date; if additions are made to the record, they should be post-dated and signed. They should be stored in a secure place, as it may be some time before they are required. However, it should be remembered that very few cases actually result in a formal disciplinary hearing or action for compensation. In such cases, if the incident happened in an NHS hospital, civil litigation will be covered by the NHS Litigation Authority (NHSLA). Membership with a defence organization is strongly recommended, as they can provide representation or advice in fatal accident inquiries (Scotland) or coroner's inquests (England, Wales, and Northern Ireland), in criminal cases, or where there is disagreement between the hospital and medical personnel. Members should inform their defence organization at an early stage if they are involved in a serious incident, as they can provide valuable advice and support.

Summary

At some point all clinicians are likely to encounter serious adverse events and error in their own practice and that of their colleagues. All events should be reported through local and, where appropriate, national reporting systems and investigated. Where an investigation is undertaken, the results should be disseminated to all those concerned; this may be at national level. Where appropriate, changes in practice should be made; it is vital that, where such changes have been recommended, there is a process in place to ensure these have been incorporated into practice and that the effect of these changes is subject to audit. Full disclosure to the patient or relatives is mandatory. The consequences of such events can be devastating for the clinicians involved and may affect their professional and personal life. It is important that clinicians recognize the potential effects on themselves and their colleagues and know how and when to seek support and, if appropriate, expert help.

Further reading

Association of Anaesthetists of Great Britain and Ireland (2005). *Catastrophes in anaesthetic practice*. Available at: <http://www.aagbi.org/sites/default/files/catastophes05.pdf>.

Flin R, O'Connor P, and Crichton M (2007). *Safety at the sharp end. A guide to non-technical skills*. Ashgate Publishing, Aldershot.

Frappell-Cooke W, Gulina M, Green K, Hacker-Hughes J, and Greenberg N (2010). Does trauma risk management reduce psychological distress in deployed troops? *Occupational Medicine*, **60**, 645–50.

Staender S and Manser T (2012). Taking care of patients, relatives and staff after critical incidents and accidents. *European Journal of Anaesthesiology*, **29**, 303–6.

St Pierre M, Hofinger G, and Buerschaper C (2008). *Crisis management in acute care settings. Human factors and team psychology in a high stakes environment.* Springer–Verlag, Berlin Heidelberg.

White S and Akerele O (2005). Anaesthetists' attitude to intraoperative death. *European Journal of Anaesthesiology*, **22**, 938–41.

Current approaches to complex colorectal surgery

Background

Laparoscopic approach to colorectal resection is increasingly common. The benefits of this approach are reduced requirement for analgesia, earlier return of bowel function, reduced blood loss, reduced wound infection rates, potentially quicker post-operative recovery, and shortened hospital stay, although this has been shown to depend on the type of analgesia used, with epidural analgesia being associated with increased length of stay. However, warnings have been issued by the National Patient Safety Agency (NPSA) regarding delayed recognition of post-operative complications, particularly concealed haemorrhage and bowel perforation.

The laparoscopic approach may not be appropriate in patients with previous surgery, due to adhesions or distorted anatomy, and in those with serious comorbidity, e.g. raised intracranial pressure (ICP), right-to-left cardiac shunts, end-stage respiratory disease, severe valvular heart disease, and severely compromised left ventricular (LV) function. The effects of pneumoperitoneum and positioning will reduce splanchnic, renal, and liver blood flow, particularly in the presence of hypovolaemia, which, in this case, would be potentially detrimental to graft function.

Learning outcomes

1 Understand different approaches for complex colonic surgery

2 Familiarity with the enhanced recovery after surgery programme

3 Appreciate the difficulties of major abdominal surgery in immunocompromised patients.

CPD matrix matches

1A01; 2A03

Case history

A 36-year-old male with ulcerative colitis, complicated by sclerosing cholangitis and cirrhosis, for which he required orthotopic liver transplantation 6 months ago, presents for total colectomy with a dysplastic lesion in his distal colon. The liver is reported to be functioning well, but the procedure was complicated by hepatic vein stenosis. As a result, he has portal hypertension and splenomegaly.

How should perioperative care be managed?

Many colorectal units have adopted the framework for enhanced recovery after surgery (ERAS) as best practice. This is a care bundle, developed from the work of Henrik Kehlet and colleagues, which has demonstrated a reduction in perioperative morbidity and length of hospital stay.

The main components of the programme are:

- Shortened preoperative fasting, with carbohydrate loading using high-calorie drinks to reduce perioperative insulin resistance
- Avoidance of bowel preparation
- Avoidance of long-acting sedative premedication
- General anaesthesia using an agent with rapid elimination and recovery profile
- Use of dynamic assessment of intravascular volume and cardiac output monitoring
- Use of epidural analgesia, in open cases, to reduce exposure to systemic opioids. In laparoscopic surgery, this may be modified to subarachnoid block, supplemented with opioid or transversus abdominal plane (TAP) block
- Avoidance of surgical drains
- Avoidance of nasogastric (NG) tube
- Early resumption of oral intake
- Early and sustained mobilization, supported by good analgesia and prompt removal of urinary catheter and intravenous (IV) lines
- Use of a clearly defined pathway and committed staff to implement the programme, including patient education, which should begin in the preoperative period
- Use of dynamic assessment of cardiac output and intravascular volume has been recommended, although this has been questioned recently, particularly in fit patients undergoing laparoscopic surgery.

In common with other care bundles, the success of this programme has been measured in the delivery of the programme as a complete package. The individual components are supported by good, or at least biologically plausible, evidence; thus, even if all the recommendations cannot be met, the general principles can be applied.

What are the key aspects of the preoperative assessment in this case history?

A standard approach to history, examination, and investigations should be followed, with particular attention given to:

- Reason for original transplant and the potential for that disease process to affect other organ systems

- The potential complications of prior hepatic failure; usually these will resolve, following successful transplantation; in this case, there is residual portal hypertension and splenomegaly

- Confirmation of normal/adequate liver function

- Current immunosuppressive therapy, including potential complications

- A management plan for the delivery of these drugs preoperatively.

The preoperative assessment and plan should involve close cooperation with the liver transplant unit.

Case update: relevant clinical history and investigations

The patient reports that he feels well; he regularly cycles 10 km. The results of the investigations are as follows:

- Haemoglobin (Hb) 120 g/L
- White cell count (WCC) 3.0×10^9/L
- Platelets (Plt) 84×10^9/L
- Sodium (Na$^+$) 139 mmol/L
- Potassium (K$^+$) 4.4 mmol/L
- Urea 7.7 mmol/L
- Creatinine (Cr) 125 micromoles/L
- Bilirubin (Bil) 17 mmol/L
- Alanine transaminase (ALT) 36 U/L
- Alkaline phosphatase (ALP) 73 U/L
- Gamma glutamyl transferase (γGT) 76 U/L

- Prothrombin time (PT) 16 s (ratio 1.4)
- Activated partial thromboplastin time (APTT) 44 s (ratio 1.4)
- Fibrinogen 2.3 g/L.

Comments on these results

PT and APTT are both increased; platelet count is low; WCC is below the lower limit of normal, but he is not neutropenic. ALT and ALP are within their normal ranges; γGT is slightly elevated.

The transplant unit report that graft function is good and liver enzymes are within acceptable limits. The PT ratio, APTT, and bilirubin have been persistently raised since transplant, and there is portal hypertension with splenomegaly and a small volume of ascites detected on ultrasound.

Comments on medications and suggested plan for perioperative management

- Prednisolone
- Azathioprine
- Tacrolimus
- Amiloride
- Spironolactone.

This combination of a calcineurin inhibitor (tacrolimus), an antiproliferative agent (azathioprine), and a steroid is common for maintenance therapy. This patient has only been on these for 6 months. Azathioprine may cause leucopenia. In the longer term, calcineurin inhibitors may predispose to diabetes, hypertension, and neurotoxicity. The complications of corticosteroid therapy are well known. Sirolimus, a newer drug which blocks the action of interleukin-2, may cause hyperlipidaemia. There is a predisposition to accelerated cardiovascular disease.

Immunosuppressive therapy must be maintained perioperatively. The simplest way to do this is via the oral route. Although tacrolimus can be given intravenously, it is difficult to manage; if this is required, expert advice should be sought. Tacrolimus levels should be measured daily. This patient has been on steroids for 6 months, and on a number of occasions prior to transplant, to control his ulcerative colitis; consequently, he should be given steroid supplementation perioperatively, which can be given intravenously.

His diuretic therapy should continue post-operatively, with close monitoring of renal function and fluid balance. Preoperative weight and post-operative daily weights are useful in assessing fluid balance.

What are the important points to consider in this patient's preoperative preparation?

What is the significance of his abnormal coagulation tests? Should they be corrected preoperatively?

- The prolonged PT and APTT in this patient, in the absence of a drug effect, could be caused by vitamin K deficiency, decreased hepatic synthesis of clotting factors, or an acquired dysfibrinogenaemia

- The use of fresh frozen plasma (FFP) to correct abnormal coagulation to prevent bleeding in patients with liver disease undergoing major surgery is reasonable. However, it should be remembered that the standard laboratory coagulation tests were designed to assess specific coagulation factor deficiencies and are performed on platelet-poor plasma and take no account of endogenous anticoagulant activity. In patients with liver dysfunction, when only mildly deranged, they do not correlate well with actual coagulation factor levels or with the propensity to bleed. The relationship between coagulation factor levels and test values for PT is non-linear; thus, initially large changes in abnormal PT can be achieved with FFP, but increasingly large volumes are required to change the PT as the normal range is approached. The need to correct mild to moderate derangements prior to surgery has been questioned, as discussed in a review by Kor, Stubbs, and Ognjen. When giving FFP, it should be remembered that the half-life of factor VII is only 3–5 hours

- Whilst vitamin K deficiency is only likely in the presence of malnutrition, biliary obstruction, impaired bile salt production or secretion, or in the presence of vitamin K antagonists (coumarins or phenindiones), it would still be reasonable to consider giving oral vitamin K 24 hours before surgery

- Functional tests of coagulation, using thromboelastography (TEG) or thromboelastometry which provide a dynamic measurement of clot formation, clot strength, and dissolution, have been widely used in cardiac, liver transplant, and trauma surgery. They can be useful to confirm normal, or identify abnormal, coagulation and target specific treatment with platelets, coagulation factors, or antifibrinolytics during major haemorrhage and transfusion. The routine use of these techniques to assess preoperative coagulation status was not recommended in a recent NHS Innovation and Technology Review. In this case, neither TEG nor thromboelastometry was available. The patient in this case study was considered to be at high risk of bleeding due to the nature of the surgery, the presence of portal hypertension, low platelets, and mildly deranged PT and APTT; therefore, appropriate therapies for this patient include:

- Vitamin K 10 mg was given
- FFP 15 mL/kg was ordered for intraoperative use. In this case, this had the secondary benefit of providing volume replacement to offset the volume shift caused by draining of the patient's ascites. It should be noted that the use of FFP primarily for this purpose or purely for volume replacement is not indicated.

What interventions should be considered for this patient's thrombocytopenia?

- European guidelines recommend a platelet count of at least 50×10^9/L for invasive surgery ($>70 \times 10^9$/L for neurosurgery). In portal hypertension with splenomegaly, the platelet function is normal, unless compromised by antiplatelet drugs or renal failure. Although there is an identified cause for thrombocytopenia, other causes of thrombocytopenia should be considered in this patient group, e.g. antiviral drugs, cytomegalovirus, and platelet antibodies.

Should there be active management of this patient's ascites?

Rapid removal of large-volume ascites at laparotomy can cause circulatory dysfunction and consequently compromise renal and hepatic perfusion. As in this case, ascites should be controlled preoperatively by limitation of salt intake and diuretic therapy, recognizing that this can sometimes be a precarious balance between hypovolaemia, with the risk of compromising renal function, and ascites accumulation. In large-volume ascites, this may be combined with staged preoperative paracentesis. However, this is not without complications: infection, bowel perforation, haemorrhage. Intraoperatively, if the volume of ascites removed is <5 L, synthetic colloid can be used for intravascular replacement; if >5 L, replacement with albumin at 8 g/L per litre of ascites is reasonable. The total Na^+ load should be borne in mind.

Given that you anticipate the potential for major blood loss, what blood conservation strategies can you employ to reduce blood loss and transfusion requirement?

1 Reducing portal venous pressure:

In patients with acute variceal bleeding, reducing the portal venous pressure can reduce bleeding. This can be achieved with IV terlipressin or octreotide. β-blockers have been used, following the acute phase, as secondary prophylaxis to prevent rebleeding and as primary prophylaxis. However, there is no evidence that attempting to reduce the hepatic vein pressure gradient with these agents reduces bleeding during elective surgery.

2 Antifibrinolytics:

Tranexamic acid and epsilon amino caproic acid are synthetic lysine analogues that inhibit fibrinolysis by preventing the formation of the active complex of tissue plasminogen activator plasminogen and fibrin. Tranexamic acid has been used successfully in major orthopaedic surgery, cardiac surgery, trauma, liver transplantation, and hepatic resection (including patients with hepatitis and cirrhosis) to reduce blood loss and transfusion requirements. Unlike aprotinin, tranexamic acid has not been convincingly shown to increase the rate of thrombosis, stroke, MI, or renal injury. However, concerns have been expressed about its use in the presence of vascular abnormalities, as in this patient with hepatic vein stenosis. Aprotinin is currently not available due to safety concerns.

3 Preoperative autologous blood donation (PAD) has not been shown to consistently reduce transfusion requirements

4 Acute normovolaemic haemodilution (ANH):

ANH in the immediate preoperative period is simpler and less expensive than PAD and may reduce allogenic transfusion requirements, although it has not been shown to do so consistently.

5 Intraoperative cell salvage:

This is effective in reducing allogenic transfusion requirements during surgery where the total blood loss is in excess of 1000 mL. It has been widely used in cardiac, orthopaedic, liver transplant, and obstetric practice. The use of cell salvage in bowel surgery and malignancy has been questioned. Studies have not shown adverse outcomes in these situations. However, the manufacturers do not recommend its use in these circumstances. In this case, the potential risk of bacterial contamination of the infusate in an immunocompromised patient, along with the general concerns expressed earlier, precluded its use.

6 Conservative approach to transfusion:

In a young patient without cardiorespiratory disease, it is reasonable to maintain the haemoglobin above 70 g/L.

Discuss your anaesthetic technique for this patient

An appropriate approach would be IV induction of general anaesthesia with endotracheal intubation, maintained using volatile agent, oxygen and air, and positive pressure ventilation (PPV).

All volatile anaesthetic agents decrease hepatic blood flow. Historically, isoflurane was the agent of choice, as it preserves the reciprocal relationship between the hepatic artery and portal venous blood flow, thereby maintaining hepatic oxygen delivery. It had the least detrimental effect; the modern agents sevoflurane and desflurane are comparable to isoflurane. Isoflurane and possibly the other volatile agents may be preferable to propofol, as it has been associated with an attenuated post-operative inflammatory response and hepatocellular injury. Atracurium, cis-atracurium, and remifentanil are not dependent on liver function for their metabolism.

Which analgesic regimen will you use?

This patient is having a laparotomy for colonic resection; although epidural analgesia is recommended as part of the ERAS protocol, both epidural and systemic analgesia, using opiates delivered via a patient-controlled system, are both reasonable choices. The potential advantages of successful epidural analgesia are:

◆ Good-quality analgesia (at rest and on movement)

◆ Earlier return of bowel function

◆ Reduced nausea and vomiting, compared with systemic opiates. This may assist in maintaining oral immunosuppressive therapy in this patient.

It should be remembered that, in clinical practice, effective epidural analgesia, throughout the perioperative period, is only achieved in 60–70% of patients at best. This patient has low platelet count and mildly deranged PT and is immunosuppressed; thus, the potential complications of epidural analgesia, including haematomas and abscesses, are increased.

After a discussion with the patient of the risks and benefits of epidural analgesia and systemic opiates using patient-controlled analgesia (PCA), this patient opted for PCA using fentanyl, supplemented with regular paracetamol.

Monitoring

Standard monitoring, as recommended by AAGBI, supplemented by intra-arterial pressure monitoring and central venous pressure (CVP) monitoring, should be used. Dynamic assessment of cardiac output and volume responsiveness is highly desirable in major colorectal surgery.

What are your concerns about haemodynamic management?

◆ Maintenance of the intravascular volume and cardiac output to preserve splanchnic and liver blood flow, in the face of significant fluid shifts (ascites) and blood loss, whilst aiming to maintain a low CVP (7–8 mmHg) during PPV, to prevent hepatic venous congestion and increased blood loss

◆ Hepatic blood flow will be reduced by hypocarbia, hypercarbia, hypoxia, and sympathoadrenal stimulation.

What potential problems, specific to this patient, should you anticipate in the post-operative period?

◆ Bleeding

◆ Nausea and vomiting or prolonged ileus, leading to interruption of tacrolimus therapy

◆ Liver (graft) dysfunction, including rejection

◆ Renal injury

◆ Accumulation of ascites

◆ Fluid retention.

What would alert you to an episode of graft rejection?

The liver enzymes (AST, ALT, ALP, γGT) and bilirubin are elevated, with eosinophilia and pyrexia.

Summary

The ERAS protocol has been shown to be an effective method of delivering perioperative care to patients undergoing colonic resection. The principles have been adapted for major surgery in other specialties. Whilst the benefits of this approach have been reported, with full implementation of the protocol in many cases, as in this one, it may not be possible or appropriate to do so. Complex patients require bespoke plans for perioperative care. This should not be considered as a failure or lead to abandonment of the entire protocol; a significant element in its success is the structured delivery of care, both intra- and post-operatively, particularly in the aim to achieve daily goals in the post-operative period. This patient underwent laparotomy for colonic resection, as described previously. Ascites (3500 mL) was drained at incision. Blood loss was 800 mL. Over the first 48 hours post-operatively, his liver enzymes became mildly deranged and his PT ratio increased to 1.4. This was not unexpected, but he was monitored closely for signs of graft rejection. These changes resolved over the next 24 hours. Subsequently, he had an uncomplicated post-operative course. He returned 9 months later for a second laparotomy for the creation of an ileo-anal pouch and was successfully managed in a similar way.

Further reading

Kor DJ, Stubbs JR, and Ognjen G (2010). Perioperative coagulation management—fresh frozen plasma. *Clinical Anaesthesiology*, **24**, 51–64.

Lassen K, Soop M, Nygren J, *et al.*, for the Enhanced Recovery After Surgery (ERAS) Group (2009). Consensus review of optimal perioperative care in colorectal surgery. *Archives of Surgery*, **144**, 961–9.

National Patient Safety Agency (2010). *Laparoscopic surgery: failure to recognise postoperative deterioration. Rapid Response Report NPSA/2010/RRR016.* Available at: <http://www.nrls.npsa.nhs.uk/EasySiteWeb/getresource.axd?AssetID=82752>.

NHS Quality Improvement Scotland (2008). *The clinical and cost effectiveness of thromboelastography/thromboelastometry. HTA Programme: Health Technology Assessment Report 11.* Available at: <http://www.healthcareimprovementscotland.org/previous_resources/hta_report/hta_11.aspx>.

Yang LQ, Tao KM, Cheung CW, *et al.* (2010). The effect of isoflurane or propofol on liver injury after partial hepatectomy in cirrhotic patients. *Anaesthesia*, **65**, 1094–110.

Further reading

Chapter 2

Trauma and resuscitation

Dr Rosie Macfadyen
Dr Christopher Hoy

Major haemorrhage

Background

Major haemorrhage is a life-threatening event. Haemorrhagic shock accounts for 50% of deaths in the first 24 hours following trauma, and 80% of deaths in the operating theatre are due to haemorrhage. Knowledge of major haemorrhage and its management is important for the anaesthetist, as the patient is critically ill, requires advanced resuscitation, and often usually requires therapeutic intervention involving general anaesthesia. This case study will highlight the issues of major haemorrhage and outline the steps required to reduce morbidity and mortality and thus optimize patient outcome.

Learning outcomes

1 Understand the pathophysiology of major haemorrhage

2 Understand the rationale of management by simultaneous resuscitation and haemorrhage control

3 Make appropriate choice of fluids, blood products, and drugs in managing major haemorrhage

4 Understand the rationale for a local major haemorrhage protocol

5 Recognize the sequelae of major haemorrhage and massive transfusion.

CPD matrix matches

2A02; 2A05

Case history

A 20-year-old man was the driver of a car that was struck side-on by a lorry travelling at approximately 60 miles/hour. Whilst entrapped in the vehicle, he remained conscious, complaining of pain in his lower abdomen. He was placed in a hard collar, had an IV cannula sited, and observations monitored before extrication, showing a respiratory rate (RR) of 18/min, an oxygen saturation (SpO$_2$) of 95%, a heart rate (HR) of 110, and a blood pressure (BP) of 90/60 mmHg. He was transferred to the emergency department (ED) within a major trauma centre. In the ambulance, his systolic BP decreased to 70 mmHg on three occasions but responded to a bolus of 250 mL 0.9% NaCl on each occasions, resulting in a systolic BP of 90–95 mmHg.

You are a member of the trauma team in the ED. Primary survey reveals a conscious, pale young man who is:

- A: talking coherently
- B: RR of 22 breaths/min, saturation of 95%, clear chest, and normal chest X-ray (CXR)
- C: pulse of 120/min, BP 75/40, capillary refill time (CRT) 4 s, heart sounds I + II, tender lower abdomen, and deformed pelvis
- D: GCS 15, pupils equal and reactive, BM 6.0
- E: temperature 35.9°C.

What features of this case suggest haemorrhage, and how can its severity be graded?

Trauma is a mechanism of injury that is associated with vascular disruption, organ rupture, and long bone fracture, leading to loss of blood from the vasculature. Haemorrhage should be suspected and actively excluded in all trauma patients. Sites for blood loss are 'the floor plus four', i.e. external, thorax, abdomen, pelvis, and femur.

The clinical signs of acute blood loss preceding the loss of pressure in the vasculature are the compensatory changes that occur to maintain oxygen delivery to body tissues, including increased ventilation, increased HR, and a reduction of perfusion initially to non-essential organs, including skin and kidneys. Then the perfusion of vital organs is reduced, e.g. reduced cerebral perfusion which is revealed by an altered conscious level. These signs occur progressively as blood loss increases and have been grouped into the four stages of hypovolaemia (see Table 2.1).

Table 2.1 The stages of hypovolaemic shock in adults

Stage	I	II	III	IV
Volume loss (mL)	<750	750–1500	1500–2000	>2000
% loss	0–15	15–30	30–40	>40
RR	14–20	20–30	30–40	>40
HR	<100	>100	>120	>140
BP	Normal	Normal	Reduced	Reduced
Skin	Pale	+ sweating	+ cold	± mottling
Urine output	>30	20–30	<20	Minimal/anuria
CNS	Normal		Confused	Drowsy

From Table 2.1, it should be appreciated that the first signs of blood loss may be subtle but denote significant loss. BP does not drop until 1.5 L have been lost and is a late sign denoting failure of compensatory mechanisms to maintain pressure in the vasculature.

Major haemorrhage has been defined by various criteria, including:

◆ Adult patients:
  • Any life-threatening bleed
  • The loss of one circulating volume in a 24-hour period

◆ Obstetric patients:
  • The loss of 1500 mL, the requirement of >4 U of red cells, or a drop in Hb concentration of 40 g/L

◆ Paediatric patients:
  • The actual or anticipated loss of 40 mL/kg of blood.

Measurement of Hb concentration is a poor indicator of blood loss in early haemorrhage, as blood remaining within the vasculature will likely have near-normal Hb concentration.

As organ perfusion and oxygen delivery worsen, cells will begin anaerobic metabolism, resulting in lactic acid production. Serum lactate and base deficit measurements are sensitive in estimating the degree of bleeding and shock.

Case update

The patient is given 500 mL of crystalloid which returns his systolic BP to 85 mmHg.

A pelvic binder device is applied, following the IV administration of 5 mg of morphine. He is not catheterized, because of blood in the urethral meatus.

He has a bedside HemoCue® performed which shows Hb 100 g/L, and an ABG shows lactate 3.0 mmol/L, base deficit 3.0 mmol/L, and hydrogen ion (H^+) of 48 nmol/L. Venous blood is drawn and sent for full blood count (FBC), urea and electrolytes (U&E), coagulation screen, and cross-match for 4 U of packed red cells (PRC). The ED consultant informs blood transfusion service (BTS) that a major haemorrhage is likely to be present.

What are the pathophysiological features of a major haemorrhage?

◆ **Hypovolaemia**: the loss of volume of blood from the vasculature results in reduced intravascular pressure and reduced organ perfusion, resulting in cellular hypoxia, acidosis, and organ dysfunction

- **Anaemia**: oxygen carriage is dependent upon Hb concentration. A low concentration of Hb results from the loss of red cell mass and physiological measures that increase water reabsorption, including the action of aldosterone and vasopressin. Volume resuscitation with clear fluids will further reduce the Hb concentration, thus reducing the oxygen-carrying capacity of the blood, contributing to cellular hypoxia and acidosis
- **Acute coagulopathy of trauma (ACoT)**: this is associated with a higher risk of mortality and may be due to several mechanisms, including:
  - Consumption
  - Dilution
  - Protein C activation
  - Hyperfibrinolysis
  - Hypocalcaemia
  - Drugs, including anticoagulants and antiplatelet medications
  - Hypothermia
- **Acidosis**: this is the end result of anaerobic metabolism. The change in pH within cells will lead to enzyme dysfunction and uncoupling of the processes which maintain ion gradients that, in turn, maintain cell activities
- **Free radical formation**: under stress conditions, there is failure of the electron transport chain to fully reduce oxygen to water. The resulting oxygen species are charged free radicals that cause irreversible damage to mitochondria.

The combination of coagulopathy, acidosis, and hypothermia is often referred to as the 'triad of death' in trauma, as they increase the risk of mortality.

What are the priorities in managing this patient with suspected pelvic fracture and major haemorrhage?

Optimal management of major haemorrhage should be aimed at the cessation of blood loss with concurrent resuscitation. This process is a continuum, beginning in the pre-hospital environment and continued in the ED, theatre, and intensive care unit (ICU). Unnecessary delays in achieving haemostasis should be avoided, as these will adversely affect outcome.

The trauma patient may have multiple life-threatening injuries, including thoracic, cervical spine, neurological, and intra-abdominal injuries, and long bone fracture. The primary survey is a means of rapidly assessing for life-threatening injuries, with an intrinsic order of prioritization that should allow recognition and management of the most pressing injury, before attention is directed to the next. It has been traditionally taught as 'ABCDE'.

In the immediate pre-hospital environment, control of catastrophic external haemorrhage has become the first priority, before cervical spine control, airway, breathing, and circulation (C-A-B-C). The Combat Application Tourniquet (CAT) is a device that can be applied rapidly to prevent exsanguination from an injured limb.

Unstable skeletal cervical spine injury may lead to devastating injury to the spinal cord, and anyone with neck symptoms, or a mechanism consistent with a cervical spine injury, should have their cervical spine immobilized. This can be achieved rapidly with two-hand manual in-line stabilization, then replaced with a rigid collar, blocks, and tape (triple immobilization).

Airway management and breathing are aimed at optimizing the oxygenation of blood and include the administration of high-flow oxygen, intubation for respiratory failure, and management of life-threatening intrathoracic injuries.

The 'circulation' aspect of the primary survey is aimed at identifying and resuscitating shocked patients, i.e. those with failure of delivery of oxygen to their tissues. Circulatory failure has four mechanisms whereby the pressure in the arterial vasculature can be diminished (see Table 2.2).

In trauma, hypovolaemia is the most common cause of shock and should be actively sought and managed as the most likely cause. The priorities in managing the hypovolaemic patient are:

1 Haemostasis: the process of stopping further blood loss, including:

  (a) Immediate measures: various methods are available to rapidly reduce blood loss. These include direct pressure over a bleeding wound, limb tourniquets, pelvic binders, and femoral traction devices (see Figure 2.1a–c). If a suitably qualified surgeon is present, abdominal packing or aortic cross-clamping may be employed, if deemed necessary

  (b) Investigation to confirm haemorrhage: the practice of ultrasonography in ED to confirm haemorrhage is growing, but CT scanning has better sensitivity and specificity, and, in the multiply injured patient, full body CT scanning is the most rapid means to achieve a definitive diagnosis of their injuries. Unstable patients with suspected haemorrhage may need immediate transfer to theatre without imaging

Table 2.2 Types of shock

Mechanism of shock	Examples
Hypovolaemia	Major haemorrhage
Cardiogenic	Myocardial contusion, arrhythmia
Obstructive	Cardiac tamponade, tension pneuomnthorax
Distributory (vasodilatory)	Septic shock, neurogenic shock

(a)

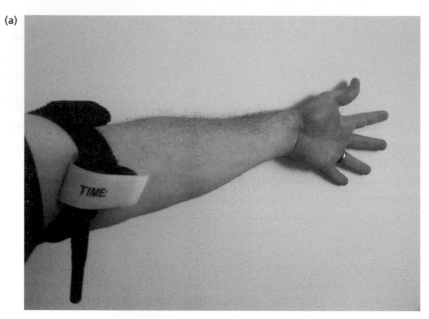

(b)

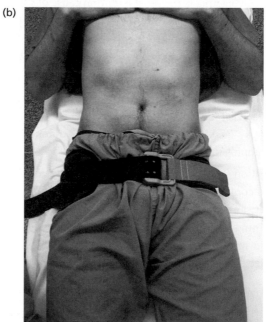

Fig. 2.1 Devices for immediate haemorrhage control, rapidly applied to reduce haemorrhage. (a) Combat Application Tourniquet. (b) Pelvic-binding device. (c) Femoral traction device.

(c)

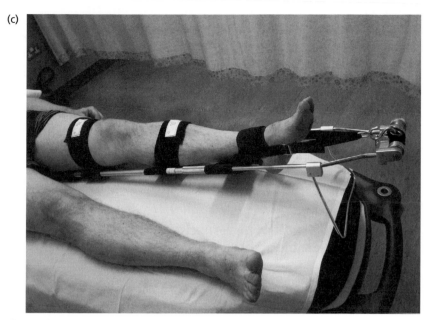

Fig. 2.1 (continued)

    (c) Definitive control: this has traditionally been performed surgically, but interventional radiology is being increasingly employed

2 Resuscitation: to occur **simultaneously with the process of confirming haemorrhage and achieving haemostasis**. The overall aim is the improvement in oxygen delivery to tissues to reduce acidosis. Resuscitation consists of:

    (a) Improving intravascular volume

    (b) Optimizing Hb concentration with red cell transfusion

    (c) Prevention and managing coagulopathy

3 Minimizing delays at all stages of the care pathway.

The patient's pelvic fracture is suspected from the mechanism of injury and clinical signs. Pelvic fracture is associated with major haemorrhage due to the associated vascular disruption of bones and pelvic vessels.

The immediate measure to reduced blood loss was achieved by the pelvic binder to reduce the volume of the pelvic cavity and encourage tamponade of the bleeding vessels. Simultaneously, resuscitation by means IV volume restoration was instituted.

Investigation of the polytrauma patient is ideally carried out by whole body imaging with CT scanning. The advantage is this allows a rapid identification of all injuries in one investigation. However, it requires the patient to have a degree of cardiovascular stability, as it requires transfer to the radiology suite and limits access to the patient during the scan. Severely unstable patients are unable to undergo CT scanning for these reasons. In such cases, the site of haemorrhage can be identified from clinical findings and bedside radiology tests, including CXR, pelvic X-ray, and focussed assessment sonography in trauma (FAST) scan. Transfer to theatre on confirming the site of haemorrhage should be prompt to minimize delays in definitive haemostatic control.

How should this patient be resuscitated in terms of fluids, blood products, and drugs?

Initial fluid and patient response

The aim of fluid resuscitation is the improvement in organ perfusion via an increase arterial pressure.

NICE guidelines recommend the administration of IV fluids in the pre-hospital setting only when the radial pulse has diminished. The loss of a radial pulse is traditionally said to occur when the systolic pressure falls below 80 mmHg. Crystalloid 250 mL boluses are advised until the return of the radial pulse. This strategy is known as **hypotensive resuscitation**, aimed at reducing the stress on fragile fibrin clots to prevent secondary haemorrhage.

Advanced trauma life support (ATLS) teaching on fluid administration advocates 1–2 L of warmed crystalloid to the hypovolaemic trauma patient. European guidelines agree with the initial use of crystalloids. A rise in BP and a reduction in HR are used to assess for improvement in response to fluid, as they reflect a reduction in the need of the cardiovascular system to compensate for low blood volume; such patients are labelled as 'fluid responders.' This response may be: (1) sustained or (2) transient, with the latter more likely to have an ongoing haemorrhage. The third group is labelled as 'non-responder,' indicating that the haemorrhage is so profound and ongoing that fluid therapy does not expand blood volume to improve BP or allow a reduction in HR. Fluid non-responders may have another reason for their profound shock, and causes such as tension pneumothorax or cardiac tamponade should be excluded. Based on fluid responsiveness, the urgency blood products and surgical intervention can be predicted (see Table 2.3).

Table 2.3 Stratifying patients according to fluid response

Response	Rapid	Transient	Minimal/ non-responding
Vital signs	Return to normal	Temporary improvement, recurrence of tachycardia and hypotension	Remain abnormal
Estimated loss	10–20%	Moderate and ongoing	Severe
Need for further crystalloid	Low	High	High
Likely blood requirement	Low	Moderate to high	Immediate
Need intervention	Possible	Likely	Highly likely
Early surgical opinion	Yes	Yes	Yes

Blood pressure target

Whilst aiming to restore an arterial pressure consistent with organ perfusion, it should be noted that overly aggressive fluid resuscitation and elevation of arterial pressure can increase bleeding by clot disruption, coagulation dilution, and hypothermia. The concepts of 'low volume' and 'hypotensive' resuscitation aim to minimize fluid administration before definitive haemostasis. Minimal volume resuscitation is preferable to aggressive volume resuscitation, before active bleeding has been controlled. There is insufficient evidence to determine an optimal BP level during active haemorrhagic shock, but European guidelines recommend a target systolic BP of 80–100 mmHg in those without traumatic brain injury. If brain injury is suspected, then maintenance of cerebral perfusion pressure (CPP) by achieving a normal mean arterial pressure (MAP) is recommended.

Blood product use

The continual administration of crystalloid or colloid fluids will expand the intravascular volume and improve BP but has no oxygen-carrying capacity and will dilute Hb, clotting factors, and platelets. Thus, with ongoing haemorrhage, the need for administration of red cells, clotting factors, and platelets becomes increasingly likely to sustain oxygen delivery and haemostasis.

Red cell replacement

Hb concentration is central in determining arterial oxygen concentration in non-hyperbaric conditions, according to the formula:

$$\text{Arterial oxygen content} = \text{Hb concentration in g/dL} \times 1.34 \times \% \text{ saturation} /$$
$$100 + (0.003 \times PO_2 \text{ in mmHg/dL})$$

(where 0.003 represents the solubility constant for dissolved oxygen in plasma, i.e. 0.003 mL oxygen/PO_2 in mmHg/dL)

The corresponding figure in kPa is 0.023, i.e.

$$\text{Arterial oxygen content} = \text{Hb concentration in g/dL} \times 1.34 \times \% \text{ saturation} / 100 \times (0.023 \times PO_2 \text{ in kPa})$$

It is not possible to determine the optimal Hb levels in patients with traumatic haemorrhagic shock, because no studies have assessed the relationship between Hb levels and the adverse outcomes in patients with traumatic haemorrhage. The European guidelines produced by the Task Force for Advanced Bleeding Care in Trauma in 2010 recommend a target Hb of 70–90 g/L. Near-patient testing can rapidly quantify Hb concentrations and reduce delays in the decision to transfuse. Fully cross-matched blood is preferable, but clinical urgency may necessitate the use of group-specific or O-negative units to optimize Hb.

Clotting factors and platelets

Monitoring and measures to control coagulopathy should be undertaken as early as possible. Traditional means of assessing coagulation have consisted of measuring PT (or international normalized ratio, INR), APTT, fibrinogen concentration, and platelet concentration. These parameters, although widely used, reflect only the early stage of clot formation, provide no information on clot strength, and provide no information on fibrinolysis. TEG is a technique that provides near-patient assessment of the kinetics, strength, and dissolution of blood clotting. It is used routinely in cardiothoracic anaesthesia to rapidly identify the likely cause of coagulopathy and guide decision making in product administration and is increasingly used in other settings, including obstetric haemorrhage, major vascular surgery, and trauma.

FFP administration should begin as soon as possible, following red cell transfusion, initially 10–15 mL/kg. Further FFP can be administered if PT ratio or APTT ratio are >1.5.

Platelet transfusion is recommended when their concentration is $<50 \times 10^9$/L, or $<100 \times 10^9$/L in traumatic brain injury.

Fibrinogen deficiency is treated with fibrinogen concentrate or cryoprecipitate. The target range for treatment during active bleeding is 1.5–2.0 g/L.

Drugs

Tranexamic acid is a drug with several mechanisms of action, including inhibition of fibrinolysis. In a large randomized controlled trial (RCT) of trauma patients (CRASH-2) it was shown to reduce mortality without increasing thromboembolic complications. It should be administered to all haemorrhagic trauma patients as a 10–15 mg/kg loading dose, followed by 1–5 mg/kg over 8 hours (1 g loading dose, followed by 1 g over 8 hours for an average-sized adult). The greatest reduction in haemorrhagic deaths is seen when the drug is administered within 1 hour of injury and is now often administered by pre-hospital trauma teams when transfer to hospital is delayed.

Recombinant factor VIIa has failed to show an improvement in the mortality rate in haemorrhagic shock but is associated with an increased risk of thromboembolic events. It has no place in the routine management of haemorrhagic shock.

Calcium chloride should be administered if ionized calcium levels are deficient.

A new approach

A novel approach to major haemorrhage has been advocated, based on the management of recent battlefield casualties. This approach has advocated the minimization of clear fluids and the early use of red cells, plasma, and platelet units in a ratio of 1:1:1 to improve outcome in trauma, although controversy exists. This evidence has been questioned by the optimum ratio effect of red cells:plasma due to 'survivor bias', i.e. that those patients who died early were much more likely to have received a higher ratio of red cells:plasma due to the time factor in thawing and administering plasma. Furthermore, the survival benefit may have been as a result of a highly organized major haemorrhage protocol where delays were minimized.

The optimum ratio of red cells:plasma remains controversial, and further research is warranted on this question. In contrast, early administration of red cells and plasma is not controversial, and the simultaneous early administration of plasma with red cells, as part of a regimented major haemorrhage protocol, likely improves outcomes in major haemorrhage.

Case update

The patient remains haemodynamically stable, with HR 110 and BP 88/50. You decide to transfer him to the radiology suite for whole body CT scanning.

The investigation shows a pelvic fracture with significant blood in the pelvic cavity. The pelvis is fractured, as shown in Figure 2.2:

The addition of IV contrast to the study reveals bleeding from a branch of the internal iliac artery.

There is no evidence of primary brain, C-spine, thoracic, intra-abdominal, or other skeletal injuries.

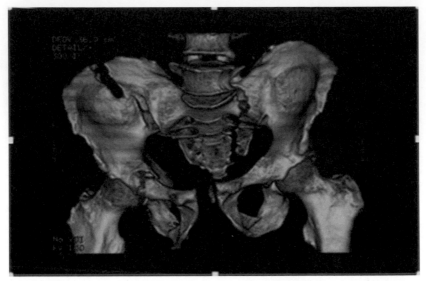

Fig. 2.2 A three-dimensional reconstruction of a complex pelvic fracture with involvement of the right ilium, right acetabulum, right ramus, pubic symphysis, and left side of the sacrum.

What are the options for definitive haemorrhage control in trauma?

The options for management in haemorrhagic trauma patients are:

1 Non-operative management:

   (a) Observation: employed for haemodynamically stable patients when organ preservation is desirable, e.g. splenic laceration

   (b) Interventional radiology (IR): a minimally invasive approach to achieve haemostasis in blunt abdominal trauma and pelvic fracture. IR procedures may involve:

   (i) Embolization of smaller vessels

   (ii) Stent graft placement in larger vessels

2 Operative management: surgical exploration and repair.

Traditionally, surgical exploration and repair have been the means of definitive haemorrhage control. However, the surgical process is a further trauma ('second hit') that will evoke a stress response, contributing to cellular dysfunction and increasing the risk of morbidity and mortality.

Benefits of minimally invasive IR include:

◆ Avoiding the stress response associated with laparotomy or pelvic exploration

◆ Better access to the retroperitoneal space and pelvic cavity.

Although originally employed only in the haemodynamically stable patients, IR has been demonstrated to be of benefit in haemodynamically unstable patients with pelvic fracture. This approach now forms part of the trauma protocol for a growing range of haemodynamically unstable injuries associated with blunt abdominal trauma in many centres. Although prospective studies have shown that the number of laparotomies performed in blunt abdominal trauma can be halved with the use of IR, the overall quality of the evidence for interventional radiological and surgical interventions in trauma is poor. The decision on intervention should be made by the consultant in surgical and radiological teams.

Case update

The consultant interventional radiologist, consultant orthopaedic surgeon, and general surgeon discuss the findings of the CT scan whilst you are transferring the patient off the CT scanner. They agree the best management strategy is to use IR to achieve definitive haemostatic control. You transfer the patient to the IR suite along the corridor where you anaesthetize him for the procedure.

During the procedure, you are phoned by the haematology laboratory, with results of FBC and coagulation screen taken just before leaving the ED. They are as follows:

+ Hb 65 g/L
+ WCC 7.5 × 10^9/L
+ Plt 100 × 10^9/L
+ PT ratio 1.7
+ APTT ratio 1.6
+ Fibrinogen 2.0 g/L
+ ABG showing base excess (BE) –4.0 mmol/L, H^+ 50 nmol/L, lactate 3.8 mmol/L.

You speak with BTS and request an emergency transfusion pack consisting of 4 U of PRC, 4 U of FFP, and 1 U of platelets.

They inform you that the red cells are ready and will be delivered immediately and they had begun thawing the plasma as soon as the patient's coagulation results were available, as the major haemorrhage protocol had been activated by the ED consultant.

How has the introduction of a major haemorrhage protocol influenced management and outcome?

The timely and comprehensive delivery of care in major haemorrhage must coordinate the efforts of front-line medical and nursing staff, laboratory biomedical scientists, BTS, and support staff, including switchboard operators and porters. The introduction of major haemorrhage protocols have been shown to improve several markers of quality of care, including reduced exposure to crystalloid, improved temperature control, and better blood product use. Systematic reviews of major haemorrhage protocols have associated full compliance of protocols with improved survival. However, full compliance with protocols has been shown to be poor. Each institution must have a locally agreed major haemorrhage protocol, given their demonstrable benefit. The anaesthetist must be familiar with the content of the local protocol to achieve full compliance and improve survival. A sample generic protocol is shown in Figure 2.3.

Case update

Over the next 40 min, the patient is transfused with the requested blood products, using a rapid infusion device with heating ability. You then send further blood samples to haematology and also an ABG sample.

Meanwhile, the interventional radiologist performs catheterization of the left internal iliac artery, as shown in Figure 2.4a. Good haemostasis is then achieved by the selective embolization of the bleeding vessel (see Figure 2.4b), and the patient remains cardiovascularly stable.

The blood results from samples taken post-transfusion of 4 U of red cells, 4 U of FFP, and 1 U of platelets show Hb 82 g/L, WCC 9.0×10^9/L, Plt 99×10^9/L, H^+ 48 nmol/L, BE –4.5 mmol/L, bicarbonate (HCO_3^-) 15 mmol/L. Despite the use of warmed IV fluids and a warming blanket, his temperature is 35.8°C.

What is 'damage control' surgery?

This concept advocates doing minimum surgical intervention to achieve stability, thus minimizing the physiological insult to the patient, who is then given a period of physiological normalization in a level 3 setting. The systemic inflammatory response to trauma and haemorrhage, although increasing oxygen delivery, leads to cellular acidosis and dysfunction. Each iatrogenic intervention, although performed to improve survival, is a further stimulus to this pathophysiological process.

Indications for damage control surgery in the severely injured patient include deep haemorrhagic shock, signs of ongoing bleeding, coagulopathy, hypothermia, acidosis, inaccessible major anatomical injury, a need for time-consuming procedures, or concomitant major injury outside the abdomen.

Following the period of correction and stabilization, the patient may be returned to theatre for more definitive correction of their injuries whilst not *in extremis*. In this particular case, the patient was acidotic, coagulopathic, and cold, immediately following definitive haemostatic control of the haemorrhage.

Major haemorrhage protocol

To trigger the major haemorrhage protocol (MHP)

1 Phone 2222 and state that there is a major haemorrhage and the location of the patient. Remain on the line whist the switchboard operator transfers your call to Blood Bank. Tell Blood Bank:

- The diagnosis, e.g. ruptured aortic aneurysm, obstetric emergency

- The patient's details: name, DOB, CHI number (A&E/ARU number for uniden-tified patients)

- What blood components are required, e.g. red cells, FFP, platelets, and how many units

- How urgently the blood components are required

- The patient's current location and planned moves

- Your name and contact details

- What samples are being sent to Blood Bank/Haematology and whether they are ready for collection (Blood Bank will inform you whether a sample for blood grouping is required).

Switchboard will inform:

- *Porters: a dedicated emergency porter will report to Blood Bank*

- *Haematology lab and on-call haematology doctor*

2 **Send the following blood samples with the major haemorrhage porter:**

- A sample for blood grouping to Blood Bank (unless Blood Bank have informed you this is not required because they already have a suitable sample)

- FBC and coagulation screen samples to Haematology.

If further blood components are required, contact Blood Bank directly. Send FBC and coagulation screen samples, as indicated. Haematology advice is avail-able from the on-call haematology doctor—via switchboard. **When the major haemorrhage is over:** inform Blood Bank directly. **Red cells can be obtained rapidly from Blood Bank without triggering the MHP.**

Contact numbers for Blood Bank in an emergency: MHP trigger 2222; Blood Bank phone 3333; Switchboard 0.

O-negative blood location: inform Blood Bank immediately if used; Blood Bank at each hospital A&E—6 U, labour ward 2 U.

Fig. 2.3 Major haemorrhage protocol example.

(a)

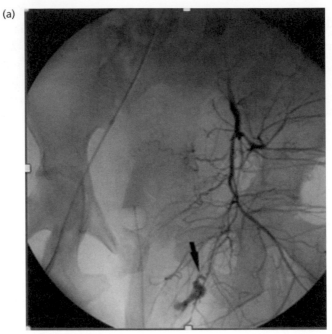

Fig. 2.4 (a) Interventional radiology: contrast-enhanced demonstration of the internal iliac artery. Black arrow indicates bleeding point from a branch of the anterior division, with characteristic 'blushing' of contrast.

(b)

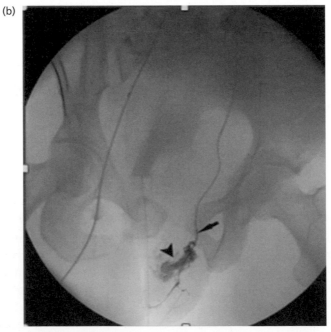

Fig. 2.4 (b) Interventional radiology: embolization of the bleeding vessel by microcatheterization.

At this point, to proceed with open orthopaedic stabilization of the trauma would involve further blood loss and a worsening of the metabolic and haematological parameters. The resulting increase of cellular dysfunction would increase the risk of multiorgan dysfunction syndrome (MODS) and death. Hence, with the minimum necessary intervention to preserve life and allow stabilization, the patient should be given a period in which normal physiology is restored to allow further surgery to be carried out under more favourable metabolic conditions.

Case update

Given the patient's metabolic acidosis, coagulopathy, and anaemia, you arrange intensive care admission with the consultant intensivist.

Over the next 18 hours, he is kept sedated and ventilated. He is warmed to normothermia, receives further blood products to achieve Hb of 8.0, PT ratio <1.5, and APTT ratio <1.5, and 10 mL of 10% calcium chloride to achieve normocalcaemia. His BE gradually returns to –2.0 mmol/L. He does not require inotropic or vasopressor support. His pelvic binder is kept on throughout this period.

The following morning, the orthopaedic trauma team plans to take him to theatre to internally fix his pelvis. This is performed with the loss of 500 mL of blood, but he remains otherwise stable. He is returned to ICU post-operatively for monitoring and correction of his haematological and acid–base disturbance. He is extubated later that day and stepped down to high dependency unit (HDU) care.

Summary

Haemorrhage in trauma is a common, time-critical injury and is responsible for half of all early deaths. The stress response following haemorrhage increases oxygen consumption, whilst reduced Hb and arterial pressure increase oxygen consumption, resulting in tissue acidosis and organ dysfunction. The priorities in the management of major haemorrhage should be directed at the identification and cessation of the bleeding site, with simultaneous resuscitation, whilst avoiding delays. Recent changes in the management of haemorrhagic shock have included the early administration of blood products in preference to clear fluids, early use of tranexamic acid, near-patient testing of Hb and coagulation function, and haemorrhage protocols. Minimizing acidosis, coagulopathy, and hypothermia by resuscitation and damage control surgery should reduce the risk of poor outcomes.

Further reading

Bouige A, Harrois A, and Duranteau J (2013). Resuscitative strategies in traumatic haemorrhagic shock. *Annals of Intensive Care*, **3**, 1.

Rossaint R, Bouillon, Cerny V, *et al.* (2010).Management of bleeding following major trauma: an updated European Guideline. *Critical Care*, **14**, R52.

Westerman RW, Davey KL, and Porter K (2008). Assessing the potential for major trauma transfusion guidelines in the UK. *Emergency Medicine Journal*, **25**, 134–5.

Zealley IA and Chakraverty S (2010). The role of interventional radiology in trauma. *BMJ*, **340**, c497.

Burns

Background

Patients presenting to the ED with burn-related injuries frequently require early input from the anaesthesia and critical care teams. In addition to thermal burns from flame contact, smoke inhalation can cause significant early and late injuries to the airway mucosa and lung parenchyma. Receiving clinicians must also be mindful of the cause of fire exposure, as, if related to vehicle accidents or explosions, additional life-threatening physical injuries may also be present and difficult to detect.

Learning outcomes

1 Identify potential emergency airway problems requiring immediate management in a burns patient

2 Have an appreciation of the detection and treatment of pulmonary injury from smoke and carbon monoxide (CO) toxicity

3 Discuss the accepted approach to fluid resuscitation in a patient with significant burn injury.

CPD matrix matches

2A02; 2A05

Case history

A 42-year-old man is brought into the ED at 11.00 p.m. Firefighters were called to his house at 10.00 p.m. and rescued him from his living room in which he had been trapped for at least 25 min. He had attempted to escape through his hallway which was on fire, and he has sustained burns to his hands, arms, torso, and legs. The paramedics attending him say he was very drowsy at the scene but has become more alert during transfer to the ED. He complains of severe pain around the sites of his burns and of dizziness and headache.

What are your immediate management priorities?

Immediate management follows the ATLS 'ABCDE' system of prioritization, with a rapid primary survey, followed by a careful secondary survey. Monitoring (electrocardiogram (ECG), non-invasive blood pressure (NIBP), and SpO_2) should be applied as soon as possible.

How would you assess and manage this patient's airway?

From the history given, there is no reason to immobilize the patient's cervical spine. Airway assessment involves a standard assessment of the airway plus additional attention to detecting symptoms and signs of upper airway thermal injury. Symptoms include hoarseness, globus, and dyspnoea. Signs include carbonaceous deposits around the nose and mouth, inspiratory stridor, and a swollen uvula on inspection of the oropharynx.

The patient has a red, raw-looking oropharynx with some mild swelling of the uvula. He sounds hoarse. There is no inspiratory stridor, and his airway examination is otherwise unremarkable.

How do you proceed?

If there is sufficient clinical suspicion of upper airway thermal injury, the patient should be anaesthetized, intubated, and ventilated. Airway oedema can develop rapidly, and a patient who may have been straightforward to intubate on initial presentation can become impossible to intubate several hours later. An uncut endotracheal tube (ETT) should be used to allow for the development of facial oedema. If possible, a tube, with an 8 mm or greater internal diameter, should be used to facilitate bronchoscopy in the ICU, should this be required.

What drugs would you use?

Suxamethonium is a safe drug in the first 24 hours post-burn. After this period, the proliferation of extrajunctional acetylcholine receptors may lead to life-threatening hyperkalaemia if succinylcholine is used, an effect which may persist for up to a year post-burn.

His pulse oximetry reading is 100% on air. Are you satisfied with this? How would you further assess breathing and respiratory function?

This patient complains of dizziness and headache. He has been trapped in a burning building for 25 min. This raises the possibility of CO poisoning. CO binds to Hb (carboxyhaemoglobin, COHb) with 200 times the affinity of oxygen, causing a leftward shift of the oxyhaemoglobin dissociation curve, and also inhibits cellular cytochrome oxidase pathways, leading to decreased cellular oxygen utilization. CO poisoning can cause cellular hypoxia in the presence of normal pulse oximetry readings, due to the 'cherry red' appearance of COHb, and is diagnosed by co-oximetric analysis of an arterial blood sample. Symptoms range from headache (10–25% COHb), dizziness and confusion (25–40% COHb), progressing to reduced level of consciousness, seizures, and coma (40–60% COHb). The half-life of COHb is 4 hours in room air, but only 1 hour when breathing 100% oxygen. There is anecdotal evidence for the use of hyperbaric oxygen therapy for CO poisoning, but, in the context of an acute burn injury, it is rarely practical. The patient should receive high-flow oxygen via a non-rebreathing face mask. ABG analysis in this patient demonstrated a COHb of 36%.

How might the circulation in a burns patient be compromised?

Burn injuries lead to an increase in evaporative losses due to the loss of skin integrity, and the associated systemic inflammatory response causes an increase in vascular endothelial permeability, leading to a loss of fluid into the interstitial space. Therefore, a patient with burns will become hypovolaemic and require fluid resuscitation. This requires calculation of the body surface area (BSA) burnt. The 'rule of nines' diagram allows rough estimation of the BSA burnt; however, a Lund and Browder chart (see Figure 2.5) should be completed at the earliest opportunity to allow a more accurate calculation of the burnt area.

This patient has estimated 28% BSA full-thickness burns. His weight is approximately 85 kg. What is his fluid requirement in the first 24 hours post-burn injury?

There exist a number of formulae to provide guidance on the volume of fluid required to resuscitate the burnt patient. They provide a guide to the volumes of fluid needed, and, in all cases, fluid resuscitation should be modified in light of the clinical response of the patient.

The most common formula used to calculate fluid requirements in burns is the Parkland formula:

$$\text{Volume of fluid required in the first 24 hours post-burn} = 4 \text{ mL/kg} \times \% \text{ of BSA burn}$$

Half of the calculated volume should be given in the first 8 hours and the remainder in the next 16 hours. Note that the calculated fluid volume commences from the time of burn, not the time of arrival at hospital. The Parkland

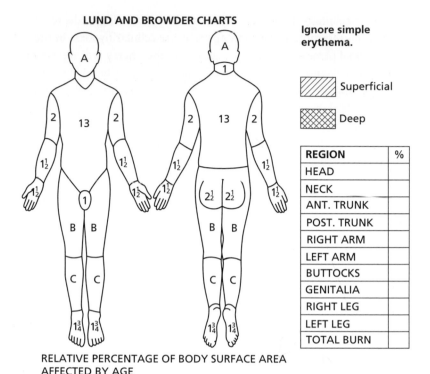

LUND AND BROWDER CHARTS

Ignore simple erythema.

Superficial

Deep

REGION	%
HEAD	
NECK	
ANT. TRUNK	
POST. TRUNK	
RIGHT ARM	
LEFT ARM	
BUTTOCKS	
GENITALIA	
RIGHT LEG	
LEFT LEG	
TOTAL BURN	

RELATIVE PERCENTAGE OF BODY SURFACE AREA
AFFECTED BY AGE

AREA	AGE 0	1	5	10	15	ADULT
A = 1/2 OF HEAD	9 1/2	8 1/2	6 1/2	5 1/2	4 1/2	3 1/2
B = 1/2 OF THIGH	2 3/4	3 1/2	4	4 1/2	4 1/2	4 3/4
C = 1/2 OF ONE LOWER LEG	2 1/2	2 1/2	2 3/4	3	3 1/4	3 1/2

Fig. 2.5 Lund and Browder chart to quantify BSA. Reprinted with permission from the *Journal of the American College of Surgeons,* formerly *Surgery Gynecology & Obstetrics*: Lund CC, Browder NC, 'The estimation of areas of burns', *Surgery Gynecology & Obstetrics*, 1944, 79, pp. 352 0150358.

formula only takes into account fluid requirements due to the burn itself and not ongoing maintenance requirements or losses from other causes. The fluid of choice is balanced electrolyte solution.

This patient would require in the region of $(4 \times 85) \times 28 = 9520$ mL of balanced electrolyte solution in the first 24 hours to cover for fluid losses from the burns themselves.

Venous access may be challenging and may require the insertion of lines through burnt skin. The interosseous route may be useful in this setting.

A urine output of >0.5 mL/kg/hour should be used as a clinical endpoint of successful resuscitation. Over-resuscitation ('fluid creep') should be avoided, as this is associated with worsening of tissue oedema, acute lung injury (ALI), and limb and abdominal compartment syndromes.

What other immediate management steps do you initiate in the emergency department?

The skin is an organ of thermoregulation, and a patient with burns will lose heat rapidly. Attention should be paid to keeping the patient warm with blankets or forced air warmers and warmed fluids, but this should not detract from the need for adequate exposure to facilitate a thorough search for other injuries.

Full-thickness burns are insensate but will be surrounded by areas of partial-thickness burns which will be exquisitely painful, and adequate analgesia should be provided. IV opioids are a suitable choice.

There is evidence to support early feeding in burns, and an NG tube should be inserted as soon as possible.

Should this man be transferred to a specialist burns centre?

The National Burn Care Referral Guidance, produced by the British Burns Association, establishes criteria for discussion or referral of burns patients to specialist burns centres. This patient has significant burns to 'special areas' (hands) and has 28% of BSA burns, with a mechanism of injury placing him at risk of inhalation injury. He should be referred to a regional burns centre for ongoing management.

The patient is now intubated and ventilated in the intensive care unit of the regional burns centre. What would make you suspect he had an inhalation injury?

Pre-existing risk factors for inhalation injury in this man include the history of being trapped in an enclosed space, unconsciousness at the scene, and a raised COHb level in the ED.

It is important to distinguish between upper airway thermal injury and lower airway inhalational injury. Upper airway thermal injury presents in the first hours after injury, as described previously. Lower airway inhalational injury ('smoke inhalation') develops in the following 24–48 hours and can cause widespread injury to the lungs. There is disruption of bronchial epithelial cells with oedema, causing airway narrowing, mucosal sloughing with cast formation, and alveolar collapse leading to impaired gas exchange. Treatment includes regular bronchoscopic lavage to clear debris.

Patients with severe burns may develop secondary acute respiratory distress syndrome (ARDS) as part of the systemic inflammatory response to burns. Treatment is supportive and centres around lung protective ventilation. Burns patients are at increased risk of ventilator-associated pneumonia (VAP), and an appropriate VAP prevention bundle should be instituted.

How should this man's nutritional needs be addressed?

Burn injury generates a hypermetabolic response in the patient and may lead to a doubling of the normal resting energy expenditure. Burns are also associated with a reduction in gut mucosal integrity. There is evidence to suggest that early feeding in the burns patient can reduce the incidence of would infection and length of hospital stay. Enteral feeding is the initial route of choice. Enteral feed supplemented with glutamine is associated with improved gut mucosal integrity, decreased hospital length of stay, and possibly decreased mortality. Hyperglycaemia is associated with increased wound infection rates and mortality and should be avoided.

Summary

The patient with major burns presents the anaesthetist with multiple management challenges. Immediate priorities follow the ABC approach, and the airway must be secured early if there is any suspicion of upper airway thermal injury. It is important to look for other signs of injury in the major burns patient presenting to the ED. Fluid management can be complex, and it is possible to over- as well as under-resuscitate in this situation. A burn is an evolving injury, which can lead to multiorgan failure. Adherence to strict infection control procedures, temperature homeostasis, and nutritional requirements are essential for a good outcome.

Further reading

Bishop S and Maguire S (2012). Anaesthesia and intensive care for major burns. *Continuing Education in Anaesthesia, Critical Care & Pain*, **12**, 118–22.

Latenser B (2009). Critical care of the burns patient: the first 48 hours. *Critical Care Medicine*, **37**, 2819–26.

Sepsis

Background

The mortality from acute bacterial sepsis in the intensive care population remains high, at around 30%, with little change over the past decade, despite considerable advances in intensive care therapies. Currently, there is a global initiative to promote the early recognition of sepsis and rapid and aggressive delivery of sepsis care 'bundles'.

Learning outcomes

1 Define the key recognition points of sepsis and septic shock

2 Understand the principles of the rapid delivery of the 'Sepsis Six' bundle

3 Outline the principles of the intensive care management of a patient with ALI secondary to pneumonia.

CPD matrix matches

2C01; 2C03

Case history

A 46-year-old man is brought into the ED by ambulance. He gives a history of gradually worsening shortness of breath and fever. His past medical history is unremarkable. He is on no medication and has no allergies. His initial observations are: HR 140 bpm, RR 35/min, BP 70/45 mmHg, and his temperature is 39.5°C. SpO_2 on 15 L/min oxygen via a non-rebreathing face mask is 90%. He seems confused. He is using his accessory muscles of breathing and is cool and clammy peripherally, and, on auscultation, he has reduced breath sounds at the left lung base extending to the midzone. His CXR is as shown in Figure 2.6.

Blood gas analysis gives the following results: pH: 7.21, PaO_2 9.2 kPa, $PaCO_2$ 3.2 kPa, HCO_3^- 16 mmol/L. The ED resident is concerned about his clinical state and calls you as the on-call ICU registrar to assist in the ongoing management of this patient.

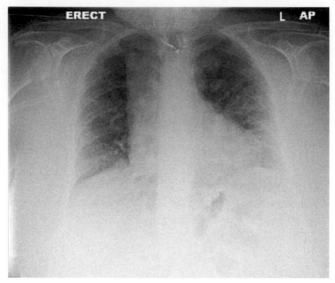

Fig. 2.6 CXR demonstrating left basal consolidation.

What are your immediate treatment priorities?

Treatment priorities for this patient should follow an ABC approach. Full minimal monitoring (SpO$_2$, NIBP, ECG) should be applied. He is already receiving high-flow oxygen via a non-rebreathing face mask. IV access should be obtained.

The presumptive diagnosis here is severe community-acquired pneumonia (CAP) which has rendered the patient, an otherwise fit and well man, very unwell with signs of severe sepsis.

Severe sepsis is part of a spectrum of physiological derangement, ranging from the systemic inflammatory response syndrome (SIRS) to septic shock, and is defined as*:

1 SIRS:

    (a) Two or more of:

        (i) Temperature >38°C or <36°C

        (ii) HR >90 bpm

        (iii) RR >20 breaths/min or PaCO$_2$ 4.3 kPa

        (iv) WCC >12 000 cells/mm^3 or >10% immature forms

---

* Data from 'American College of Chest Physicians/Society of Critical Care Medicine Consensus Conference: Definitions of sepsis and organ failure and guidelines for the use of innovative therapies in sepsis', *Critical Care Medicine*, 20, 6, 1992.

2 Sepsis:

  (a) SIRS with evidence or clinical suspicion of infection

3 Severe sepsis:

  (a) Sepsis associated with organ dysfunction or hypoperfusion

4 Septic shock:

  (a) Sepsis with the presence of end-organ hypoperfusion despite adequate fluid resuscitation.

In recent years, there has been increasing emphasis on early recognition and goal-directed treatment of sepsis. A UK initiative (available at: <http://survivesepsis.org>) defines the 'Sepsis Six' as six tasks to be completed within 1 hour following the recognition of sepsis:

♦ Give high-flow oxygen

♦ Take blood cultures

♦ Give IV antibiotics

♦ Start IV fluid resuscitation

♦ Check Hb and lactate

♦ Monitor accurately hourly urine output.

Implementation of these tasks has been shown to reduce mortality from sepsis.

Going through the 'Sepsis Six' bundle, what would be an appropriate choice of antibiotic for this patient?

This man has a CAP. The British Thoracic Society guidelines for the management of CAP recommends a broad-spectrum β-lactamase stable antibiotic, such as co-amoxiclav, together with a macrolide, such as clarithromycin, as initial IV antibiotic therapy.

How much fluid do you give him, and what fluid do you give?

Resuscitation should commence with a 20 mL/kg bolus of IV fluid. There is some evidence to suggest 4.5% human albumin solution may have a mortality benefit in patients with severe sepsis, but its availability and cost are such that other fluids are more likely to be used. Balanced electrolyte solutions, as they are physiologically balanced solution, is less likely to cause iatrogenic hyperchloraemic metabolic acidosis, compared to resuscitation with normal saline. The patient's clinical response to the initial bolus (peripheral perfusion, HR, BP, mental state, urine output) should be used as a guide to ongoing fluid resuscitation therapy.

What is the rationale behind measuring Hb and lactate in patients with severe sepsis?

Sepsis and severe sepsis are defined by the presence of end-organ hypoperfusion. Lactate is a by-product of anaerobic respiration, and, in the context of sepsis, lactic acidosis can be a measure of tissue hypoxia due to inadequate oxygen delivery. This is known as a type A lactic acidosis. Measurement of lactate gives an indication of tissue hypoxia and can be used as a guide to effectiveness of resuscitation efforts. There is evidence that failure to clear lactate in the first 6 hours of resuscitation is associated with increased mortality.

Oxygen delivery (DO_2, in mL/min) is estimated by:

$$DO_2 = \text{Cardiac output} \times \text{Oxygen content of arterial blood}$$

The oxygen content (CaO_2) of arterial blood is described by the equation:

$$CaO_2 = (1.34 \times Hb \times SaO_2) + (0.023 \times PaO_2 \text{ in kPa})$$

Thus, an anaemic patient will have reduced oxygen delivery, even in the face of an adequate cardiac output and adequate oxygenation. The Surviving Sepsis campaign, a set of evidence-based guidelines on early goal-directed sepsis therapy, recommends transfusing patients with a haematocrit of <0.3.

Case update

The patient's HR and BP improve with fluid resuscitation and are now 120 bpm and 90/45 mmHg, respectively. He becomes increasingly drowsy and more tachypnoeic with a RR of 40 breaths/min. His SpO_2 on 15 L/min oxygen deteriorates to 85%. You decide to anaesthetize and intubate this man before transferring him to the ICU.

Three days later, his CXR demonstrates changes, as shown in Figure 2.7.

His ABG shows a PaO_2 of 8.3 kPa. He is receiving an inspired fraction of inspired oxygen concentration (FiO_2) of 0.9.

Comment on his chest X-ray and arterial blood gases

This patient has developed ARDS.

The American-European Consensus Conference (AECC) definition of ALI and its most severe subset ARDS is[*]:

1 ALI:

 (a) Acute onset

 (b) Bilateral infiltrates on frontal CXR

---

[*] Data from Bernard GR et al., 'The American-European Consensus Conference on ARDS. Definitions, mechanisms, relevant outcomes, and clinical trial coordination', *American Journal of Respiratory Critical Care Medicine*, 1994, 149, 3 Pt 1, pp. 818–824.

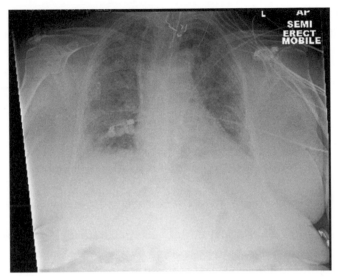

Fig. 2.7 Bilateral interstitial infiltrates.

(c) PaO_2/FiO_2 ratio <300 mmHg (40 kPa)

(d) Pulmonary artery occlusion pressure (PAOP) ≤18 mmHg (or no clinical evidence of left atrial hypertension if PAOP not measured)

2 ARDS:

(a) As for ALI, except: PaO_2/FiO_2 ratio <200 mmHg (27 kPa).

These definitions of ALI/ARDS were updated in 2011. The 'Berlin definition' of ARDS was designed to address a number of issues with the AECC definition, including a lack of clear definition of acute onset, the influence of ventilator settings on PaO_2/FiO_2 ratio, the clinical difficulty of distinguishing hydrostatic pulmonary oedema from other causes of pulmonary oedema, and variability on CXR definition of infiltrates. The Berlin definition removes the term ALI altogether and instead defines ARDS as mild, moderate, or severe by the degree of oxygenation defect.

The Berlin definition of ARDS is:

◆ Onset within 1 week of a known clinical insult, or new or worsening respiratory symptoms

◆ Bilateral opacities on chest imaging: not fully explained by effusions, lobar or lingular collapse, or nodules

◆ Respiratory failure not fully explained by cardiac failure or fluid overload. Need objective assessment (e.g. echocardiography) to exclude hydrostatic oedema if no risk factors present

- Oxygenation defect:
  - Mild: 200 mmHg < PaO_2/FiO_2 ratio ≤300 mmHg, with positive end-expiratory pressure (PEEP) or continuous positive airway pressure (CPAP) ≥5 cmH_2O
  - Moderate: 100 mmHg < PaO_2/FiO_2 ratio ≤200 mmHg, with PEEP ≥5 cmH_2O
  - Severe: PaO_2/FiO_2 ratio ≤100 mmHg, with PEEP ≥5 cmH_2O.

What ventilator settings would you use in this man?

This patient is at risk of ventilator-associated lung injury (VALI). This may manifest as:

- Barotrauma: the use of large tidal volumes results in the generation of high transpulmonary pressures, especially in the presence of pulmonary pathology, causing reduced pulmonary compliance such as ARDS. This may result in the rupture of alveoli, with gas tracking along the perivascular sheaths and breaching the mediastinal pleura, leading to the development of pneumothoraces, pneumomediastinum, and surgical emphysema

- Volutrauma: overdistension of alveoli by excessively high tidal volumes leads to damage of the alveolar–capillary barrier. Increased pulmonary vascular permeability leads to the alveolus becoming flooded with proteinaceous material, and the reduction in surfactant production by the damaged type 2 pneumocytes results in reduced pulmonary compliance, alveolar collapse, and impaired gas exchange due to increased venous admixture and physiological dead space

- Atelectrauma: repetitive recruitment and derecruitment of alveoli during the respiratory cycle can lead to diffuse alveolar damage. Loss of physiological PEEP due to endotracheal intubation, reduction in surfactant production by damaged type 2 pneumocytes, and the lung pathology itself (e.g. pneumonia) all contribute to alveolar derecruitment and thus predispose the lung to atelectrauma

- Biotrauma: damage to the alveolar–capillary interface by injurious mechanical ventilation leads to an influx of cytokines and other inflammatory mediators into the alveolar space. This leads to an intense inflammatory reaction within the lung parenchyma itself, and spillover of inflammatory mediators into the systemic circulation may result in a SIRS-type response.

The ARDSNet group published a trial in 2000 comparing low (6 mL/kg, end-inspiratory plateau pressure <30 cmH_2O) and high (12 mL/kg, end-inspiratory plateau pressure <50 cmH$_2$O) tidal volume strategies. To date, lung-protective ventilation using low tidal volumes is the only intervention shown to improve survival in ARDS, and it has become standard practice in ICU for patients with, or at risk of developing, ARDS.

Other strategies used in dealing with ALI/ARDS include:

- Permissive hypercapnia
- PEEP
- Restrictive fluid strategies
- Prone ventilation
- High-frequency oscillatory ventilation
- Extracorporeal membrane oxygenation (ECMO).

What strategies are used in your intensive care unit to reduce the incidence of ventilator-associated pneumonia?

VAP is associated with increased duration of mechanical ventilation, ICU length of stay, and mortality. Most ICUs in the UK have implemented care bundles to reduce the incidence of VAP.

A care bundle may be defined as a group of evidence-based interventions relating to a particular condition or event. When used together, the elements of the bundle will lead to better outcomes, compared to when the elements are used separately. The 'Sepsis Six' care bundle has already been described.

Components of a VAP prevention bundle typically include:

- Daily sedation holds, if appropriate
- Nursing patient in semi-recumbent (30–45° head-up) position: this reduces the passive regurgitation of gastric contents into the oropharynx
- Selective decontamination of the digestive tract (SDD) and selective oral decontamination (SOD): the rationale behind these interventions is to reduce the pathogenic colonization of the oral cavity and digestive tract without disrupting the normal gut flora. SOD involves the application of topical pastes to the mouth, containing a mixture of antibacterial and antifungal agents (e.g. tobramycin, amphotericin B, and colistin). SDD includes 4 days of IV broad-spectrum antibiotic administration (e.g. cefotaxime), in addition to the oral SDD regimen
- Oral decontamination with topical antiseptics such as chlorhexidine paste 1–2% (if SDD or SOD not used).

Summary

Sepsis, regardless of the aetiology, carries a high mortality. This can be ameliorated by early recognition, appropriate investigations, and treatment, including source control, if possible. Goal-directed therapy in sepsis involves attempting to maximize tissue oxygen delivery by manipulating cardiac output and arterial oxygen content. The definition of ALI has recently been modified to better reflect current imaging practice and ventilation strategies. It is important to remember that mechanical ventilation can be lifesaving, but injudicious ventilation can result in worsening lung injury. Lung-protective ventilation strategies are mandatory in a patient with ALI.

Further reading

British Thoracic Society. Available at: <https://www.brit-thoracic.org.uk/guidelines-and-quality-standards/community-acquired-pneumonia-in-adults-guideline/>.

Finfer S, Bellomo R, Boyce N, French J, Myburgh J, and Norton R; the SAFE Study Investigators (2004). A comparison of albumin and saline for fluid resuscitation in the intensive care unit. *New England Journal of Medicine*, **350**, 2247–56.

Horner DL and Bellamy MC (2012). Care bundles in intensive care. *Continuing Education in Anaesthesia, Critical Care & Pain*, **12**, 199–202.

Hughes M and Black R, eds (2011). *Advanced respiratory critical care*. Oxford University Press, Oxford.

Nguyen HB, Rivers EP, Knoblich BP, *et al.* (2004). Early lactate clearance is associated with improved outcome in severe sepsis and septic shock. *Critical Care Medicine*, **32**, 1637–42.

No authors listed (2000). Ventilation with lower tidal volumes as compared with traditional tidal volumes for acute lung injury and the acute respiratory distress syndrome. The Acute Respiratory Distress Syndrome Network. *New England Journal of Medicine*, **342**, 1301–8.

Rubenfeld GD, for the ARDS Definition Task Force (2012). Acute respiratory distress syndrome—the Berlin definition. *Journal of the American Medical Association*, **307**, 2526–33.

Society of Critical Care Medicine. *Surviving sepsis campaign*. Available at: <http://www.survivingsepsis.org>.

Case 2.4

General anaesthesia for major trauma

Background

Trauma is a pathology that is common and is associated with significant mortality and long-term morbidity in survivors. Management of the patient with multiple injuries requires the teamwork of several medical and surgical specialties. Injuries must be prioritized and dealt with in a timely manner. The anaesthetist will be involved in managing trauma patients throughout the patient's journey and has a central role not just in anaesthetizing for surgical procedures, but also in optimizing the conditions that will improve the likelihood of survival and recovery.

Learning outcomes

1 Understand the role of the anaesthetist in reducing trauma-related mortality

2 Understand the need to prioritize management of injuries in a polytrauma patient

3 Consider the global picture of organ support when anesthetizing the polytrauma patient

4 Understand how trauma can impact upon the conduct of anaesthesia.

CPD matrix matches

2A02; 2C01

Case history

You are the on-call anaesthetist called to the ED, as part of the trauma team. A 35-year-old motorcyclist was involved in a collision with a car. The paramedics hand over to the ED team leader whist the gentleman is being assessed by the emergency medicine registrar, establishing that the gentleman has:

+ An absence of C-spine symptoms: triple C-spine immobilization and a spinal board are *in situ*

+ A patent airway with no signs of obstruction

- RR of 24/min, SpO$_2$ 95% on high-flow oxygen through a 'trauma mask.' Chest examination reveals pain on the left side of the chest
- HR 110 bpm, BP 95/55 mmHg, CRT 3 s, cool hands. An IV cannula is inserted, venous blood drawn, and 500 mL of warmed Hartmann's solution administered, resulting in the HR falling to 100 bpm and an increase in BP to 100/60 mmHg
- His eyes are open, and he obeys commands, but his speech is confused. His pupils are equally reactive to light. Witnesses reported that he was initially unconscious but spontaneously recovered before the ambulance arrived. His blood sugar is 6.0 mmol/l.
- His temperature is 36.1°C. His abdomen is tender and guarded, and he has an obviously deformed, painful right thigh.

Why is the anaesthetist crucial for the management of a trauma patient?

There are approximately 5 million trauma deaths per year worldwide. In western countries, trauma is the fourth leading cause of death, and the incidence is highest in younger patients. In addition, for every trauma death, there are two survivors with long-term health issues. Worldwide, traumatic injuries account for 12% of the world's health burden. The ultimate aims of trauma care are to:

1 Reduce the likelihood of early death

2 Prevent complications that cause late deaths and impair the quality of life in survivors.

Deaths in trauma occur in a trimodal distribution over time, according to the pathology involved (see Figure 2.8).

Peak 1 represents death occurring seconds to minutes following trauma and generally involves severe injuries of the airway, myocardium, great vessels, or brain. It is unlikely that medical care, however prompt, could prevent these deaths.

Peak 2 is accounted by deaths occurring minutes to hours following trauma. Injuries may be in the thorax, abdomen, cranium, or skeleton and are usually associated with haemorrhage. To improve the likelihood of survival, these patients require rapid assessment to identify injuries, with simultaneous resuscitation, followed by early intervention to correct the injuries, which may consist of surgery or IR.

The third 'peak' of deaths occurs days to weeks following trauma, even after definitive correction of the traumatic injuries has occurred. The pathology associated with these deaths includes sepsis and multiorgan failure. Aspects of care provided at all stages of the pathway will impact on the likelihood of infection or organ failure.

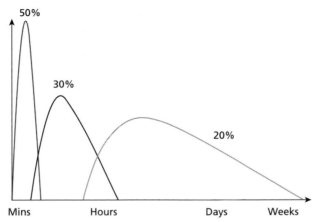

Fig. 2.8 The trimodal distribution of death following major trauma. From Trunkey DD. Trauma Sci Am 1983; 249(2): 20–7.

Trauma management is a core skill of the anaesthetist who may be involved in the care of the trauma patient at the following stages:

- Pre-hospital: advanced airway management and resuscitation
- ED: primary survey, airway management, ventilation, cardiovascular support, IV access, advanced monitoring, haemorrhage management
- Transfer: intrahospital transfer to radiology or theatre, or interhospital transfer to a tertiary care facility
- Intraoperative: provision of anaesthesia and organ support
- Post-operative: provision of organ support and re-establishment of homeostasis in level 2/HDU or level 3/ICU.

Case update

The patient remains tachypnoeic, and a CXR shows some left-sided rib fractures and left upper lobe opacification. He requires 500 mL of Hartmann's solution to maintain a systolic BP above 80 mmHg. His bladder is catheterized.

An X-ray of his femur shows a displaced mid-shaft fracture. He has a femoral nerve block performed, and his leg is placed in a femoral traction device.

He is transferred to the radiology department where a full body CT scan is performed. Findings on CT scanning are:

- Right frontal lobe contusion with small subdural collection
- No evidence of C-spine injury
- Left-sided pulmonary contusions
- Small bowel thickening and extraluminal gas, suggesting disruption
- Right femoral mid-shaft fractures.

The orthopaedic surgeon is keen to proceed with nailing of the femoral fracture, and the general surgeon is keen to proceed with laparotomy. The neurosurgical opinion is that no operative intervention is required.

How should the treatment of these injuries be prioritized?

The trauma patient will often have multiple injuries that require input from different surgical specialties. A global view of the patient must be taken to avoid inappropriate or disordered surgical procedures. Interventions to deal with injuries must be both prioritized and timely to facilitate favourable patient outcome.

Prioritization of operative procedures can be achieved by considering:

- Which injuries will lead to death most quickly
- Which injuries must be addressed to allow stabilization
- Which injuries can be delayed until stabilization has occurred.

Table 2.4 outlines a model of triage for surgical correction when dealing with multiple injuries in polytrauma.

Historically, it was recognized that trauma patients would experience a 'second hit' if they had operative management, i.e. a worsening of their clinical condition despite surgery. For this reason, penetrating abdominal trauma was managed expectantly until the first World War, and skeletal injuries were

Table 2.4 Timing of surgical intervention

Timing	Rationale	Examples
Immediate	Necessary to prevent early death Allows physiological stabilization	Haemorrhage control: • Vascular repair
		Cavity decompression: • Craniotomy
		Cavity decontamination • Bowel repair
	Physiological correction	
Early (day 1)	Can be delayed to allow physiological stabilization	Fracture stabilization: • Femoral nailing
		Soft tissue debridement: • Burns debridement
Late	Reconstructive surgery	

managed by immobilization until 1970s. This 'second hit' in now recognized as further activation of the neurohormonal stress response associated with oxidative dysfunction within the mitochondria.

Surgical management of the trauma patient has moved from 'expectant/non-operative' management, through a period of 'early total care' when all injuries would be corrected at an early stage. This approach saw unwell trauma patients exposed to insults that could have been delayed until they were physiologically stabilized.

Currently, all procedures that are necessary to sustain life and prevent early death are performed immediately. These are procedures without which stabilization cannot occur and include arresting of haemorrhage, decompression of the brain, and decontamination of cavities.

Case update

Following these procedures, the patient who has undergone multiple insults, and at risk of anaemia, coagulopathy, acidosis, hyperthermia, and other metabolic derangements, can have their physiology normalized in intensive care. When they have been stabilized, further necessary, but not life-threatening, procedures can be carried out. This approach is known as damage control.

The subject patient has two injuries requiring surgical attention. The fractured femur requires an intramedullary nail, and the small bowel injury necessitates a laparotomy. A fractured femur can be a life-threatening injury, as it can cause haemorrhagic shock, due to the associated blood loss. The bowel injury will cause soiling of the abdominal cavity and lead to septic shock, unless it is repaired. Of these injuries, addressing the fractured femur would be prioritized over the abdominal injury, according to the 'ABCDE' approach to triage. However, with the femur in traction and immobilized externally, the haemorrhage associated with the injury will be contained, and operative management can be delayed. This means the abdominal injury should be addressed immediately, and the general surgeons have priority to proceed.

What are the issues when considering anaesthetizing this patient?

- Airway and C-spine management:
  - The patient is unfasted and at risk of aspiration of gastric contents
  - The C-spine cannot be clinically 'cleared', and so CT radiological evidence of injury must be absent before removing the collar–blocks–tape immobilizing devices. Intubation will require manual in-line stabilization and may be difficult

- Respiratory:
  - The patient will require PPV in the presence of a pulmonary injury
- Cardiovascular.
  - The patient is at risk from hypovolaemia and sepsis. Optimizing oxygen delivery will be aided by attention to:
  - Advanced monitoring: an arterial line will allow continuous BP measurement. Cardiac output monitoring (such as the Cardio-Q® oesophageal Doppler, LidCCO®, LidCCO Rapide®) is a non-invasive means for stroke volume variation, cardiac index, and systemic vascular resistance, which provide evidence of fluid filling status, contractility, and vascular tone, respectively
  - Hb: the vehicle of oxygen carriage should be monitored, as there has been significant blood loss and clear fluid administration
  - Coagulation: given the trauma, blood loss, and risk of sepsis, the patient is at risk of coagulopathy
  - Lactic acidosis: an objective measure of cellular anaerobic metabolism is provided by monitoring pH/H^+, BE, and lactate
- Neurological:
  - The patient has a mild head injury, but this could worsen in the perioperative period. Attention should be paid to neuroprotective measures
- Renal:
  - The patient has risk factors for developing an acute kidney injury. Intraoperative renal support should consist of optimizing perfusion of the kidneys by attaining an adequate MAP for renal perfusion, minimizing exposure to renal toxins, and monitoring urine output
- Hepatic:
  - The shocked patient may develop a delayed hepatic dysfunction. Intraoperatively, hepatic perfusion of oxygenated blood at normal MAP will support hepatic function
- Metabolic:
  - In addition to the acid–base disturbance, this patient may develop hypocalcaemia, hypomagnesaemia, hypokalaemia, and hypophosphataemia in the post-operative period
- Sepsis:
  - The abdominal cavity is likely to be soiled and the immune function reduced by the stress response. Treatment-dose antibiotics covering intestinal aerobic and anaerobic organisms should be given, according to local protocols

* Temperature:
  * There are risk factors for perioperative hypothermia. An indwelling temperature probe should be placed. Heating blankets and warmed IV fluids should be used to minimize heat loss
* Anaesthesia:
  * Choices of drugs for induction, neuromuscular blockade, and maintenance will need to be rationalized and adjusted, given the risks of hypovolaemia, hypothermia, sepsis, and neurological injury
* Analgesia:
  * Intraoperative analgesia will allow reduction of anaesthetic drug dosages and reduce the risk of developing chronic pain. Post-operative pain management should be planned. The risk and benefits of regional analgesia can be considered.

How should the airway be managed for this general anaesthetic? Are there any anticipated difficulties?

This patient should receive an RSI of general anaesthesia, with the placement of a cuffed ETT. The elements of RSI are pre-oxygenation, cricoid pressure on loss of consciousness, a tilting table, and the availability of suction. There are numerous risk factors for aspiration of gastric contents that can lead to physical obstruction of the airway or pneumonitis. The risk factors for aspiration present here are:

* Major trauma: sympathetic activity inhibiting gastric motility
* Opioid use
* 'Unfasted' status
* Intra-abdominal injury: producing gastric stasis
* Head injury: obtunding laryngeal reflexes.

As with any general anaesthetic, unanticipated difficult laryngoscopy may be encountered, and the strategy of airway management should be decided upon before induction of anaesthesia. In this case, since an RSI has been determined necessary, should the anaesthetist fail to intubate the trachea on three attempts, they should proceed with awakening the patient whilst maintaining oxygenation and ventilation.

How should general anaesthesia be induced and maintained?

The aims of induction are to:

* Rapidly achieve adequate anaesthesia and neuromuscular block
* Allow tracheal intubation

- Prevent aspiration of gastric contents
- Prevent hypoxia and cardiovascular instability.

As mentioned, this patient mandates an RSI. There are several drugs that could be used to achieve this end. The pharmacokinetics of the drugs and the patient's condition should be considered when choosing agents.

Induction agents

- Thiopentone: this barbiturate is classically used in an RSI at 3–5 mg/kg. Thiopentone has the advantage of acting in one arm–brain circulation with a definitive endpoint, and it is a potent suppressor of seizure activity. However, in hypovolaemia, cardiac output is diverted to the vital organs such as the heart, lungs, and brain, and so proportionally more of the drug will be distributed to these organs. As a result, a smaller dose is required to induce anaesthesia, and hypotension secondary to reduced contractility and vasodilation will occur at smaller doses than in the normal patient. In addition, in the acidotic patient, a greater portion of the administered drug will be available in an unionized form and therefore have a more profound effect. Thus, in the presented case, thiopentone should be used cautiously and at a smaller dose. It is not possible to calculate an accurate dose reduction that will induce anaesthesia and yet avoid cardiovascular collapse
- Propofol: this phenol derivative has largely replaced thiopentone in routine anaesthetic practice at a dose of 2–3 mg/kg. Its endpoint is not as definite as thiopentone but will induce anaesthesia rapidly. In the shocked patient, cardiac output and drug distribution will be preferentially to the vital organs, and so smaller doses than normal will induce anaesthesia and cardiovascular compromise
- Etomidate: this imidazole derivative is useful, as it does not cause cardiac depression and vasodilation associated with thiopentone or propofol, when used in normal doses of 0.2 mg/kg. Thus, an accurate dose can be rapidly administered without impairing oxygen delivery. There are concerns regarding etomidate in that it temporarily inhibits the adrenal synthesis of glucocorticoids required to mediate the stress response. Infusion of the drug for sedation is associated with increased mortality in ICU patients; however, a single dose for induction has not been associated with worse outcome
- Ketamine: induction using this agent at 1–2 mg/kg is less rapid, yet it generally confers cardiovascular stability due to anticholinergic and sympathetic activity. It will temporarily increase the ICP and has traditionally been avoided in head-injured patients. However, the agent has neuroprotective properties, and the maintenance of cardiovascular stability and oxygen delivery may outweigh the transitory effect of increase in ICP

- Midazolam: this benzodiazepine is the slowest agent, if used singularly. Although it causes minimal cardiovascular disturbance, it is useful to supplement induction when used with thiopentone or propofol, as it allows dose reduction of the drugs associated with cardiovascular disturbance

- Opioids: used alone, these agents will not cause rapid loss of consciousness, but, as the effect of agents is additive, they are useful as co-induction agents and cause minimal cardiovascular disturbance. Fentanyl and alfentanil bolus dose before induction will allow dose reduction of thiopentone or propofol. Alternatively, infusion of remifentail can be used. The latter has the advantages that it can be infused according to body mass or titrated to the desired plasma or 'effect' site concentration, according to kinetic modelling infusion devices. In addition, opioids will obtund the sympathetic response to laryngoscopy, reducing surges in ICP.

Neuromuscular blockade

The choice of agent to achieve 'paralysis' to facilitate intubation and ventilation is between suxamethonium and rocuronium.

- Suxamethonium: this is an agent traditionally used in RSI at 1–2 mg/kg, as it provides intubating conditions in 45 s. As it will temporarily increase ICP, co-induction with opioids should be carried out. Other serious potential risks with suxamethonium are anaphylaxis and malignant hyperthermia. In addition, hyperkalaemia may occur in those with chronic neuromuscular conditions, as well as those with severe burns or immobility of >48 hours' duration. Normally, a short-acting second agent is needed to maintain neuromuscular blockade. If pseudocholinesterase deficiency is present, a prolonged effect may occur

- Rocuronium: if used for RSI, a dose of 1 mg/kg will achieve intubating conditions in 60 s. Rocuronium is associated with a risk of anaphylaxis but is not associated with malignant hyperthermia or hyperkalaemia. Unlike suxmethonium, rocuronium is not a short-acting agent, and a dose of 1 mg/kg will provide up to an hour of effect.

Maintenance of anaesthesia in the trauma patient case can be achieved by inhalational of volatile anaesthetic or total intravenous anaesthesia (TIVA). Evidence to support one technique over another in a trauma patient is absent.

It should be remembered the trauma patient may be hypovalaemic. This is significant for two reasons:

1 The cardiovascular system will be attempting to compensate by tachycardia and vasoconstriction to maintain BP. Anaesthetic agents, with the exception of ketamine, will suppress the cardiovascular system, and a normal dose may cause

decompensation and worsen tissue perfusion. Lighter doses of volatile (0.7–1.0 minimum alveolar concentration, MAC) or lower target-controlled infusion (TCI) of propofol (3.0–4.0 micrograms/mL) may be needed to avoid this

2 In shock, splanchnic, renal, skeletal, and skin perfusion is reduced; the cardiac output is diverted to the heart, lungs, and brain. Thus, proportionally more anaesthetic will be distributed to the brain and heart. This allows a reduced dose of the administered agent to achieve anaesthesia, and fortunately a reduction in the cardiovascular depression.

Methods to reduce the anaesthetic dose, whilst maintaining cardiovascular stability, include:

- Opioid administration
- Benzodiazepine administration
- Regional analgesia preoperatively: the femoral nerve block will reduce afferent pain stimulation of the cerebrum and reduce sedation requirement. Central neuroaxial blockade is a risk to the trauma patient who is hypovolaemic, as it may provoke cardiovascular collapse, and unrecognized coagulopathy may result is epidural haematoma.

Inappropriate methods in this patient due to the aim of neuroprotection are:

- Nitrous oxide: will increase cerebral oxygen consumption
- Ketamine infusion: will increase ICP.

Whichever technique is chosen, it should be noted that emergency/trauma anaesthesia has been associated with an increased risk of awareness. This is possibly because lighter doses of anaesthesia are used to avoid cardiovascular depression in the hypovolaemic–acidotic patient. In addition, the use of TIVA and continuous neuromuscular blockade have also been associated with increased risk of awareness. In patients with an increased risk of awareness, the bispectral index (BIS) can provide an indication of the depth of anaesthesia. This dimensionless number, derived from frontotemporal electroencephalograms (EEGs), indicates cortical activity, with 100 being normal and 0 being isoelectric. A BIS of 40–60 is associated with a low probability of conscious recall and can be used to titrate anaesthetic dose. It should be noted that there is considerable interindividual variability with BIS and conscious level, and there is conflicting evidence on the efficacy of BIS in reducing the risk of awareness.

What are the issues with ventilation of this patient?

The overall aim of cardiorespiratory support is cellular oxygenation to meet metabolic demands and avoidance of anaerobic metabolism and acidosis. Intraoperative ventilation should be aimed at:

- An adequate PaO_2 that achieves saturation of Hb
- Low to normal $PaCO_2$
- Minimizing the risk of ventilator-induced lung injury (VILI).

The role of the respiratory system is to develop a partial pressure of oxygen in the pulmonary capillaries that will saturate the Hb molecules within erythrocytes, thus optimizing arterial oxygen content. An inadequate partial pressure of oxygen in capillary blood will reduce the percentage of Hb that is saturated with oxygen, risking inadequate arterial oxygen content and subsequent lactic acidosis. Appropriate monitoring of the respiratory system of this patient intraoperatively consists of continuous pulse oximetry and intermittent arterial blood analysis of PaO_2. Monitoring of pulmonary capillary blood is not possible, but arterial PaO_2 is the best surrogate indicator.

The ventilator parameters that can be adjusted to improve PaO_2 are:

- Minute ventilation (MV): the product of tidal volume (Vt) and RR. Tidal volume can either be controlled directly (volume-controlled ventilation) or indirectly by varying the inspiratory pressure (pressure-controlled ventilation)

- FiO_2

- PEEP: general anaesthesia, supine position, and alveolar pathology will predispose to alveolar collapse which can be overcome by PEEP. Studies in ALI in intensive care patients have shown no adverse outcome when comparing higher levels of PEEP to lower levels.

The ventilator parameters of inspiratory pressure, tidal volume, PEEP, RR, and FiO_2 can be adjusted to achieve appropriate oxygenation.

The other role of the respiratory system is the excretion of carbon dioxide. This product of aerobic metabolism is a volatile acid. Hypercarbia contributes to cellular acidosis and will cause an increase in cerebral blood volume by cerebrovasodilation, risking a rise in ICP in head injury. Conversely, hypocarbia ($PaCO_2$ <4.0 kPa) will cause cerebrovasoconstriction and impair oxygen delivery in the brain. For these reasons, it is considered neuroprotective to target a $PaCO_2$ of 4.0–4.5 kPa. There is an inverse linear relationship between alveolar PCO_2 and MV; so, in order to reduce $PaCO_2$, MV must be increased.

PPV is a means to achieve oxygenation and normocarbia, but it is not without risk. The physical forces involved in PPV induce inflammatory changes within the lung, known as VILI. In patients with ALI, a lung-protective ventilation strategy of restricting the tidal volume to 6 mL/kg (ideal bodyweight) and the inspiratory plateau pressure to 30 cmH_2O is associated with a reduction in mortality. The inflammatory changes associated with PPV are known to occur early in the ventilation period in normal lungs, not as a late consequence. Given the presence of the pulmonary contusions and the possibility of post-operative ventilation, lung-protective ventilation is a strategy that may reduce the likelihood of post-operative respiratory complications.

The process of cellular oxygen utilization to produce adenosine triphosphate (ATP) involves several enzyme-dependent steps during the citric acid cycle and the electron transport chain. Under conditions of stress, including trauma, the utilization of oxygen can become dysfunctional and lead to the incomplete reduction of oxygen to water, generating charged free radical species that cause irreversible mitochondrial damage. High levels of oxygen supplied to the dysfunctional cell will fuel the formation of these free radicals, and so the lowest FiO_2 consistent with an adequate Hb saturation should be used.

What influence does a head injury have on the management of a trauma patient?

Although this patient does not require neurosurgery, he nonetheless has a significant primary brain injury. The principle in management of this injury is the prevention of secondary brain injury throughout the perioperative period. This is achieved by ensuring cerebral oxygenation and prevention of a rise in ICP. The following factors should be addressed to achieve this end:

- Airway: laryngoscopy and the presence of an ETT will evoke a sympathetic response, increasing the cerebral blood volume and pressure, as will coughing or straining. These responses can be reduced by adequate doses of anaesthetic and opioids, and the maintenance of neuromuscular blockade. In addition, the ETT should be secured with tape, not a tie which can reduce jugular venous drainage

- Gas exchange: hypoxia and hypercarbia will cause cerebral vasodilation and an increase in ICP. The patient should be ventilated to achieve a PaO_2 >10 kPa and $PaCO_2$ 4–4.5 kPa. PEEP should be minimized to prevent elevation in jugular venous pressure (JVP)

- CPP is required to perfuse the brain (CPP = MAP – ICP). Normally, CPP is constant over a range of MAP, from 50 to 150 mmHg, because of autoregulation, i.e. cerebrovasodilation in response to hypotension and cerebrovasoconstriction in response to hypertension. In brain injury and under anaesthesia, autoregulation is obtunded, and so perfusion becomes dependent on the MAP. For this reason, normotension should be targeted and hypotensive resuscitation avoided

- Hb concentration
- Anaesthesia: volatile agents will reduce the cerebral demand for oxygen, protecting against hypoxia. However, it will also cause dose-dependent cerebrovasodilation, which increases ICP. On balance, a MAC of 0.7–1.0 should allow adequate anaesthesia, without raising ICP. Opioids will supplement anaesthesia, in addition to analgesia, obtunding laryngeal reflexes, e.g. remifentanil infusion. Ketamine has traditionally been associated with increasing ICP.

Case update

The general surgeons perform a laparotomy and find two full-thickness disruptions of the jejenum. They perform two short resections and end-to-end anastomoses of the small bowel and lavage the abdominal cavity. No other injuries are found, and the abdomen is closed within an hour of beginning the procedure.

The patient remains stable throughout the procedure.

Table 2.5 shows the results of the intraoperative arterial and venous blood analysis performed intraoperatively.

Given the patient's stability and lack of metabolic derangement, it is decided to proceed with the insertion of an intramedullary nail to the fractured femur. General anaesthesia is continued for this procedure, during which the patient loses approximately 750 mL of blood and requires 1 L of Hartmann's solution.

Table 2.5 Intraoperative arterial and venous blood results

Parameter (normal range)	Result
H^+ (35–45 nmol/L)	44
HCO_3^- (22–28 mmol/L)	21
Lactate (0.0–2.0 mmol/L)	2.0
BE (–2.0 to 2.0)	2.0
PaO_2 (11–13 kPa)	11 (FiO_2 0.4)
$PaCO_2$ (4.0–6.0 kPa)	4.5
Hb (12–17 g/dL)	9.0
WCC (4.0–9.0 x 10^9/L)	5.0
Plt (150–400 x 10^9/L)	200
PT ratio (1.0)	1.2
APTT ratio (1.0)	1.2
Fibrinogen (1.5–3.5 g/dL)	2.0

The procedure takes 90 min. Towards the end of the procedure, a near-patient HemoCue® shows a Hb of 7.0 g/dL. An ABG shows H^+ 50 nmol/L, BE −4.0 mmol/L, and lactate 3.0 mmol/L.

Should this patient be extubated following the surgical procedure, or should ventilation continue in the post-immediate post-operative period?

The advantage of extubation following surgery is that the patient is no longer exposed to the risks of PPV, i.e. physical forces that induce inflammation and dysfunction of the respiratory membrane, known as VILI. Ventilation is also associated with barotrauma, wasting of the respiratory muscles, VAP, impairment of haemodynamics, and inflammatory changes in distant organs.

To minimize the risks of mechanical ventilation, patients should be extubated and returned to spontaneous negative pressure ventilation as soon as it is likely they will not develop respiratory failure post-extubation.

Patients at risk of respiratory failure should be identified before extubation. The Difficult Airway Society has produced an extubation guideline (see Figure 2.9) to assist with stratifying patients into low-risk or high-risk groups for adverse events post-extubation and forming a strategy for managing the high-risk group.

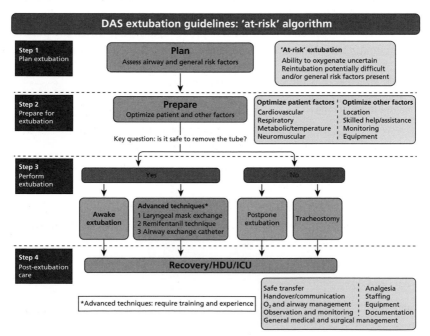

Fig. 2.9 Difficult Airway Society extubation guideline. Reproduced with permission from V. Mitchell et al., 'Difficult Airway Society Guidelines for the management of tracheal extubation', *Anaesthesia*, 67, 3, pp. 318–340, © 2012 The Association of Anaesthetists of Great Britain and Ireland.

Extubation is a high-risk stage in the perioperative period that can lead to complications. In our subject case, the most likely complications following extubation are aspiration and respiratory failure. The general risk factors for respiratory failure are:

◆ Cardiovascular:

- The patient has undergone a major trauma followed by two surgical procedures of intermediate risk. Each of these contributes to the stress response, increasing oxygen demand and placing demands on the cardiovascular system to increase oxygen delivery. The stress response is known to continue for 48 hours following a major surgery. Continued sedation and ventilation in the immediate post-operative period will reduce oxygen consumption

◆ Respiratory:

- The patient has pulmonary contusions that are at risk of worsening during the intraoperative period. An assessment of the function of the respiratory membrane can be made by comparing the partial pressure of oxygen of arterial blood to that of inspired gas (P/F ratio)

◆ Neurological:

- Brain injury: the patient's preoperative mild brain injury may have worsened despite neuroprotective measures. On emergence from anaesthesia, this may manifest as acute confusion, causing ineffective ventilation

- Pain: untreated pain is a risk factor for post-operative respiratory failure. Similarly, excessive use of opioid may cause hypoventilation

◆ Metabolic:

- Metabolic acidosis creates an oxygen debt for which the respiratory system will try to compensate. On emergence from anaesthesia, this may cause a rapid, inefficient ventilation and respiratory failure

- Disturbance of calcium and magnesium homeostasis may result in inefficient respiratory muscle activity

- Hypothermia: the expenditure of energy in shivering and cerebral dysfunction in the hypothermic patient may contribute to post-operative respiratory failure.

Case update

It is decided that the patient should be kept sedated and ventilated, and admission to the ICU is organized.

Over the next 12 hours, he is ventilated with a lung-protective strategy; he has his Hb kept above 8.0 g/dL with red cell transfusion, and his BE returns to normal. His PaO_2 is kept above 10 kPa with an FiO_2 of 0.3, PEEP of 5 cmH_2O, and the inspiratory support is weaned. He is extubated and maintains an SpO_2 of 95% on FiO_2 of 0.4, with no signs of respiratory distress. Serial CXRs show a gradual resolution of the pulmonary contusion.

The patient resumes oral intake of nutrition and is discharged to the orthopaedic ward on day 2 post-operatively.

Summary

Trauma is a common pathology that is associated with significant mortality and morbidity in survivors. Those surviving the initial injury are at risk of dying early due to their injuries, or dying later as a result of multiorgan dysfunction and sepsis. Following an initial assessment and resuscitation measures, potential injuries should be suspected. If the patient is stable, a whole body imaging will allow diagnosis and the prioritized management of underlying injuries. Cardiovascular instability is an indication for surgery directed at haemorrhage control before diagnosing and managing other injuries. The anaesthetist should aim to maintain adequate cellular oxygenation to limit anaerobic metabolism and acidosis, to support other organ systems, and to minimize the potential for sepsis. A multisystem model of care will allow the support of vital organs. Anaesthesia should be conducted, respective of the patient's past medical history and their acute injuries and physiological status. All supportive therapies, from oxygen administration to ventilation, inotropic/vasopressor support, and renal replacement therapy (RRT), carry an inherent risk of iatrogenic injury and should be de-escalated, when appropriate, to minimize this risk.

Further reading

American College of Surgeons Committee on Trauma (2008). *ATLS Student Course Manual*, 8th edn. American College of Surgeons, Chicago (ISBN 978–1–880696–31–6).

Difficult Airway Society. *DAS extubation guidelines*. Available at: <http://www.das.uk.com/content/das-extubation-guidelines>.

Kilpatrick B and Slinger P (2010). Lung protective strategies in anaesthesia. *British Journal of Anaesthesia*, **105** (suppl 1), 108–16.

National Confidential Enquiry into Patient Outcome and Death (2007). *Trauma:who cares?* Available at: <http://www.ncepod.org.uk>.

Nicola R (2013). Early total care versus damage control: current concepts in the orthopedic care of polytrauma patients. *ISRN Orthopedics*, 2013, article ID 329452.

Patel P (2005). An update on neuroanesthesia for the occasional neuroanesthesiologist. *Canadian Journal of Anesthesia*, **52**, 6.

Chapter 3

Day case anaesthesia

Dr Alasdair Waite
Dr Mark Ross

Post-operative nausea and vomiting

Background

With an increased drive to day-surgery procedures across the NHS, anaesthetists are being increasingly challenged to provide safe and effective perioperative care that also facilitates a rapid post-operative recovery. After inadequate analgesia, post-operative nausea and vomiting (PONV) is the commonest reason for unplanned overnight admission.

Learning outcomes

1 Effectively assess a patient at risk of PONV

2 Consider alternative anaesthetic and analgesic strategies to minimize risk of PONV

3 Outline the different classes of antiemetic agents.

CPD matrix matches

1A02; 2A03

Case history

It is 8.15 a.m., and you meet a 44-year-old lady presenting for elective wire-guided wide local excision of breast tumour, with sentinel node biopsy. She is ASA 1, takes no medication, and has no allergies. She has a history of PONV.

What further information would you like during the preoperative assessment?

◆ Height and weight/body mass index (BMI)

◆ Presence or absence of reflux

◆ Fasting status

◆ Presence or absence of carer at home

◆ Further details about her PONV.

Case update

Your patient is 1.70 m tall and weighs 60 kg, giving a BMI of 21 kg/m^2. She has no reflux and is fasted for solids overnight, though she had a cup of black coffee at 7.00 a.m. She is chewing gum when you meet her.

Your patient had three previous operations: a tonsillectomy at age 12, a laparoscopy and excision of skin lesions under general anaesthetic at age 39. She was sick after all operations, despite telling the anaesthetist about her PONV prior to her laparoscopy. She was assured she would get anti-sickness drugs and a 'special' anaesthetic last time, but she vomited post-operatively and had to stay in hospital for 4 days post-operatively following the laparoscopy and 3 days following the skin lesion excision.

Will her fasting status delay her operation?

Not necessarily. She requires to go to the radiology department to have ultrasound-guided wire insertion. This means it should be unlikely she will be first on the list. The commonly accepted preoperative fasting in adults undergoing elective surgery is 'the 2–6 rule':

- '2': intake of water up to 2 hours before induction of anaesthesia
- '6': a minimum preoperative fasting time of 6 hours for food (solids, milk, and milk-containing drinks).

Would you consider her recent cup of coffee or gum chewing in breach of fasting guidelines?

She had black coffee. This does not contain fat or solids, so many anaesthetists would treat this as equivalent to water and accept a 2-hour period of fasting as acceptable. If there were other concerns or she had milk in her coffee or food at 7.00 a.m., she would need to wait until 1.00 p.m. before proceeding to surgery.

Chewing gum may be allowed up to 2 hours prior to surgery, as suggested by the AAGBI in 2010. It is now 8.15 a.m., so her procedure should not be carried out before 10.15 a.m.

She does not have a carer at home. Is she suitable for day case surgery?

No. She should have a carer at home who is able to look after her for 24 hours post-operatively.

Is her history of post-operative nausea and vomiting significant?

Yes. She needed to stay in hospital as a result of vomiting for 4 days following her last two procedures. It is not uncommon for patients to be sick following tonsillectomy if they swallow some blood in the immediate post-operative period. This causes gastric irritation, nausea, and vomiting. Published rates of PONV following tonsillectomy range from 0% to as high as 44%.

Laparoscopy is also regarded as relatively high risk for PONV, with 41% of patients requiring some form of antiemetic in the post-anaesthetic care unit (PACU) following gynaecological laparoscopy if they received only placebo. This can be reduced to 2% with multimodal antiemetic prophylaxis.

Skin lesion excision would be expected to be a low-risk procedure for PONV. It is body surface surgery and can usually be analgesed effectively without the use of opiates. Her history suggests she is at high risk of PONV, and her breast surgery procedure is likely to be more emetogenic than her last procedure.

Is there any other information you would like?

+ What analgesics has she taken in the past?
+ Are there particular drugs which cause her to be nauseated?
+ Can she tolerate non-steroidal anti-inflammatory drugs (NSAIDs)?
+ Does she suffer from travel sickness?
+ Are there any medications she takes for travel sickness that she finds effective?
+ Were there any antiemetics she found helpful following her last operation?

Can this procedure be carried out under local or regional anaesthesia?

Wide local excision could be carried out under local infiltration, but axillary node sampling is unlikely to be tolerated. Paravertebral block is used by many centres for breast surgery and could be considered. Some centres will use this technique for day case surgery. An epidural covering dermatomes C8–T5 could, in theory, be used (insertion C7/T1). There are a number of risks involved in epidural analgesia, and careful balancing of the risks and benefits would be needed. The authors are unaware of any institutions where cervical/thoracic epidural anaesthesia for day case procedures is routinely carried out.

How are you going to provide anaesthesia and analgesia for this lady, given she refuses a regional technique?

+ Use a technique and drugs that will minimize the risk of nausea
+ Avoid drugs that have emetic effects, if possible, and use multimodal antiemetics
+ Use drugs with half-lives that maximize the chance of same-day discharge.

Preoperatively

- Avoid long preoperative fasting, and hence dehydration, so limit fluid fasting to 2 hours for water or clear fluids
- Early on morning or afternoon list with 6-hour solids fasting
- Premedication: consider hyoscine patch, omeprazole 20–40 mg if history of dyspepsia, benzodiazepine anxiolysis only if absolutely necessary as may decrease chance of same-day discharge.

Intraoperatively

- Airway: laryngeal mask airway (LMA) or tracheal tube—both acceptable
- Breathing: spontaneous ventilation or intermittent positive pressure ventilation (IPPV)—both acceptable. Muscle relaxant is not required for surgical reasons. IPPV will increase risk of PONV if gas is forced into the stomach
- Induction: ideally use propofol TIVA. Thiopental and etomidate should be avoided, as they may be emetogenic. Remifentanil is an ideal agent to cover airway manipulation without long-lasting opioid effects and could be used. Nitrous oxide should be avoided. Bag-and-mask ventilation should aim to minimize inflation of the stomach. Short-acting opiate may be required to aid LMA/ETT placement. Fentanyl and alfentanil can be considered, though fentanyl has the advantage of being less likely to cause apnoea when using an LMA, yet being redistributed prior to emergence if used in a small enough dose
- Maintenance: the optimal choice for this patient's procedure is propofol, delivered by TCI
- Analgesia: minimally emetogenic, analgesic options include:
  - Clonidine: 75–150 micrograms IV, but this will result in significant postoperative sedation and will make same-day discharge unlikely
  - Ketamine: 0.15 mg/kg IV, following induction, will provide excellent analgesia, but with likely side effects of hallucinations and sedation which will prevent same-day discharge
  - Paracetamol: 1 g either pre- or intraoperative
  - Bupivicaine: 2 mg/kg infiltration by surgeon at end of case
  - Oxycodone can be considered and has been found to be less emetogenic than other opiates in our unit
  - Tramadol is not minimally emetogenic. Some patients may tolerate its emetic side effects if it is given prior to emergence, though this is not reliable.

- Antiemetics: combination antiemetic therapy is vital for this patient. The mainstay would be a 5-HT$_3$ antagonist such as ondansetron, granisetron, or dolasetron. An H$_1$-antagonist (antihistamine) would commonly be added, e.g. cyclizine 50 mg. Adjuncts include: dexamethasone, an anticholinergic such as a hyoscine transdermal patch, or an antidopaminergic agent such as piperizine, prochlorperazine, droperidol. There is conflicting evidence regarding the antiemetic efficacy of metoclopramide
- Acupuncture and acupressure are also reported to be useful in some patients.

Post-operatively

- Regular paracetamol, oral 1 g 6-hourly
- NSAIDs, e.g. ibuprofen 400 mg qds or diclofenac 50 mg tds, are usually avoided in the first 24 hours following breast surgery, due to a perceived increased risk of haematoma. Consider gastric protection, such as ranitidine or lanzoprazole, if longer duration therapies of NSAIDs are used
- Tramadol 50 mg is unlikely to be better tolerated than dihydrocodeine 30 mg as take-home analgesia for breakthrough pain, but there is some interindividual variation. Ask if the patient has prior experience and any preference
- Oxycodone can be considered and may be less emetic than other opiates.

Would you give IV fluids?

Yes. There is some evidence that the administration of IV fluid in the perioperative period decreases PONV.

Are you aware of any other effective antiemetic drugs? In what way might they be beneficial?

Palonosetron is a second-generation 5-HT$_3$ blocker with a 40-hour half-life. It may be more effective for post-discharge nausea and vomiting. It does not seem to prolong QTc.

Would the administration of this combination of drugs give you any concerns about post-operative sedation?

Yes, a number of these drugs have sedative effects and long half-lives and, when combined, can produce marked sedation which may last a number of hours. The patient would need to be observed in the recovery area (PACU), prior to returning to a ward environment where staff would need to be informed that longer-acting drugs had been used and to be vigilant for signs of sedation. The aim is for same-day discharge, so the use of sedating drugs with long half-lives is to be avoided.

If this lady manages to arrange for a carer at home, would she be suitable as a day case?

She may still be suitable if some longer-acting drugs were used, though this would depend on the rate and nature of her recovery. Performing her surgery earlier in the day would allow time for her to recover and being fit for discharge on the day of surgery. The priority is to provide safe and effective anaesthesia and antiemesis. Day of surgery discharge should be aimed for, but not to the extent of compromising care. Careful anaesthesia and a 1-night post-operative stay are preferable to a poorly considered technique and a 4-day inpatient stay.

Summary

There has been an increasing drive towards day case surgery. Certain criteria must be fulfilled for this to be done safely. This includes the patient having the necessary domestic support before they can be discharged. In addition, they can only be discharged home when they are comfortable and any PONV is adequately treated. Analgesia will usually involve a multimodal approach.

Although the management of PONV is important in any field of anaesthesia, it is especially important in day case surgery, due to the effect this will have on discharge.

The anaesthetist has an important role in both the management of post-operative analgesia and the prevention and treatment of PONV.

Further reading

Apfel1 CC, Meyer A, Orhan-Sungur M, Jalota L, Whelan RP, and Jukar-Rao S (2012). Supplemental intravenous crystalloids for the prevention of postoperative nausea and vomiting: quantitative review. *British Journal of Anaesthesia*, **108**, 893–902.

Carlisle JB and Stevenson CA (2006). Drugs for preventing postoperative nausea and vomiting. *Cochrane Database of Systematic Reviews*, **3**, CD004125.

Lee A and Fan LTY (2009). Stimulation of the wrist acupuncture point P6 for preventing postoperative nausea and vomiting. *Cochrane Database of Systematic Reviews*, **2**, CD003281.

Scuderi PE, James RL, Harris L, and Mims GR 3rd (2000). Multimodal antiemetic management prevents early postoperative vomiting after outpatient laparoscopy. *Anesthesia & Analgesia*, **91**, 1408–14.

Verma R, Alladi R, Jackson I, *et al.* (2011). Day case and short stay surgery: 2. *Anaesthesia*, **66**, 417–34.

Day case dental anaesthesia

Background

Anaesthesia for dental surgery would routinely be considered a day case procedure. However, many patients may be scheduled for such procedures, occasionally by non-physicians, without appreciation for the impact of their comorbidity on the day surgery process. This case highlights a planned routine dental extraction in a patient with considerable comorbidity and discusses the suitability or not for this to be performed as a day case.

Learning outcomes

1 Assess a patient with complex comorbidity listed for an outpatient anaesthetic procedure
2 Acknowledge potential perioperative complications in an adult with congenital heart disease
3 Discuss the anaesthetic technique for such patients.

CPD matrix matches

2A03

Case history

You are anaesthetizing for an adult dental day case in a dental hospital. An 18-year-old male presents for elective removal of all four wisdom teeth. He weighs 60 kg. He has Eisenmenger's syndrome.

What is Eisenmenger's syndrome?

Eisenmenger's syndrome is a syndrome of right-to-left cardiac shunt as a result of pulmonary hypertension. The initial shunt is left to right, due to an intraventricular, intra-atrial, or aortopulmonary defect. Over time, pulmonary hypertension develops and is described as Eisenmenger's syndrome when the shunt reverses and becomes right to left or bidirectional.

What problem does this present?

The patient may be cyanosed, dyspnoeic, and polycythaemic, and he may have signs and symptoms of ventricular strain. Patients with Eisenmenger's syndrome are at increased risk of supraventricular arrhythmias, sudden death, thrombosis, bacterial endocarditis and clots, and air emboli. He may also be warfarinized. Decreasing afterload will increase shunt and worsen hypoxia.

How would you go about anaesthetizing this gentleman?

You would involve an anaesthetic consultant immediately.

You are the consultant. How would you go about anaesthetizing this gentleman?

You need to break down this case into components relating to the surgery, clinical condition, suitability of the location, and mode of anaesthesia. These need to be discussed with the dental surgeon and the safest course of action followed.

Does he need this surgical procedure?

This will have been carefully considered by the referring dentist and by the accepting surgeon, but it does no harm to ask. The dental radiographs can be reviewed and surgery reconsidered. If the patient has had pain and infection around impacted wisdom teeth, then they are at risk of bacterial endocarditis, and the dental infection is likely to return in the future. The shunt will continue to worsen with time, so delaying the procedure may mean the same procedure is carried out when patient fitness has worsened.

Does he need a general anaesthetic?

It may be that the wisdom teeth may be relatively straightforward to remove under local anaesthetic block, avoiding the need for general anaesthesia. The teeth may not all need to be removed at the same time, though the patient is keen to limit the extractions to one visit. Significant anxiety on the patient's part will increase circulating catecholamines and increase the risk of arrhythmia, decreasing cardiac function. This may be attenuated by careful conscious sedation.

Case update

Whilst two teeth look to be very straightforward to extract, two look particularly difficult, and having a general anaesthetic will make the procedure significantly easier for the surgeon. The additional time to remove the straightforward teeth will be relatively small, so, on balance, it is probably safer to remove all four teeth in one operation, rather than two. This was the reason for his addition to a general anaesthetic dental list.

This gentleman has regularly been followed up by the local cardiology services, and a recent clinic letter should be available. If there have been any changes or deterioration since his last cardiac review, then a discussion with the patient's cardiologist is advisable, in case a change in drug management would improve cardiac function. This gentleman saw his cardiologist 2 weeks ago and has not noticed any changes in his condition in the last year.

Is a remote dental hospital a suitable site?

Any operating location outwith a theatre suite is regarded as remote. This would include a physically distant single theatre in a large hospital complex or a single theatre in a separate hospital. The authors regard any location where it is not possible to receive qualified anaesthetic help by shouting from the theatre door should be classified as remote for the purposes of anaesthesia.

This dental hospital may be on a larger hospital site or a number of miles from general hospital critical care facilities. Whilst the standard of care should not differ from any other operating theatre, this gentleman has a higher than average chance of perioperative complications and help may be required. It would be advisable to carry out this gentleman's procedure in a theatre suite where immediate help would be available, and he should be referred to the nearest maxillofacial surgery unit. A general anaesthetic should not be carried out in this remote location.

Would you provide conscious sedation for this gentleman in this location if all the dental extractions were thought to be straightforward?

The authors feel that, whilst this may be uneventful, should perioperative problems develop, the level of support immediately available may not be sufficient. This gentleman would be best treated in a maxillofacial unit within a theatre suite environment.

What anaesthetic would you give this gentleman?

This anaesthetic requires being carried out carefully, with attention to managing systemic and pulmonary vascular resistance (PVR). A drop in systemic vascular resistance (SVR) will decrease pulmonary perfusion by increasing right-to-left shunt. A rise in PVR will also increase right-to-left shunt and worsen oxygenation. PVR is difficult to reduce, and SVR is the variable that is likely to change the most with administration of anaesthesia. The circulating volume needs to be maintained, and dehydration should be avoided.

Bradycardia and high-pressure IPPV should be avoided. Where possible, techniques involving spontaneous ventilation should be used.

What induction agent would you use?

The choice of induction agent is probably less important than the familiarity of the anaesthetist with the agent and their ability to administer it in a safe and controlled manner.

What analgesia would you use?

Analgesia will be provided by the dentist's administration of local anaesthetic. Use of an octapressin-containing local anaesthetic solution, rather than an adrenaline-containing solution, should be considered to avoid adrenaline-related tachycardia and arrhythmia. Careful use of short-acting opiates, such as fentanyl, to dampen any stimulation from airway manipulation by the dental surgeon or anaesthetist would be advisable.

Would you intubate and ventilate this gentleman?

This procedure requires sharing of the airway and involves potential blood loss into the mouth, but this does not necessarily require intubation, and the procedure can be safely carried out using a flexible LMA. A throat pack can be used to secure the airway, though precautions must be in place to ensure it is not left *in situ* at the end of the case.

The authors would aim to use a spontaneously ventilating technique with a flexible LMA, if possible, to avoid increasing PVR. If IPPV is unavoidable, then low inflation pressures should be used. Nitrous oxide increases PVR, PONV, and the size of any air emboli, and it should therefore be avoided.

What monitoring would you use?

Standard monitoring of ECG, SpO_2, end-tidal carbon dioxide ($ETCO_2$), and end-tidal agent monitoring would be necessary. A secure IV access is also needed. The authors would use intra-arterial BP monitoring in this situation.

Are there any other features of your anaesthetic you wish to mention?

- High oxygen levels may cause pulmonary vasodilation
- Vasopressors, such as the alpha adrenergic agonists metaraminol, phenylephrine, and noradrenaline, can be used to maintain SVR. They may, however, also increase PVR and cause bradycardia
- Hypovolaemia should be avoided, and antithrombotic prophylaxis should be considered

- Anticholinergics, such as atropine and glycopyrrolate, can be used to prevent bradycardia
- Histamine-releasing drugs may increase PVR
- Special care needs to be taken to ensure air bubbles are not introduced during IV administration of drugs and fluids due to the risk of paradoxical embolus
- Thromboprophylaxis may need to be considered if polycythaemia is present and mobility is limited.
- Cardiology and Haematology specialists may need consulted.

Would you use antibiotic prophylaxis?

Until 2008, all patients like this in the UK would have received antibiotic prophylaxis. The Working Party of the British Society for Antimicrobial Chemotherapy guidelines in 2006 and NICE guideline CG64 in 2008, whilst recognizing this population group as being at higher risk of developing bacterial endocarditis, stated they would not recommend antibiotic prophylaxis in this particular situation. These recommendations are supported by guidelines from the American Heart Association and European Society of Cardiology.

The issue is that available evidence suggests that dental treatment per se does not increase the risk of infective endocarditis.

The Working Party of the British Society for Antimicrobial Chemotherapy recommends prophylaxis for dental procedures only for those patients with a history of previous endocarditis, cardiac valve replacement, or those with a surgically constructed systemic or pulmonary shunt or conduit.

If this gentleman was undergoing surgery at a site that was infected, e.g. one or more of the teeth to be removed were infected at the time of surgery, then these recommendations suggest using antibiotics that cover the organisms that cause infective endocarditis. It is also important to note that these groups differ in their recommendations relating to antibiotic prophylaxis for certain non-dental surgical operations.

Is this gentleman suitable as a day case patient?

If the procedure is carried out first on the morning theatre list, there are no surgical or anaesthetic complications, and he returns to his preoperative state quickly, there is the potential for same-day discharge. His physiology would need to have returned to baseline; he would need to meet all standard discharge protocols, and he would need to live close to the hospital.

The authors, however, would prefer such a patient to remain overnight in hospital for observation, whilst recognizing there may not be an evidence base for this recommendation.

Summary

Current practice has moved dental anaesthesia away from isolated sites towards theatre complexes such as dental hospitals and hospitals with dental services.

Due consideration must be given to the suitability of some cases to be done as day cases, as there may be significant comorbidities.

Consideration must be given as to whether cases can be done entirely as local anaesthetics, with or without sedation, or as a full general anaesthetic.

Antimicrobial chemoprophylaxis may still be required for some patients.

Further reading

Habib G, Hoen B, Tornos B, *et al.* (2009). Guidelines on the prevention, diagnosis, and treatment of infective endocarditis (new version 2009): the Task Force on the Prevention, Diagnosis, and Treatment of Infective Endocarditis of the European Society of Cardiology (ESC). Endorsed by the European Society of Clinical Microbiology and Infectious Diseases (ESCMID) and the International Society of Chemotherapy (ISC) for Infection and Cancer. *European Heart Journal*, **30**, 2369–413.

Jayaraman L, Sethi N, and Sood J (2009). Anaesthesia outside the operating theatre. *Update in Anaesthesia*, **25**, 37–41.

National Institute for Health and Clinical Excellence (2008). *Prophylaxis against infective endocarditis (CG64)*. Available at: <http://guidance.nice.org.uk/CG64>.

Solanki SL, Vaishnav V, and Vijay AK (2008). Non cardiac surgery in a patient with Eisenmenger Syndrome—Anaesthesiologist's challenge. *Journal of Anaesthesiology Clinical Pharmacology*, **26**, 539–40.

Chapter 4

Regional anaesthesia

Dr Omair Malik

Lower limb anaesthesia

Background

Regional anaesthesia plays an important role in the intra- and post-operative care of trauma patients. The availability and advancement of ultrasound technology as a core skill has allowed the safer delivery of regional anaesthesia, not only by experts, but also by those who are enthusiastic about the field.

Learning outcomes

1 The benefits and risks of regional anaesthesia in the trauma patient
2 The innervation of the lower limb
3 Understanding the numerous lower limb regional techniques and how to select the correct one
4 Nerve location techniques, including ultrasound
5 Delivery of safe regional anaesthesia.

CPD matrix matches

2G02; 2G03

Case history

You are the named anaesthetist for the emergency (CEPOD) list. The orthopaedic surgeon tells you of a case he wishes to do. The patient is a previously healthy 25-year-old man who has suffered a displaced fracture of his distal right tibia and fibula whilst playing rugby. He requires an open reduction and internal fixation under anaesthesia.

What are the benefits and risks of regional anaesthesia?

Analgesia

The greatest benefit of regional anaesthesia is the post-operative analgesia the patient will be afforded. Regional anaesthesia, as part of a multimodal analgesic strategy, provides improved analgesia, compared with systemic analgesia alone. The use of a regional technique may reduce/avoid the need for opioid analgesia.

The benefits of an opioid-free analgesic strategy are numerous, including less sedation, reduced nausea, and a decreased incidence of opioid-induced ileus.

Rehabilitation

Patients who have a regional anaesthesia technique, as part of their orthopaedic/trauma surgery, are quicker to mobilize than those receiving systemic opioid analgesia. In addition to quicker mobilization, the shorter convalescence leads to a reduced time to discharge.

Mortality and morbidity

It has long been thought that regional anaesthesia may impact on mortality. Although there seems to be some improvement in short-term mortality (1 month), this does not continue into the long term. Regional anaesthesia also appears to reduce the incidence of deep vein thrombosis (DVT), although this effect is somewhat masked by the widespread use of thromboprophylaxis.

Risks

Regional anaesthesia is a core skill but is highly operator-dependent. If the correct structures are located and the local anaesthesia placed in the correct vicinity, the incidence of serious complications is very low.

Motor nerve blockade is seen in the majority of regional techniques. Although this may not be a desired effect, it should be viewed as a side effect, rather than a complication, and the patient should be made aware of this. The most common complication is analgesic failure of nerve block. This can range from 5% to 25%, depending on the difficulty of the technique.

Familiarity with the anatomy and technique helps to reduce the incidence of 'failed' block. During a difficult block, more damage is likely to occur with multiple attempts to locate the target with a needle.

There is an argument that regional anaesthesia masks the pain of limb compartment syndrome, although this has not been shown in evidence.

Less common temporary complications include vascular puncture, nerve damage, local anaesthesia toxicity, and infection. The risk of permanent damage or death is extremely low. All frequently occurring and major complications must be explained to the patient before undertaking regional anaesthesia. A safe and methodical technique must be used to ensure the patient receives maximum benefit and minimal risk.

Case update

You see the patient preoperatively. After taking a history and examination, you explain your intraoperative plan. The patient agrees to receive a regional anaesthesia technique as part of his care. Prior to commencing any regional technique, it is important to have detailed anatomical knowledge of the specific region.

Describe the main nerves innervating the lower limb

See Figure 4.1.

◆ The innervation of the lower limb originates from the sacral plexus (giving rise to the sciatic nerve) and the lumbar plexus (giving rise to the lateral cutaneous nerve of the thigh and the femoral and obturator nerves)

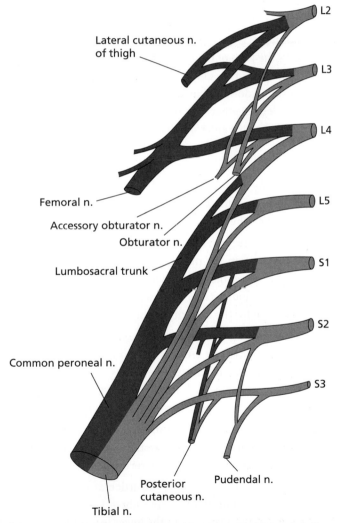

Fig. 4.1 The lumbosacral plexus. (Reproduced from Graeme McLeod, Colin McCartney, and Tony Wildsmith, *Principles and Practice of Regional Anaesthesia*, Fourth Edition, 2012, Figure 18.1, page 188, with permission from Oxford University Press.)

- The lumbar plexus arises from the 12th thoracic nerve to the 5th lumbar nerves. The plexus gives rise to the innervation of the lateral thigh (the lateral cutaneous nerve) and the anterior aspect of the thigh (femoral nerve), extending to the anteromedial aspect of the lower leg (saphenous nerve)

- The femoral nerve arises from the ventral rami of L2–4. It pierces the psoas muscle, then passes downward between the psoas and iliacus. The nerve enters the thigh, running deep to the inguinal ligament. It lies lateral to the femoral artery and deep to the fascia iliaca. Approximately 4 cm inferior to the inguinal ligament, the femoral nerve splits into anterior and posterior (containing the saphenous nerve) branches

- The saphenous nerve is the largest cutaneous branch of the femoral nerve. It initially follows the path of the femoral artery, before descending vertically down the medial part of the knee between the gracilis and sartorius muscles. The nerve continues down the medial aspect of the knee and anteromedially down the lower leg, together with the saphenous vein. The saphenous nerve provides sensation to the anteromedial aspect of the lower leg, including the medial malleolus

- The lateral cutaneous nerve of the thigh arises from the dorsal divisions of L2 and L3. It emerges from the lateral border of the psoas muscle, passing laterally and inferiorly towards the anterior superior iliac spine, before coursing underneath the inguinal ligament

- The sacral plexus arises from the anterior rami L4–S4. It supplies the motor and sensory innervation for the posterior thigh and the majority of the lower leg and foot. Essentially, the sciatic nerve is two separate nerves, the tibial and common fibular (also known as the common peroneal nerve), which run in unison for the majority of their course in the upper leg

- The sciatic nerve exits the pelvis through the greater sciatic foramen, usually inferiorly to the piriformis. It crosses the short external rotator muscles to run posteriorly in the thigh between the biceps femoris and the semimembranous muscles. Just below the level of the mid-thigh, the nerve bifurcates into its tibial and common fibular branches, which innervate the lower leg

- After bifurcation, the tibial nerve continues in a straight path down the popliteal fossa, lying close to the tibia as it continues its descent. It runs posterior to the medial malleolus, before entering the foot

- The sural nerve is an amalgamation of an articular and a cutaneous branch of the tibial nerve, in addition to some fibres from the common fibular nerve. It descends posterolaterally in the lower leg, running behind the lateral malleolus. The nerve is purely sensory, providing innervation to the posterolateral aspect of the lower leg and the lateral foot

- The common fibular nerve descends obliquely to run on the lateral side of the popliteal fossa. The nerve winds round the head of the fibula, soon dividing into superficial (providing sensation to the lateral aspect of the calf and the majority of the dorsum of the foot) and deep branches that supply sensory innervation to the webbing between the 1st and 2nd digits.

Case update

You are in the anaesthetic room, setting up for your list. The orthopaedic surgeon tells you he intends to make two longitudinal incisions, one along each side of the ankle, after which he intends to insert plates and screws to stabilize the fracture. He will also require a tourniquet to be placed.

Which nerve blocks can be considered to provide regional anaesthesia and analgesia for this type of surgery? Which blocks are the most appropriate for this patient?

In essence, regional anaesthesia will be achieved if a suitable amount of local anaesthetic is placed in close proximity to the nerve supplying the area in question. However, there are specific areas in which the nerves are more easily accessible; these sites provide the landmarks for the most commonly used regional blocks. Purists may argue that blocking the nerve at the most immediately proximal point is best (as it will preserve movement of more proximal joints). When undertaking a regional technique, it is best to select one with which the operator is familiar. Operator experience is a major factor in regional technique success.

In this case, to obtain satisfactory regional anaesthesia, the distal branches of both the sciatic (tibial and common fibular) and femoral (or saphenous) nerves need to be blocked. As the surgeons are going to make longitudinal incisions, which will extend above the malleoli, the traditional ankle block is not suitable.

The options for a regional block of the ankle include:

- Spinal anaesthesia alone
- Lumbar plexus block
- Femoral or saphenous nerve block.

In addition to:

- Sciatic or popliteal nerve block.

Any of those options listed will successfully block the nervous supply to the ankle. However, there are benefits and limitations to all techniques. It is preferable to preserve proximal limb movement to allow for better mobilization and prevent complications such as pressure sores. As stated, it is advisable to use a familiar technique, but also one which is more simplistic. To this end, the lumbar plexus block does require a significant level of expertise and therefore is best done by those experienced in it.

A femoral nerve block is more likely (than saphenous block) to aid in the tolerance of tourniquet-induced pain, which can be a factor, even in the well-anaesthetized patient. Due to the size of the sciatic nerve, it can be blocked from a number of sites. Proximal approaches include anterior and posterior; more distal approaches include lateral and the popliteal nerve block (which often means blocking the tibial and common fibular separately).

Certain nerve blocks have benefited from the introduction and widespread uptake of ultrasound technology. The target nerves in both the femoral and popliteal nerve blocks are easily visualized with ultrasound. To this end, an ultrasound-guided femoral and popliteal nerve block offers an efficacious and safe option, requiring a moderate level of expertise.

Case update

You have requested for the patient to be sent to theatre. The operating department assistant asks you what method you would like to use in locating the target nerves for your regional blocks.

What methods are available for locating the target site for local anaesthesia injection in order to obtain a successful block? Which methods would be suitable in this case?

Target-locating methods in regional anaesthesia include the following:

1 Subcutaneous infiltration, e.g. in digital ring blocks

2 Blind injection: as used in peribulbar blocks for cataract surgery

3 Change in resistance: usually reserved for 'field blocks' where the target is not an individual nerve, but rather an area in which the nerve supply crosses, e.g. the abdominal wall blocks (ilioinguinal, TAP, and posterior rectus sheath) and neuraxial blocks

4 Nerve stimulation

5 Ultrasound guidance.

Nerve stimulation has long been considered the gold standard for nerve location in regional anaesthesia. A small current (0.5–1.0 mA) passed down a regional block needle produces an impulse when in close proximity of the nerve. This allows the operator to deliver the local anaesthetic agent close to the nerve, whilst reducing the risk of intraneural injection.

Ultrasound has the advantage of allowing the visualization of the needle tip and local solution deposition, thus allowing the detection of inadvertent intraneural injection and optimal local anaesthetic spread. It can be argued that ultrasound is now the gold standard approach to regional anaesthesia. However, success is operator-dependent. Clinicians carrying out ultrasound-guided blocks must have the requisite training and experience. Inexperienced individuals must be supervised to ensure successful regional anaesthesia. As ultrasound is still relatively new, there will be those clinicians who are experienced in the nerve stimulation technique, but not so with ultrasound. An acceptable and safe method for this cohort is to use a combination of nerve stimulation and ultrasound to locate the nerve.

The connective tissue within nerves reflects ultrasound waves. Nerves are best visualized with a high-resolution (8–14 MHz) ultrasound probe, perpendicular to the nerve axis. The disadvantage of high-resolution probes is the shallow penetrative depth they offer. Depending on their structure, nerves can appear hypo- or hyperechoic (dark or bright). The characteristic pattern is of a circular/oval hypoechoic (dark) area surrounded by a brighter hyperechoic rim.

Once the ultrasound probe has successfully located the target nerve, the needle can be introduced and advanced in either the transverse axis (out of plane) or the longitudinal axis (in plane). The out-of-plane approach relies on the operator discerning 'bouncing' tissues as the needle is advanced to act as a guide to the needle tip position. The in-plane method is preferable, as it allows the visualization of the entire needle along its course, thus ensuring the needle tip position. The needle has to travel a greater distance in the in-plane method, and it is most probably an unfamiliar approach to those inexperienced with ultrasound.

With the needle in the correct position, in close proximity to the nerve, the injectate can be visualized with ultrasound. This allows greater confidence that the local anaesthetic solution is surrounding the nerve and has not been misplaced. Ultrasound technology allows for fine 'tweaking' of the needle position to ensure optimal placement of the local anaesthetic, often leading to a decrease in total volumes required.

Case update

You decide upon an ultrasound-guided femoral and popliteal nerve block under general anaesthesia as your intraoperative plan.

How do you go about safely administering regional anaesthesia?

Inserting a needle loaded with local anaesthetic is simply one action in what should be a process, beginning with your preoperative visit and sometimes ending up to 72 hours after the procedure (if a catheter technique is used). To deliver safe and effective regional anaesthesia, it is best to adopt a structured approach.

Preoperatively

First, it is vital to discover the correct surgical site from the surgical consent form; the patient must also confirm this. It should then be decided if the patient would benefit from a regional technique. Consent for the block must be obtained. The technique, its benefits, side effects, and risks must be explained and documented.

Perioperatively

1 Identity and checks.

In theatre, prior to induction of anaesthesia, it is obligatory for the team to pause and conduct a surgical checklist. This allows the confirmation of the patient identity, procedure, correct surgical site, and the marking of the site. The World Health Organization (WHO) surgical checklist has been implemented to reduce the incidence of wrong-site surgery.

2 Prepare the patient.

Two of the major risks of attempting a regional block include inadvertent intraneural injection and intravascular injection, leading to possible local anaesthetic toxicity. Performing a regional block on the awake/lightly sedated patient offers the greatest margin of safety. Blocks are widely performed on asleep patients, but this renders them incapable of alerting the operator to pain/paraesthesiae (intraneural injection) or the early signs of local anaesthetic toxicity.

3 Position and asepsis.

The patient must be positioned correctly to facilitate needle insertion. The distal part of the limb should be exposed, if attempting to discern 'twitches' by nerve stimulation. The landmarks should be examined (femoral crease and proximal popliteal fossa) and marked, if required (see Figure 4.2). The block should be performed in aseptic conditions; therefore, the area must be cleaned with a skin disinfectant. It is important to avoid contact of the disinfecting agent with the local anaesthetic solution or equipment. The disinfectant must be allowed to dry (allowing time to prepare equipment), and any remaining fluid discarded.

4 Stop before you block.

The Royal College of Anaesthetists recommends a brief pause before needle insertion to double-check the correct side of block with the anaesthetic assistant. It is also prudent to remind yourself of the maximum volume of solution you are able to give at this point.

5 Nerve location, needle insertion, and injection.

The nerve is visualized by ultrasound (see Figure 4.3). Once the target nerve has been identified, subcutaneous local anaesthesia can be placed

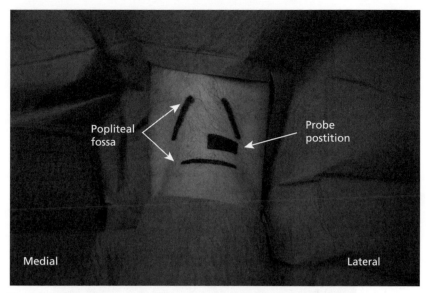

Fig. 4.2 Surface probe positions for popliteal ultrasonic nerve visualization.

under direct vision, in order to make the remainder of the procedure painless. The regional needle is then loaded with local anaesthetic solution and guided (in-plane), until it is in close proximity to the nerve (at this point, nerve stimulation can be used, if required). The needle is attached to the local anaesthetic syringe via a flexible extension. The syringe is aspirated, and 1–2 mL of solution injected; this should result in the body of the nerve being displaced away from the needle. The nerve structure should be seen to remain intact. If the local anaesthetic solution has been deposited in the desired area, the remainder of the local anaesthetic may be carefully injected (with frequent aspiration), at all times under direct vision. The needle can be removed, and the patient prepared for general anaesthesia.

The operator must be vigilant of the signs of local anaesthetic toxicity at all times. Care must be taken in the positioning of the insensate limb. Clues regarding a successful or an unsuccessful block may become apparent during surgery through verbal and non-verbal responses.

Post-operatively

In the post-operative period, the patient should be reviewed to ensure the block is working as planned. Care must be taken to protect the insensate limb. The patient should be seen post-operatively and be reviewed regularly by the acute pain service.

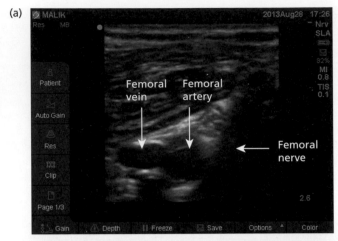

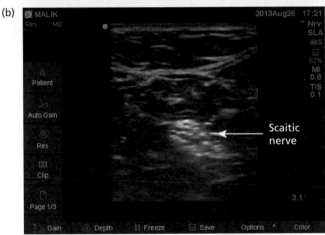

Fig. 4.3 Ultrasound images of (a) femoral and (b) popliteal nerves.

Summary

Regional anaesthesia offers an excellent method of analgesia for patients undergoing fracture surgery. Patients must be made aware of the risks and benefits of regional anaesthesia. Operator experience and knowledge are important factors in regional block success. Ultrasound technology has made regional anaesthesia a more accessible modality and has increased its safety. Clinicians must adopt a structured approach to performing regional anaesthesia.

Further reading

Bonnet F and Marret E (2005). Influence of anaesthetic and analgesic techniques on outcome after surgery. *British Journal of Anaesthesia*, **95**, 52–8.

Capdevila X, Barthelet Y, Biboulet P, Ryckwaert Y, Rubernovitch J, and d'Athis F (1999). Effects of perioperative analgesic technique on the surgical outcome and duration of rehabilitation after major knee surgery. *Anesthesiology*, **91**, 8–15.

Grant CRK and Raju PKBC (2013). Practical aspects of ultrasound-guided regional anaesthesia. *Anaesthesia & Intensive Care Medicine*, **14**, 137–41.

Grant CRK and Raju PKBC (2013). Lower limb nerve blocks. *Anaesthesia & Intensive Care Medicine*, **14**, 149–53.

Mar GJ, Barrington MJ, and McGuirk BR (2009). Acute compartment syndrome of the lower limb and the effect of postoperative analgesia on diagnosis. *British Journal of Anaesthesia*, **102**, 3–11.

Richman JM, Liu SS, Courpas G, *et al.* (2006). Does continuous peripheral nerve block provide superior pain control to opioids? A meta-analysis. *Anesthesia & Analgesia*, **102**, 248–57.

Royal College of Anaesthetists (2009). *Major complications of central neuraxial blocks in the United Kingdom: NAP 3, the 3rd National Audit Project of the Royal College of Anaesthetists*. Available at: <http://www.rcoa.ac.uk/system/files/CSQ-NAP3-Full_1.pdf>.

Unwin SC, Parker MJ, and Griffiths R (2000). General versus regional anaesthesia for hip surgery: a meta-analysis of randomized trials. *British Journal of Anaesthesia*, **84**, 450–5.

World Health Organization. *Surgical safety checklist.* Available at: <http://who.int/patientsafety/safesurgery/tools_resources/SSSL_Checklist_finalJun08.pdf>.

Upper limb regional anaesthesia

Background

Analgesia for patients undergoing orthopaedic surgery can be challenging. Regional anaesthesia techniques offer an excellent method of maintaining patient comfort without sedation or other side effects seen with systematic analgesia. Regional anaesthesia can be considered to be a pain-relieving modality but can also be used as the main method of intraoperative anaesthesia.

Learning outcomes

1 To appreciate and understand the role of regional anaesthesia in orthopaedic surgery
2 The innervation of the upper limb
3 Understanding the numerous upper limb regional techniques and how to select the correct one
4 Nerve catheter techniques.

CPD matrix matches

2G02; 2G03

Case history

You are to anaesthetize a 55-year-old labourer for a left elbow arthroplasty. He has a history of well-controlled hypertension and has a BMI of 32. He states he has a fear of going to sleep for the procedure.

Which intraoperative anaesthetic options are available?

The options include general anaesthesia, with or without regional anaesthesia, or regional anaesthesia with sedation.

General anaesthesia will certainly give good intraoperative conditions. However, post-operatively, the patient will require stronger systemic analgesia, which may cause nausea and sedation and prolong hospital stay. General anaesthesia may be combined with a regional anaesthesia technique to ensure optimal intra- and post-operative comfort. Regional anaesthesia can also be the sole method of anaesthesia in such case, usually combined with sedation for intraoperative patient comfort.

Regional anaesthesia plays a key role in the care for patients undergoing orthopaedic procedures. Orthopaedic patients who are admitted as day cases and inpatients both benefit from the advantages of regional techniques. The bony pain and nausea from orthopaedic surgery can be a post-operative challenge for the acute pain team. Traditional systemic analgesic options include NSAIDs and opioids. Opioid analgesia is infrequently effective against bony pain and often leads to sedation, nausea, constipation, and respiratory depression, all factors which can delay discharge. If a PCA pump is required post-operatively, this can also have implications for early mobilization. Regional anaesthesia decreases the reliance on post-operative opioid analgesia, thus negating the side effects; it is also more effective against bone pain.

Describe the origins of the nervous supply of the upper limb

See Figure 4.4.

The complete nervous supply to the upper limb is derived from the ventral rami (roots) of C5–T1, which amalgamate after emerging from the intravertebral foramina to form the three trunks of the brachial plexus.

Trunks

The roots of C5 and C6 unite to form the upper trunk. C7 continues as the middle trunk, leaving C8 and T1 to form the lower trunk. The upper trunk gives rise to the suprascapular nerve. The trunks pass between the anterior and middle scalene muscles.

Divisions

As the trunks pass behind the clavicle, they each divide into an anterior and posterior division.

Cords

The cords are formed by amalgamation of the divisions of certain trunks. They are named by their relation to the axillary artery. The anterior divisions of the upper and middle trunks form the lateral cord. The medial cord continues from the anterior division of the lower trunk. Finally, the posterior divisions of all three trunks unify to form the posterior cord. The cords pass over the first rib and continue under the clavicle, in close relation to the subclavian artery.

The main nerves supplying the upper limb arise from the cords, usually as the subclavian artery becomes the axillary artery.

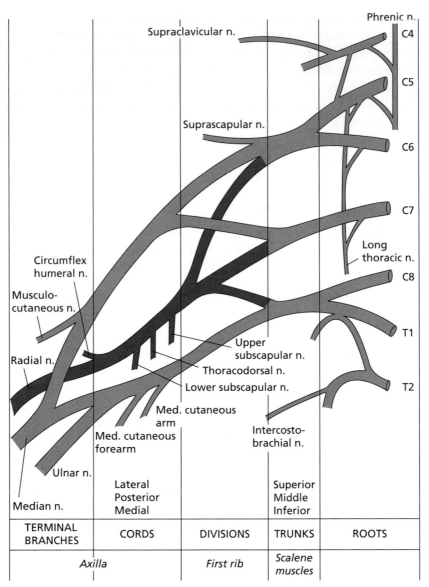

Fig. 4.4 The brachial plexus. (Reproduced from Graeme McLeod, Colin McCartney, and Tony Wildsmith, *Principles and Practice of Regional Anaesthesia*, Fourth Edition, 2012, Figure 17.1, page 171, with permission from Oxford University Press.)

The lateral cord gives rise to the musculocutaneous nerve (C5, 6, 7), which leaves high in the axilla, passes through the coracobrachialis muscle, and becomes the lateral cutaneous nerve of the forearm.

The medial cord gives rise to the medial cutaneous nerve of the arm, the medial cutaneous nerve of the forearm, and the ulnar nerve (C8, T1), respectively.

The ulnar nerve descends medially down the arm to carry cutaneous sensation from the medial one and half digits.

The remainder of the medial and lateral cords unites to form the median nerve. This nerve descends medially in the arm, in close relation to the brachial artery, until the cubital fossa. The median nerve then descends down the forearm to enter the carpal tunnel, providing sensory innervation to the lateral three and half digits.

Nerves originating from the posterior cord include:

- The upper subscapular nerve
- The thoracodorsal nerve
- The lower subscapular nerve
- The axillary nerve: which leaves the brachial plexus to travel inferoposteriorly to the axillary artery. It provides motor innervation to the deltoid and teres minor; it gains cutaneous sensation laterally, just below the shoulder
- The radial nerve: also descends inferoposteriorly to the axillary artery. Initially, it is in the posterior aspect of the arm, moving more anteriorly as it descends. It passes anterior to the lateral epicondyle as it continues into the forearm. It is responsible for the extensor muscles of the elbow, wrists, and fingers and the sensory innervation from the dorsum of the hand.

Case update

During your preoperative visit, you decide to discuss regional anaesthesia as an option for post operative analgesia.

Which regional blocks are possible for upper limb anaesthesia? Which are suitable for elbow surgery? Which technique would you choose for this patient and why?

The upper limb innervation can be blocked from a number of sites. These include (from proximal to distal):
Brachial plexus blocks:

1. Interscalene block
2. Supraclavicular block
3. Infraclavicular block
4. Axillary block

Individual nerve blocks of the forearm (median and ulnar)
Bier's Block

Brachial plexus blocks are the most suitable regional techniques for elbow surgery. The most appropriate block should be chosen on a patient-to-patient basis, taking the risks and benefits into account. An elbow arthroplasty is a painful procedure, which has high post-operative analgesic requirements.

The interscalene block is ideally used for shoulder surgery; it anaesthetizes the majority of the upper limb (sparing C8–T1 in 50% of cases), in addition to the side of the neck. Such widespread motor and sensory block leads to reduced proximal muscle movement and potentially greater patient dissatisfaction. The block also commonly infers phrenic nerve paralysis, leading to a 25% reduction in lung function, which would be poorly tolerated in the overweight patient. For these reasons, the interscalene would not be the optimal regional technique.

Supraclavicular or axillary blocks are more suitable for anaesthesia of the elbow alone. The close proximity of the nerves in the supraclavicular approach lends itself to be suitable for the insertion of a nerve block catheter; thus allowing prolonged analgesia. As the patient has a fear of general anaesthesia, a supraclavicular nerve catheter technique plus IV sedation allows us to offer optimal intra- and post-operative analgesia, whilst ensuring patient tolerance and satisfaction.

Case update

The patient is grateful you have taken his fears regarding general anaesthesia into account. He consents to a regional technique and IV sedation.

How do you place a nerve catheter, and how can you ensure good intra- and post-operative analgesia?

Preparation

The preparation for a regional technique with sedation begins preoperatively. The patient must be made aware of the sensations which he may perceive (pressure, movement) and that these are not a sign of technique failure. He must be reassured that there will be someone close by, monitoring him at all times. Anxious patients should be offered premedication, prior to leaving for theatre.

Preoperatively

Placing a nerve catheter is a two-stage technique.

The first stage is location of the nerve and deposition of the local anaesthetic solution safely around it. This stage is identical to that described in the previous case. Sterility must be ensured, the surgical site confirmed, and full monitoring be in place. A nerve catheter placement block needle kit should be used.

The block can be done with the patient in a semi-sitting position, with his head turned away from the surgical site and his arm straight down by his side. Sedation is commenced, propofol TCI being an excellent option. The ultrasound probe is placed in the transverse axis (see Figure 4.5) in the pocket created by the superior aspect of the clavicle. The trunks of the brachial plexus should be visualized as hypoechoic circular structures, lateral to the subclavian artery (see Figure 4.6). Lidocaine 1% is injected subcutaneously under ultrasound vision for patient comfort. In-plane block needle advancement is from lateral to medial, with the aim to pierce the brachial plexus sheath. Proximity to the brachial plexus can be confirmed by upper limb twitches elicited by nerve stimulation. The local anaesthetic solution is then deposited in a safe manner around the trunks; 10 mL of 0.5% levobupivacaine should be sufficient for intraoperative anaesthesia.

The second stage is the placement of the nerve catheter through the block needle into the 'reservoir' of local solution. The catheter is usually advanced 2–3 cm beyond the tip of the needle, under dynamic ultrasound guidance. Care must be taken in removing the block needle without displacing the catheter. The catheter is then secured (usually by adhesive tags supplied with the nerve catheter kit) (see Figure 4.7) and clearly labelled.

The block is tested at 5-min intervals, checking for loss of temperature and fine touch. Operative anaesthesia should be achieved within 30 min. The TCI can be increased for patient comfort and the block supplemented, as required.

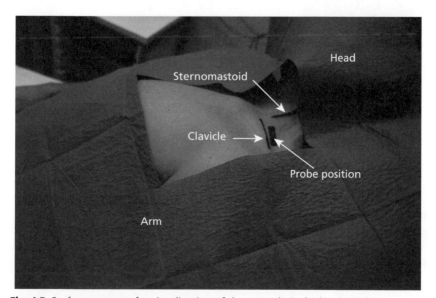

Fig. 4.5 Surface anatomy for visualization of the supraclavicular brachial plexus.

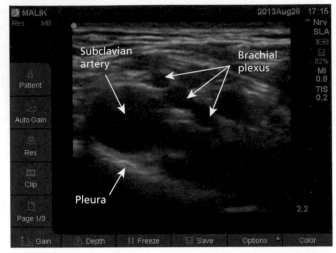

Fig. 4.6 The hypoechoic elements of the supraclavicular plexus, situated lateral to the subclavian artery.

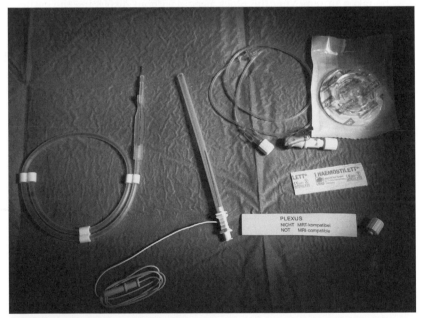

Fig. 4.7 An example of a Sonoplex® nerve catheter kit. (Reproduced with kind permission from Pajunk.)

Post-operatively

The patient should be prescribed simple analgesia, as part of his post-operative regime. If the block has been successful intraoperatively, then it should also infer excellent post-operative pain relief.

An infusion of local anaesthetic solution is commenced via the nerve catheter. A standard regimen is 5 mL/hour of 0.25% or 0.5% levobupivacaine, with a maximum dose of 0.5 mg/kg/hour. The drug can be administered via an electronic pump or an elastomeric device (e.g. PainBuster®). When attaching the infusion to the nerve catheter, the pump and its contents must be checked with a second person to prevent inadvertent IV infusion. It is prudent to implement similar observations as those afforded to patients who have continuous neuraxial blocks prescribed for post-operative analgesia. Nerve catheters are usually removed within 48–72 hours.

Summary

Regional anaesthesia has an important role in patient comfort and satisfaction, both during and after orthopaedic surgery. An understanding of the benefits and limitations of the different upper limb blocks is vital in order to offer the best option to patients. Nerve catheter techniques provide a useful means to offer prolonged post-operative analgesia.

Further reading

Coventry DM and Raju PKRC (2013). Upper limb blocks. *Anaesthesia & Intensive Care Medicine*, **14**, 154–8.

Ellis H (2013). Applied anatomy for upper limb nerve blocks. *Anaesthesia & Intensive Care Medicine*, **14**, 133–6.

Urmey W and McDonald M (1996). Hemidiaphragmatic paresis during intersaclene brachial plexus block: effects on pulmonary function and chest wall mechanics. *Anesthesia & Analgesia*, **83**, 747–51.

Regional anaesthesia in the elderly patient

Background

There are approximately 10 million people (16% of the total population) over the age of 65 living in the UK; this figure is projected to double by 2050. Elderly patients contribute to a large proportion of the NHS workload.

Learning outcomes

1 Physiological changes in the elderly patient

2 Preoperative management and optimization

3 Methods of delivering safe anaesthesia to the elderly trauma patient

4 Care of the insensate limb.

CPD matrix matches

2A03; 2G01, 2G02

Case history

You are to anaesthetize an 85-year-old lady who sustained a fractured left neck of femur after having fallen yesterday morning. She is to undergo a left dynamic hip screw (DHS). She is the first patient on your list this morning.

What are the relevant physiological changes seen in elderly patients?

Ageing affects all the systems within the body. Changes to the cardiovascular, respiratory, and renal systems have the greatest relevance to anaesthesia.

Cardiovascular

There is a linear decline in cardiac function. An 80-year-old has half the cardiac output of a 20-year-old. Decreased sensitivity to catecholamines and increased myocardial stiffness decrease contractility, and a progressive stiffening of the thoracic aorta leads to increased afterload. These factors, combined, lead to an overall reduction in stroke volume.

Large and medium-sized vessels stiffen with age, resulting in increased systolic and diastolic blood pressure. The raised SVR may lead to LV hypertrophy and strain. Hypertension is the most common cardiovascular manifestation of ageing. The autoregulation curve is shifted to the right (as a result of hypertension), rendering the elderly less tolerant of low MAPs. Autonomic and baroreceptor downregulations mean there is an impaired/blunted response to hypotension.

There is a greater proportion of coronary artery disease in the elderly population; however, this may not manifest symptomatically, as the patients may not be able to exert themselves to such an extent. Arrhythmias are commonplace also, due to a decrease in the number of cardiac-conducting cells and increased fibrous tissue deposition. Atrial fibrillation (AF) has a prevalence of 5.5% in the over 65s; it is an important comorbidity to be aware of, as it further reduces cardiac output by 30%. Arrhythmias are more commonly seen in those with heart valve lesions.

Respiratory

Vital capacity, forced expiratory volume in 1 s (FEV_1), and forced vital capacity (FVC) all decrease with advancing age; residual capacity and closing capacity both increase. The increased closing capacity encroaches upon an unchanged functional residual capacity by the age of 65, leading to dependent airway closure and ventilation/perfusion (V/Q) mismatch. Chest wall and lung compliance is reduced, resulting in decreased peak flows.

A V/Q mismatch, along with decreased mucociliary clearance, leads to atelectasis, secretion pooling, and a greater incidence of pneumonia. Immobilization and dehydration are factors in developing pulmonary emboli (PEs) perioperatively. Blunted ventilatory responses to hypoxaemia and hypercapnia make both of these complications more common post-operatively. The edentulous airway may make manual bag–mask ventilation challenging.

Renal

Reductions in cardiac output, coupled with increased atherosclerotic disease, lead to a linear decrease in renal function with age. Creatinine (Cr) clearance falls; however, due to reduced Cr production, serum Cr remains unchanged. Handling of renally cleared drugs (aminoglycosides, penicillins, digoxin) is impaired, lengthening their half-lives.

Care must also be taken with fluid balance. Elderly patients are often hypovolaemic preoperatively, increasing the risk of complications such as intraoperative hypotension and venous thromboembolism (VTE). Vigorous IV fluid administration may be poorly tolerated, due to poor cardiorespiratory reserve, leading to accumulation within the lungs and pulmonary oedema.

Central nervous system

Declining cognitive function can make obtaining consent challenging. Often a patient with impaired cognition may not be compliant with treatment, as they are incapable of understanding the nature of their condition.

The changes brought about by illness and a change of environment can lead to cognitive decline. Post-operative cognitive dysfunction (POCD) is a common phenomenon, affecting approximately 25% of patients over 60 years undergoing major surgery. POCD is multifactorial, with anaesthetic agents and sedatives having been implicated. However, there is no difference in incidence between those undergoing general and regional anaesthesia.

Case update

You see the patient preoperatively. She is moderately confused, with a background of mild dementia. She states she takes some tablets for her heart (aspirin, bisoprolol, bendroflumethiazide, simvastatin, and irbesartan). Her pain score is 3/10 at rest, after having received some opioid analgesia. On auscultation of her chest, you hear a previously undiagnosed non-radiating ejection systolic murmur and an irregular pulse of 110 bpm.

Outline the key principles in your preoperative work-up for this patient

The overriding principle is to ensure the patient is optimized for safe surgery in the most prompt manner by avoiding unnecessary delay. This is achieved by:

1 Evaluation of the patient and their comorbidities

2 Prompt instigation of the required investigations

3 Ensuring analgesia

4 Prevention of other further comorbidity (VTE, pressure sores, infection).

In addition to their presenting complaint, elderly patients will commonly present to hospital with a number of other comorbidities. Often these comorbidities are well established, and records relating to their management and history can be obtained (collateral histories, GP or hospital records). Undiagnosed cardiac conditions, such as this patient's murmur, are not uncommon events, especially as elderly patients often cannot exert themselves to the point of becoming symptomatic.

A thorough evaluation of the patient must be made to ascertain whether they are fit for surgery. It is important to know the patient's main comorbidities and be able to judge if these are stable. Any delay in surgery must be justifiable and be seen to confer some advantage to the patient. Unnecessary delays increase the duration of immobilization, which may lead to pulmonary infection, pressure sores, and VTE.

Most inpatients with a fractured neck of femur will undergo the important investigations soon after admission. Routine bloods (including coagulation profile), a CXR, and an ECG will be sufficient in most patients.

Murmurs are a common finding in the elderly. Aortic sclerosis is by far the most common anomaly causing an ejection systolic murmur. The availability of a rapid echocardiography is an important factor. An asymptomatic patient with a recent echocardiogram is unlikely to benefit from a repeat scan and may come to harm from a delay to surgery. However, if aortic stenosis is suspected, an echocardiography is recommended to confirm diagnosis and stratify risk.

Maintaining patient comfort can be challenging, especially for the immobilized patient. Patients may have had their affected limbs placed in traction by the surgeons; this measure was intended to relieve pain, although there is no evidence of any analgesic benefit. Therefore, limb traction is not recommended in patients with hip fractures. Careful titration of IV opioids remains the best analgesic option preoperatively. Peripheral nerve blocks can be used preoperatively, but it is unclear if this exerts any reduction in opioid administration.

Hip fracture patients are at increased risk of other significant morbidities. Hospital-acquired respiratory tract infections (HAI) and VTE contribute to increased duration of hospital stay, morbidity, and mortality. Prophylactic antibiotics are recommended, not only for surgical site infections, but also to help prevent HAIs.

The use of pharmacological thromboprophylaxis reduces the incidence of VTE to 1.34%. The regime used is dependent on local guidelines. Enoxaparin can be commenced soon after admission, stopped 12 hours prior to surgery, and recommenced 6 hours post-operatively. Fondaparinux compares favourably to enoxaparin; this can be commenced 6 hours post-operatively. There is benefit seen if thromboprophylaxis treatment is extended to 28–35 days after surgery. Mechanical compression devices should also be considered if the patient tolerates them.

A thorough preoperative work-up not only decreases the risk of untoward events in the perioperative period, but also has positive implications for earlier discharge and decrease morbidity and mortality once out of hospital. Surgery must not be delayed for investigations that are not vital or are unlikely to change management.

Case update

You are happy the patient has been adequately optimized for surgery. You were able to get an echocardiographic scan without delay, which showed the patient has aortic sclerosis and moderate LV function.

Describe your intraoperative plan

The options available include general anaesthesia, with or without a regional technique, or regional anaesthesia coupled with conscious sedation. There is little evidence that one technique has significant advantages over the other. However, regional anaesthesia does decrease the amount of IV opioid required post-operatively and may reduce post-operative cognitive deficit; for these reasons, the use of regional anaesthesia is commonplace for hip surgery in the elderly.

Regional anaesthesia is best attempted with the patient awake and able to respond to any paraesthesiae or pain on injection, alerting the operator to possible intraneural injection. However, needle phobia and pain at the injection site understandably cause anxiety to the patient. This, plus the likelihood of confusion/disorientation in the elderly patient, means that conscious sedation plays an important role in delivering safe and satisfactory treatment.

There are multiple sedating agents available. Sedation requires IV access to be obtained and is normally commenced prior to block placement. The ideal sedative should have rapid onset/offset, be easily titratable, have minimum 'hangover' effect, in addition to having anxiolytic, amnesic, and analgesic properties. Although no absolutely perfect sedative exists, midazolam and propofol are the two agents which appear to have the most favourable properties. Midazolam offers excellent amnesia and is easily administered by careful bolus. However, it does cause respiratory depression and can cause paradoxical reaction. Propofol offers excellent sedation, is easily titrated by TCI, and has a rapid offset. The amnesia offered by propofol is dose-related and less effective than that seen with midazolam. Local policy and protocol will likely decide which agent is used.

Commonly, the regional technique recipe is with a low-dose spinal (e.g. 1.5–2 mL of 0.5% levobupivacaine), done with the patient in decubitus position, followed by a femoral nerve block (e.g. 0.5% levobupivacaine, up to a maximum total dose of 2 mg/kg). The spinal confers early operative analgesia, until the nerve block is fully effective, which subsequently ensures continuing intraoperative and post-operative analgesia. This technique allows for an opioid-free anaesthetic. Other options are also available, such as femoral nerve block combined with lateral cutaneous nerve block and placement of femoral nerve catheters (see Figure 4.7).

Full monitoring is required to detect any haemodynamic compromise. Oxygen therapy is commenced by face mask, preferably with $ETCO_2$ monitoring. Verbal contact with the patient should elicit a response at all times. Antibiotics, simple analgesia, and antiemetics should all be given, as per local policy. Blood loss and fluids infused should be recorded and post-operative instructions clearly documented.

Case update

The patient remains comfortable throughout the procedure and is safely transferred to recovery. At the end of the list, you go to the ward to see her. The femoral block you have placed seems to be working well, and she is still comfortable. The left leg is still immobile and numb.

What measures can be taken to care for the insensate limb?

Patients may poorly tolerate the motor and sensory block caused by regional anaesthesia. It is important to brief the patient preoperatively regarding the expected duration of the block to alleviate any concern they may have. It is also important to ensure surgeons and nursing staff are aware of the details of the block.

Local protocols should include regular observation of the insensate limb, checking for sensory block and limb movement. An increasing level of block is always a cause for concern, and a clinician should be informed immediately.

The limb must also be checked for pressure areas. The development of pressure sores in patients who may have pre-existing malnourishment can lead to marked comorbidity and hospital stay. Patients should be cared for on low-pressure, foam-based mattresses and pressure areas relieved regularly.

As the insensate limb is usually immobile, VTE prophylaxis should be commenced in a timely manner. Pharmacological prophylaxis should be prescribed 6 hours post-surgery.

Early mobilization is a priority, once the motor function and sensation have returned to the limb. Initial mobilization must be taken with care, as there may be some residual block remaining. Two members of staff must help mobilize the patient, in case she fails to weight-bear.

Any concerns about the nerve block must be referred to the acute pain service or anaesthesia staff.

Summary

Caring for elderly patients in the perioperative period can be challenging. They will often present with several comorbidities. A key part of your role is to ensure they are fit for surgery, whilst minimizing unnecessary delay.

Further reading

Bjorvatn A and Kristiansen F (2005). Fondaparinux sodium compared with enoxaparin sodium: a cost-effectiveness analysis. *American Journal of Cardiovascular Drugs*, **5**, 121–30.

Furberg CD, Psaty BM, Manolio TA, Gardin JM, Smith VE, and Rautaharju PM (1994). Prevalence of atrial fibrillation in elderly subjects (the Cardiovascular Health Study). *American Journal of Cardiology*, **74**, 236–41.

Hanning CD (2005). Postoperative cognitive dysfunction. *British Journal of Anaesthesia*, **95**, 82–7.

Höhener D, Blumenthal S, and Borgeat A (2008). Sedation and regional anaesthesia in the adult patient. *British Journal of Anaesthesia*, **100**, 8–16.

Mak JCS, Cameron ID, and March LM (2010). Evidence-based guidelines for the management of hip fractures in older persons: an update. *Medical Journal of Australia*, **192**, 37–41.

Murray D and Dodds C (2004). Perioperative care of the elderly. *Continuing Education in Anaesthesia, Critical Care & Pain*, **4**, 193–6.

National Institute for Health and Clinical Excellence (2010). *Venous thromboembolism: reducing the risk. NICE clinical guideline 92.* Available at: <http://www.nice.org.uk/nicemedia/pdf/CG92NICEGuidelinePDF.pdf>.

NHS National Services Scotland (2008). *Clinical decision-making: is the patient fit for theatre? A report from the Scottish Hip Fracture Audit.* Available at: <http://www.shfa.scot.nhs.uk/Theatre_Delay_Report.pdf>.

Otto CM, Lind BK, Kitzman DW, Gersh BJ, and Siscovick DS (1999). Association of aortic-valve sclerosis with cardiovascular mortality and morbidity in the elderly. *New England Journal of Medicine*, **341**, 142–7.

Parker MJ, Griffiths R, and Appadu BN (2002). Nerve blocks (subcostal, lateral cutaneous, femoral, triple, psoas) for hip. *Cochrane Database of Systematic Reviews*, **1**, CD001159.

Rosencher N, Vielpeau C, Emmerich J, Fagnani F, and Samama CM; ESCORTE group (2005). Venous thromboembolism and mortality after hip fracture surgery: the ESCORTE study. *Journal of Thrombosis and Haemostasis*, **3**, 2006–14.

Ross GR and Seeqmiller JE (1981). Age-related physiological changes and their clinical significance. *Western Journal of Medicine*, **135**, 434–40.

Scottish Intercollegiate Guidelines Network (2009). *Management of hip fracture in older people. A national clinical guideline.* Available at: <http://www.sign.ac.uk/pdf/sign111.pdf>.

Chapter 5

Obstetric anaesthesia

Dr Linzi Peacock
Dr Vicki Clark

Major obstetric haemorrhage

Background

Obstetric haemorrhage is a major cause of maternal morbidity and mortality worldwide. It is responsible for approximately a quarter of the 350 000 maternal deaths each year due to childbirth. The vast majority of these deaths occur in the developing world.

In the 2006–08 CMACE (Centre for Maternal and Child Enquiries) report on UK maternal deaths, haemorrhage was responsible for nine deaths, making it the 6th commonest cause of direct maternal death. Anticipating which patients are likely to bleed can be difficult. As a rule, the aetiology can be related to abnormalities of one or more of the four basic processes: tone, tissue, trauma, or thrombin (the four Ts). The commonest cause of obstetric haemorrhage is uterine atony, followed by retained products of conception, extension of the uterine incision at Caesarean section, placenta praevia and abruption.

Learning outcomes

1 Understand appropriate investigations in a parturient at risk of obstetric haemorrhage

2 Have an awareness of non-pharmacological options in the management of the atonic uterus

3 Have a core understanding of the management of major obstetric haemorrhage.

CPD matrix matches

2B02; 2B05

Case history

A 32-year-old woman, parity 2 + 1, has been listed for elective Caesarean section. Her first delivery was an emergency Caesarean section for failure to progress at 8 cm dilation, performed 5 years ago. She then had an elective Caesarean section at term 2 years ago for her second child. Both her children were large at birth, with weights of 4.2 kg and 4.4 kg. She has had an uneventful antenatal course, although she has measured large for dates. She has no significant past medical history and has not had a general anaesthetic previously. Both her Caesarean sections were performed under spinal anaesthesia. She is not on any medication, although she has been given ranitidine prior to your assessment; she has no known allergies and is a non-smoker. Her airway assessment does not predict difficulty, and her BMI is 23 kg/m². She has had a group and save sample sent to the blood transfusion laboratory. Her haematology results demonstrate a Hb of 113 g/L, WCC 12.4×10^9/L, and Plt 210×10^9/L.

What other investigations should this lady have had?

She should have had a growth scan, in view of her measuring large for dates, to assess the size of the fetus. Ultrasound imaging of her placenta is indicated, as a history of two previous Caesarean sections increases the risk of placenta praevia and placenta accreta. Colour flow Doppler imaging is the first-line test for the morbidly adherent placenta, and, if this investigation is suggestive of placenta accreta, then a magnetic resonance imaging (MRI) should be recommended.

How would you anaesthetize this lady?

A regional technique would be appropriate for surgical delivery. The procedure may take longer than average, in view of her two previous Caesarean sections, so a combined spinal–epidural technique may provide the optimal options for surgical anaesthesia. An epidural alone could be used, but the block will take longer to be effective and may spare the sacral segments.

What medications would you have ready?

+ Vasopressor, e.g. phenylephrine
+ Glycopyrrolate
+ Antibiotic: this lady requires prophylactic antibiotics, prior to the commencement of surgery. IV cefuroxime or cefotaxime would be appropriate. Co-amoxiclav is contraindicated by NICE
+ Syntocinon®: IV bolus 5 IU to be given after cord clamping. In view of the history of high birthweight babies and the likelihood that this baby is also large, then a Syntocinon® infusion of 40 IU in 500 mL of normal saline should be ready to infuse at 125 mL/hour, as this lady is at risk of post-partum haemorrhage.

Case update

Five minutes following the delivery of what appears to be a large baby, the mother's heart rate increases to 120/min, and her BP drops from 105/65 to 96/68 mmHg. She has already received 750 mL of crystalloid and 5 IU of Syntocinon®. The obstetricians suggest she is bleeding, because the uterus is atonic.

How do you assess the amount of blood lost?

Assess the volume of fluid in the suction reservoir, and confirm with the obstetricians or scrub team as to how much of the volume is liquor. Request that the volume of blood absorbed in the surgical swabs is estimated by swab weighing.

The changes in the patient's physiology suggest that she has lost 15–30% of her circulating volume, which, in a pregnant woman at full gestation, can be calculated as 100 mL/kg.

As the majority of the obstetric population are young and fit, they will respond with efficient vasoconstriction in response to blood loss, hence maintaining BP for longer in the face of ongoing haemorrhage. Tachycardia, tachypnoea, pallor, light-headedness, oliguria, and delayed capillary refill are better indicators of significant loss.

The blood loss is 1200 mL. What actions should now be taken?

It is important to communicate with the patient and partner that she is losing more blood than is usual and may be feeling nauseated or light-headed as a result of this.

The fluid infusion rate should be increased, and a second dose of 5 IU of Syntocinon® should be administered.

A second large-bore venous cannula should be sited and a near-point testing blood sample taken (such as a HemoCue® or a venous blood sample put through a co-oximeter) to get a Hb result quickly and a sample for near-patient coagulation testing, if available. An FBC and coagulation screen should also be sampled. If available, the rapid fluid infuser should be prepared at this stage and should be used in preference for volume administration, as fluids will be warmed. A standard emergency infusion in this situation is of the magnitude of 2 L of crystalloid quickly, followed by 1 L of colloid, depending on the Hb result.

An infusion of 40 IU Syntocinon® should be commenced. If a cell salvage device is available, this should be prepared at this stage in the procedure and set to collect only in the first instance.

Despite the measures taken, the uterus remains atonic and the blood loss is now 1800 mL. Which drugs are used as uterotonics during a Caesarean section, and what are their dosages and contraindications/major side effects?

- Syntocinon®: 5 IU as an IV bolus and then repeated once, if required. This causes systemic vasodilatation with a drop in BP. Syntocinon® should be given as an infusion of 10 IU in 100 mL of normal saline over 20 min to patients with significant cardiac disease. An infusion of Syntocinon® 40 IU in 500 mL of normal saline, given over 4 hours, is often commenced for mild uterine atony

- Ergometrine: 500 micrograms. This increases BP and is contraindicated in pre-eclampsia. Its major side effect is nausea and vomiting which can prove quite disruptive during the surgical procedure. The concurrent administration of an antiemetic, such as ondansetron, is recommended. Cyclizine is best avoided, as the tachycardia which can accompany it may lead to misinterpretation of cardiovascular signs in the face of ongoing haemorrhage

- Carboprost: 250 micrograms intramuscular (IM) injection into either the deltoid or quadriceps muscle. Until recently, this was injected by the surgeon directly into the uterus, but this is no longer recommended due to the risk of intravascular injection. This is contraindicated in asthmatics, as it can cause bronchospasm, pulmonary oedema, and hypertension. It can be given up to eight times at 15-min intervals

- Misoprostol: 1000 micrograms per rectum (PR). This is a cheap and easily administered agent which is of great use in areas of the world lacking refrigeration and qualified midwifery or medical staff. However, misoprostol may cause gastrointestinal (GI) upset and pyrexia.

Case update

The blood loss continues, and the obstetricians say that, despite the further uterotonic agents, the uterus remains atonic and the blood loss is at 2.2 L and ongoing. The patient is getting anxious, and proceedings are now at 55 min since administering the spinal anaesthesia.

What are the recommended types and volumes of fluid for resuscitation?

- 2 L of crystalloid and 1–2 L of colloid, run through a rapid infuser that is capable of warming the fluids

- Red blood cells should be given to maintain Hb above 80 g/L.

What actions should be taken in view of the ongoing blood loss?

A major haemorrhage alert should be activated in view of the volume of blood lost and because it is ongoing. It would be appropriate to ask for 4 U of red blood cells and 2 U of FFP as an initial resuscitation pack, although each hospital may have differing predefined emergency blood packs.

If not already present, the consultant obstetric anaesthetist should be informed and asked to attend, as should the consultant obstetrician. It would be appropriate at this stage to discuss with the patient and her partner about a general anaesthetic, as surgery is ongoing with the possible need for further surgical intervention. If this course of action is agreed, the patient should be given sodium citrate, pre-oxygenated, and a standard RSI with cricoid pressure carried out using thiopentone and suxamethonium.

Insertion of an arterial line should be considered at this stage to allow for invasive BP monitoring, repeated ABG, and haematology sampling. Near-patient coagulation testing, HemoCue® (or similar), or thromboelastography should be utilized, if available.

Case update

The blood loss is now at 2.8 L. The patient's BP is 75/40 and is requiring boluses of vasopressor to support it. Four litres of fluid have been infused, and spot Hb results are 68, 72, and 71 g/L. An FBC and a clotting screen have been sent to the laboratory, and the results are awaited. A blood transfusion should be initiated at this stage. If cell salvage is available, the centrifuge section should have been brought into use, and significant volumes of blood will now have been salvaged. Processing and re-infusion of this salvaged blood should commence if bleeding is persistent; however, it is important to remember that salvaged blood contains no coagulation factors.

The obstetricians are continuing to struggle with haemostasis. Blood loss is now at 3.5 L, despite repeated uterotonics.

What actions could the obstetricians take to stop the bleeding?

+ Mechanical: fundus rubbing, bimanual uterine compression
+ Surgical: balloon tamponade, e.g. Bakri balloon, haemostatic brace suturing (B Lynch suture), bilateral uterine artery ligation, bimanual internal iliac ligation, aortic cross-clamping, hysterectomy.

Case update

The results are back from the bloods sent when the blood loss stood at 2.8 L:

- Hb 65 g/L, WCC 8.4×10^9/L, Plt 75×10^9/L
- APTT 53 s, APTT ratio 1.7, PT 16 s, INR 1.4, fibrinogen 1.2 g/L.

What management should be initiated, based on these blood results?

Red cells should be transfused to maintain Hb above 80 g/L (according to the greentop guideline 52 of the Royal College of Obstetricians and Gynaecologists (RCOG)). Another 1–2 U of blood should be transfused, and a spot Hb check requested.

The coagulation screen is deranged, so it would be appropriate to transfuse 2 U of FFP and prime the blood transfusion laboratory to have a further 2 U available. Products should be transfused to maintain the APTT ratio <1.5 and INR <1.5, fibrinogen >1.0 g/L, and platelets >50 $\times$ 10^9/L (according to the RCOG guidelines).

Case update

The obstetricians have placed a haemostatic suture into the uterus, but unfortunately the bleeding has not been arrested, and the loss now stands at 4.3 L. Further formal bloods were sent, following the previous transfusion, and an ABG has been performed:

- ABG: H^+ 52.4 nmol/L, $PaCO_2$ 4.2 kPa, PaO_2 28.3 kPa, HCO_3^- 18.3 mmol/L, BE −6.1, lactate 2.6
- Bloods: Hb 68 g/L, K^+ 4.5 mmol/L, Ca^{2+} 0.98 mmol/L, Cl^- 116 mmol/L.

Comment on what these blood results show. What should be done to treat these results?

The patient has a metabolic acidosis with slight respiratory alkalosis. She is well oxygenated, secondary to supplemental oxygen being administered. There is evidence of tissue hypoperfusion, as the lactate is elevated.

Despite transfusion, the Hb remains low, and a further 1–2 U of red cells should be transfused. The Ca^{2+} is low and should be treated with a bolus of Ca^{2+} as it is an essential cofactor in coagulation and also improves BP. The Cl^- is elevated which is likely to be secondary to the infusion of chloride-containing fluids.

Case update

The blood loss now stands at 5 L, with no evidence that the bleeding is reducing in rapidity.

What action should the obstetricians take?

The patient should have a subtotal hysterectomy performed. This decision should be made sooner rather than later. It is recommended that a second consultant should be involved in the decision for hysterectomy, although this will depend on the availability of a second person which may not always be the case in smaller units. In some centres, the consultant gynaecologist is involved earlier in cases of major obstetric haemorrhage.

The surgery is completed with a total blood loss of 6.4 L. What is your post-operative plan?

The patient should be transferred to the ICU. It would be appropriate for this patient to remain intubated to allow for a period of haemodynamic stability prior to extubation.

The patient would have received intrathecal diamorphine at the start of the procedure for post-operative analgesia. However, as the surgery has been more extensive, it would be appropriate for the patient to have an opioid infusion and regular paracetamol, until she is awake and capable of using a PCA. If an epidural catheter was *in situ*, then it would be possible to give local anaesthetic via this route. This catheter should not be removed until blood results are available showing normal coagulation and platelets over 80×10^9/L.

NSAIDs should be withheld, as should prophylactic low-molecular-weight heparin (LMWH), until blood results are normalized.

Summary

Most patients with massive obstetric haemorrhage stabilize quickly and return to their base maternity unit within 24–48 hours. If hysterectomy has been performed, they usually require extensive debriefing by the obstetric staff to reduce the likelihood of post-traumatic stress disorder.

Further reading

Kayem G, Kurinczuk JJ, Alfirevic Z, Spark P, Brocklehurst P, and Knight M (2011). Specific second-line therapies for postpartum haemorrhage: a national cohort study. *British Journal of Obstetrics and Gynaecology*, **118**, 856–64.

Knight M (2007). Peripartum hysterectomy in the UK: management and outcomes of the associated haemorrhage. *British Journal of Obstetrics and Gynaecology*, **114**, 1380–7.

Royal College of Obstetricians and Gynaecologists (2008). *Blood transfusions in obstetrics. Green-top guideline No. 47*. Available at: <http://www.rcog.org.uk/files/rcog-corp/uploaded-files/GT47BloodTransfusions1207amended.pdf>.

Royal College of Obstetricians and Gynaecologists (2009). *Prevention and management of postpartum haemorrhage. Green-top guideline 52.* Available at: <http://www.rcog.org.uk/files/rcog-corp/GT52PostpartumHaemorrhage0411.pdf>.

Wise A and Clark V (2011). Management of major obstetric hemorrhage. In: McConachie I, ed. *Controversies in obstetric anesthesia and analgesia*, pp. 56–71. Cambridge University Press, New York.

Pre-eclampsia

Background

Pre-eclampsia is a multisystem disease, typically featuring hypertension and proteinuria occurring after 20 weeks' gestation in a previously normotensive woman. It occurs in 5–8% of pregnancies.

It is caused by failure of placental implantation early in pregnancy, resulting in endothelial damage and dysfunction. This is thought to cause the release of vasoactive substances that promote vasoconstriction and organ hypoperfusion. Pre-eclamptic women also have increased sensitivity to circulating catecholamines and an imbalance in the thromboxane:prostacyclin ratio.

Pre-eclampsia can progress to HELLP (a syndrome encompassing haemolysis, elevated liver enzymes, and a low platelet count) and eclampsia. Eclampsia occurs in 1–2% of patients with pre-eclampsia in the UK, and it may be the first presentation of the condition. Forty per cent of eclamptic fits may occur post-delivery.

The only cure for pre-eclampsia is delivery of the fetus and placenta. As a consequence, pre-eclampsia is associated with prematurity of the neonate. However, the decision for delivery is for maternal indications. Treatment of hypertension does not alter the course of the underlying disease process, but it may reduce the morbidity and mortality caused by uncontrolled hypertension.

There is a significant risk of pre-eclampsia recurring in subsequent pregnancies (one in four if severe pre-eclampsia), and NICE have recommended the use of aspirin 75 mg daily from the 12th week of gestation until birth to reduce the recurrence.

Learning outcomes

1 Discuss the recognition and initial management of pregnancy-induced hypertension

2 Outline different anti-hypertensive therapies in the parturient

3 Discuss the operative management and post-operative care of the eclamptic patient.

CPD matrix matches

2B02; 2B05

Case history

A 28-year-old primigravida presents at 27 + 5 weeks' gestation, with hypertension (160/95 mmHg) and 3+ proteinuria. She is usually fit and well and has had an uncomplicated pregnancy thus far. She takes no medications, has no allergies, and is a non-smoker. Her BMI is 26, and airway examination does not indicate any potential difficulties. A BP profile done on the day assessment unit confirms her hypertension. She feels well and has no complaints on systemic enquiry.

What is the most likely diagnosis and risk factors for this condition?

The combination of hypertension and proteinuria is indicative of pre-eclampsia, risk factors for which include:

+ Primigravida patients
+ Family history of pre-eclampsia
+ New partner
+ Chronic hypertension
+ Multiple pregnancy
+ Previous pre-eclampsia
+ Glucose intolerance and diabetes
+ Obesity
+ Molar pregnancy
+ Antiphospholipid syndrome

What investigations would be appropriate and why?

+ Cardiotocography (CTG): assessment of fetal well-being
+ Departmental ultrasound scan (USS) to assess Doppler flow in the umbilical artery and to assess fetal growth. Pre-eclampsia is associated with intrauterine growth restriction (IUGR) and prematurity
+ Blood samples:
  • FBC: thrombocytopenia may be present
  • Coagulation screen: disseminated intravascular coagulation (DIC) can occur

- Biochemistry: renal impairment may exist; elevated urate levels is a marker of pre-eclampsia; deranged liver function as a component of HELLP syndrome can occur
- Urine: proteinuria is defined as >0.3 g of protein in a 24-hour urine collection. Urinary Alb:Cr ratio ≥30 mg/mmol may be used also to predict for pre-eclampsia.

At what level of systolic and diastolic pressures should antihypertensives be initiated?

Absolute values of systolic pressure over 140 mmHg or diastolic pressure over 90 mmHg or an increase in BP by >30 mmHg, compared to booking BPs. The BP should be raised on two separate occasions before treatment is initiated. An isolated reading of diastolic BP >110 mmHg is also an indication to commence treatment.

The obstetricians want to commence antihypertensive therapy. Which drugs are commonly used?

- Labetalol
- Oral nifedipine
- Methyldopa

Case update

Her hypertension settles on treatment, and her blood results are normal, except for a urate of 0.41 mmol/L. She is discharged home but is readmitted at 28 + 6 weeks gestation, with a BP of 180/100 mmHg and 4+ proteinuria. She is now symptomatic, and biochemistry results demonstrate that her urate has now risen to 0.5 mmol/L. FBC shows Hb 102 g/L, WCC 12.4×10^9/L, Plt 113×10^9/L, down from a previous value of 247. Her urea is 5.6 mmol/L, and liver function tests (LFTs) and coagulation screen are normal.

What are the common symptoms and signs associated with her condition?

- Cerebral: headache, visual disturbance, hyperreflexia, altered consciousness, clonus
- Respiratory: dyspnoea, cyanosis, pulmonary oedema, hoarseness
- Liver: epigastric, right upper quadrant pain/vomiting
- Renal: oliguria
- Generalized oedema

- Biochemistry: elevated urate, urea, creatinine
- Deranged LFTs
- Thrombocytopenia
- DIC
- Severe constant uterine pain, secondary to placenta abruption

Case update

She receives several doses of antihypertensive agents, but her BP remains elevated at 166/102 mmHg, although her symptoms seem to have improved.

What other treatments are available to manage her BP?

- Labetalol infusion
- Hydralazine: this can be given IV as 5 mg boluses or initiated as an infusion. Hydralazine may cause a marked drop in BP, as the patient is often intravascularly volume-deplete. It may also cause tachycardia and cause the patient to feel tremulous.

What additional interventions should be considered for the optimal management of this patient's condition?

The patient should ideally be managed in a high dependency setting, with an arterial line sited to monitor the efficacy of antihypertensive therapy and to facilitate frequent blood sampling. She should be catheterized, and hourly urine volumes should be documented. Typically, fluid intake is restricted to around 80 mL/hour to minimize the risk of pulmonary oedema developing. Neurological observations, including ankle reflexes for the development of clonus, should be monitored hourly. Regular ranitidine should be prescribed, and due consideration given as to the need to fast the patient in the event that emergency surgery is required. Regular blood tests, typically 6-hourly, should be taken, assessing for deterioration in renal function and possible further fall in platelets.

Fetal issues should be discussed with the neonatologist, including the optimal time of delivery and the administration of steroids for lung maturation, as necessary, to optimize the outcome of such a preterm infant. As the patient is likely to require imminent delivery, magnesium sulphate should be considered for neural protection of the fetus, as it is under 30 weeks' gestation. This will also be useful in treating the mother, as she has severe pre-eclampsia.

Case update

Over the course of the next 12 hours, this lady starts to complain of severe frontal headache and abdominal pain. She appears jittery and agitated. Her BP is controlled at 148/96 mmHg. This woman has severe pre-eclampsia, and discussion around urgent delivery is required.

What treatment would you consider at this stage, and how should this be given?

Magnesium sulphate, 4 g IV loading dose, should be administered over 15–20 min, then 1 g/hour for 24 hours from its commencement, as this has been demonstrated to reduce the incidence of eclampsia by 50%.

Case update

The decision is made to deliver this lady urgently by Caesarean section. Her most recent bloods show a further fall in her platelets to 64×10^9/L.

How would you manage this lady for her operation?

This case should involve a consultant anaesthetist due to the risks of haemorrhagic and neurological complications. In view of her platelet count, regional anaesthesia is relatively contraindicated, and therefore general anaesthesia is favoured.

Conduct of general anaesthesia for an emergency Caesarean section

- Anti-aspiration prophylaxis: IV ranitidine and oral sodium citrate
- Pre-oxygenate for 3 min
- Obtund pressor response to laryngocopy: opioid cover is commonly given during pre-oxygenation: either alfentanil 7–10 micrograms/kg bolus or remifentanil infusion with bolus of 1 microgram/kg. Other options are labetalol 10–20 mg, fentanyl 1–4 micrograms/kg, or magnesium sulphate 30 mg/kg
- RSI with thiopentone and suxamethonium
- Be prepared for potentially difficult intubation, due to laryngeal oedema, with smaller tracheal tubes, e.g. 6.0 and 6.5 mm, as well as the usual adjuncts for anticipated difficult intubation
- Consider a lower dose of a non-depolarizing neuromuscular blocker, as a patient who has had magnesium sulphate therapy has a prolonged action of muscle relaxants. A nerve stimulator should be used prior to reversal and waking the patient

- Uterotonics: IV Syntocinon® bolus 5–10 IU at delivery. Ergometrine is contraindicated, due to its hypertensive effects. An IV Syntocinon® infusion 40 IU over 4 hours, as there is a higher risk of haemorrhage in women with pre-eclampsia, exacerbated by co-existing thrombocytopenia
- Antibiotics should be given to the mother, following cord clamping, as she is at <32 weeks' gestation
- A longer-acting opiate should be given for post-operative analgesia, following delivery of the fetus
- Fluid restrict: give the volume of fluid lost as a bolus, then maintain at 80 mL/hour
- TAP blocks are relatively contraindicated in view of thrombocytopenia
- Prior to extubation, you should assess for a leak around the tracheal tube, as laryngeal oedema may be considerable, necessitating the patient being admitted to intensive care for elective ventilation until this resolves.

What would be your post-operative plan?

Assuming the patient was extubated uneventfully, she should be ideally cared for in a high dependency setting. Antihypertensives should be continued, and magnesium sulphate should continue for a total of 24 hours from commencement. In the face of normotension, fluid restriction to 80 mL/hour should be continued, with hourly measurements of urine volumes.

A standard post-operative analgesic regimen includes regular paracetamol and morphine PCA. NSAIDs should be avoided, as these can cause renal dysfunction.

Post-operatively, she is oliguric. How should this be managed?

This should be managed initially with a fluid challenge of 250 mL of crystalloid. This should only be given once, as repeated boluses may precipitate pulmonary oedema. Colloid is avoided, as this may precipitate pulmonary oedema because the larger molecules pass into the pulmonary interstitial space.

She fails to respond to your treatment. What would you do next?

A central venous catheter (CVC) should be inserted to guide subsequent fluid management. If the CVP is <4 mmHg, further 250 mL fluid boluses should be titrated in, until the CVP is in the 4–8 mmHg range; then subsequent urine output should be assessed. If the CVP is >8 mmHg, a single dose of furosemide should be considered.

Summary

Patients with pre-eclampsia benefit from regional anaesthesia for labour and delivery. Regional anaesthesia cannot be performed, however, if the platelet count is $<80 \times 10^9$/L. If regional anaesthesia is possible, the dosage of drugs may need to be adjusted in relation to the gestation. The smaller the fetus, the less aortocaval compression, and the less subsequent compression of the cerebrospinal fluid (CSF) and epidural space. Larger local anaesthetic doses are therefore required to achieve adequate block height in earlier gestations. Vasopressors are less likely to be required and should be given in a lower dose than normal, as the patients are more sensitive to catecholamines (e.g. phenylephrine dose of 20 micrograms, compared to 40 micrograms in normal women).

Further reading

Altman D, Carroli G, Duley L, *et al.* (2002). Do women with pre-eclampsia, and their babies, benefit from magnesium sulphate? The Magpie Trial: a randomised placebo-controlled trial. *Lancet*, **359**, 1877–90.

Anonymous (1995). Which anticonvulsant for women with eclampsia? Evidence from the Collaborative Eclampsia Trial. *Lancet*, **345**, 1455–63.

Morbid obesity in obstetrics

Background

Obesity is one of the most commonly occurring risk factors in obstetric practice. The prevalence has increased markedly from 9–10% of the obstetric population in the early 1990s to 16–19% in the 2000s. The significance of obesity as a risk factor was highlighted in the 2003–2005 Confidential Enquiry into Maternal and Child Health (CEMACH) report, and this has resulted in the consensus guidelines from CMACE and the RCOG. Obese women should receive pre-conception counselling to explain the risks of pregnancy, the requirement for increased monitoring antenatally, and the problems of intrapartum management. They should receive dietary and exercise advice. Obesity is a significant risk factor for anaesthesia-related maternal mortality, and, as a result, it is recommended that women with a BMI $\geq$40 kg/m^2 are assessed by a consultant obstetric anaesthetist antenatally. It is especially important that this assessment identifies women with both difficult backs and difficult airways, as discussions with obstetric staff are essential to plan for a safe delivery.

Learning outcomes

1 Define different degrees of obesity in pregnancy and their respective anaesthetic and obstetric implications

2 Discuss the difficulties of regional anaesthesia in the obese parturient

3 Outline the manual handling and positioning issues during operative delivery.

CPD matrix matches

2B01; 2B03; 2B04

Case history

A 23-year-old primigravida attends her appointment with the midwife to book at estimated gestation of 10 weeks. She has a history of depression and is a smoker. She has no allergies and is not taking any medication at present. She has had a general anaesthetic at age 15 for dental extractions which was uneventful.

The midwife notes that her height is 1.56 m, and she weighs 115 kg. Her BMI is calculated at 47.2 kg/m^2.

How would you classify her BMI?

This lady is obese class 3 (formerly called morbid obesity), using the following accepted definitions*:

+ Class 1 is BMI 30–34.9
+ Class 2 is BMI 35–39.9 (5% of the UK population)
+ Class 3 is BMI ≥40 kg/m^2 (2% of the UK population).

The midwife carries out a routine booking and arranges for a booking ultrasound. What other appointments should be arranged for this lady?

Any patient with a BMI ≥40 kg/m^2 should be referred for antenatal consultation with a consultant obstetric anaesthetist. Women with a BMI ≥35 kg/m^2 should be referred to a consultant obstetrician to have an informed discussion regarding the intrapartum complications associated with an increased BMI.

What are the adverse outcomes associated with obesity in pregnancy?

Fetal/neonatal

+ Miscarriage
+ Fetal congenital anomaly: neural tube defects, omphalocele, and heart defects. Maternal size means that antenatal ultrasound diagnosis is technically difficult
+ Macrosomia
+ Stillbirth
+ Neonatal death
+ Breastfeeding difficulties.

Maternal

+ Thromboembolism
+ Gestational diabetes
+ Pre-eclampsia: this patient has two moderate risk factors for pre-eclampsia, with a BMI ≥35 kg/m^2 being a primigravida. Optimal management should include the administration of aspirin 75 mg from 12 weeks' gestation

---

* Data from World Health Organization, 'Obesity: Preventing and managing the global epidemic', 2000, p. 9.

- Caesarean section rates are 2–3 times higher in obese women
- Post-partum haemorrhage
- Wound infections.

The 2003–2005 CEMACH report suggested that obesity is a risk factor for maternal death, as 28% of mothers who died were obese, compared to a prevalence of 16–19% in the population.

What pre-existing conditions are more likely in obese parturients?

- Diabetes
- Hypertension
- Ischaemic heart disease
- Secondary pulmonary hypertension and chronic right ventricular failure.

What screening should be performed on this lady between 24 and 28 weeks?

Patients with a BMI ≥30 kg/m^2 should have screening for gestational diabetes with a 2-hour 75 g oral glucose tolerance test between 24 and 28 weeks' gestation.

At 32 weeks, this lady attends the antenatal anaesthetic clinic at the hospital. What should be assessed in this clinic?

- Obstetric history and plans for the mode of delivery
- Past medical history, with systemic enquiry regarding cardiorespiratory disease, diabetes, and snoring/sleep apnoea
- Anaesthetic history
- Medications and allergies
- Airway assessment
- Difficulty of venous access
- Assess the back for difficulty of regional anaesthesia ± lumbar spine ultrasound to assess the depth of the epidural space
- Further investigations might include ECG, echocardiogram, oxygen saturations, CXR, pulmonary function tests.

What should be discussed with this lady at this stage, and what would you recommend?

Women with a BMI ≥35 kg/m^2 should be delivered in a consultant-led obstetric unit. Many would suggest that women with a BMI ≥50 kg/m^2 should be delivered in tertiary referral centres. She should have 6-hourly ranitidine orally during labour, as symptomatic reflux occurs in nearly all obese, pregnant women.

The lady should have early venous access (ideally two cannulae), due to the potential difficulty of insertion and the increased risk of post-partum haemorrhage. An intraosseous needle should be available for emergency access. An arterial line may be required if there are difficulties with NIBP monitoring, as very large cuffs are required and these may not be available.

An early epidural or combined spinal/epidural (CSE) technique for labour should be advised, due to the difficulty that there may be in siting this, the increased chance of requiring an operative delivery, and the initial higher failure rates (up to 42% in one hospital study). There is also an increased rate of accidental dural puncture and the need for re-siting an epidural with increasing BMI.

Case update

The consultant anaesthetist documents that her airway does not predict difficulty but that her venous access is difficult, and she has no palpable landmarks on assessing her back. Ultrasound of her back identifies the midline and estimates her epidural space at 7.5 cm.

This lady's pregnancy continues, and she is induced at 41 + 5 weeks for being post-dates. She is admitted to the labour ward following an artificial rupture of membranes at 2 cm dilatation.

Who should be informed of this patient's admission?

The duty anaesthetist for the labour ward should be advised of the admission of any woman with a BMI $\geq$40 kg/m^2. This allows them to review the anaesthetic and obstetric plan for the lady.

The obstetric staff should be made aware of this lady. It is recommended that senior obstetric and anaesthetic staff are available for women with a BMI $\geq$40 kg/m^2.

Case update

The lady makes slow progress in labour, and it is decided that she should be commenced on a Syntocinon® infusion to augment her labour. She decides that she would like an epidural.

What problems are there in siting and managing an epidural in a woman with a raised BMI?

There is likely to be significant difficulty in palpating the landmarks for regional anaesthesia. Ask the patient if you are palpating her hips and the middle of her back, whether it feels like you are pressing on a bone or a space. A second assistant may be beneficial to retract fat pads. It may be advisable to insert the epidural in theatre where conditions are better, in terms of lighting and bed, than the labour ward, and the anaesthetic assistant can help in positioning the patient. There is the potential for requiring longer needles, e.g. 10–12 cm long, although standard 8 cm long Tuohy needles can be used in the majority of cases.

There may be fat indentation when inserting the epidural, such that the markings on the Tuohy needle underestimate the actual depth of the epidural space. It is therefore advisable to leave more catheter in the space, e.g. 5–6 cm in the space. Asking the patient to sit upright, prior to securing the catheter in place, allows for it to be pulled inwards. There is the potential for a higher block than in non-obese women, so top-up doses should be administered incrementally and with caution. CTG monitoring during epidural insertion may be impossible, so a fetal scalp electrode may be required.

Aortocaval compression occurs in all, but full upright and lateral, positions, so patient positioning during labour is important.

Case update

An epidural is inserted by a senior anaesthetic trainee and functions well, with regular epidural review taking place. Despite augmentation with Syntocinon®, this lady fails to progress beyond 4 cm dilatation, and the decision is made to take the lady for emergency Caesarean section. Her epidural has been working well, and the decision is made to top it up for the section.

What are the differences in the management of an epidural top-up in this lady, compared to someone with a normal BMI?

Less local anaesthetic is required to achieve a block to T4 bilaterally in the obese patient. It is therefore advisable to give a smaller volume and assess the block.

What are the anaesthetic problems of managing this lady in theatre?

Ensure that the operating table is capable of taking the patient's weight; a specialized bariatric table may be required. There are several considerations relating to the manual handling and positioning of this patient:

- Use a head-up tilt, with a pillow ramp or a propriety device such as the Oxford Help pillows, even with regional anaesthesia. This will prevent the block from spreading too cephalad and also places the patient in an ideal ramped position, should she require a general anaesthesia
- The patient's arms need to be out on arm boards for venous and potential arterial access
- Lateral tilt of the operating table to 15° or wedging the patient to reduce aortocaval compression
- She may require lateral support if the pannus swings to the left
- Carefully protect pressure areas with appropriate gel pads
- All obese patients should have a 40 IU Syntocinon® infusion commenced at delivery
- If there is difficulty in measuring BP, consideration should be given to the insertion of an arterial line.

In the event that a general anaesthetic is required, the difficult airway trolley should be brought into theatre, and several laryngoscopes, particularly the polio blade, may be required. PEEP is usually necessary to maintain oxygenation.

What post-operative complications is this woman more at risk of, and how are these prevented?

- Post-partum haemorrhage: 40 IU Syntocinon® infusion
- VTE: aim for early mobilization; large TED stockings. Higher doses of LMWH are required when the weight exceeds 90 kg at booking. It is also advisable for patients with a BMI ≥40 kg/m² to have thromboprophylaxis for a minimum of 1 week post-partum, irrespective of the mode of delivery
- Wound infection: antibiotics given prior to commencing surgery. The obstetricians may alter where they make their incision, e.g. supraumbilical. Often staples and extra compression sutures are used on the skin
- Hypoxia: nurse the patient sitting up. Avoid hypothermia wherever possible, as shivering increases oxygen consumption. Oxygen saturations and RR should be monitored. If a general anaesthetic had been required, then supplemental oxygen should be administered for 24 hours, and chest physiotherapy may be beneficial. Very obese patients should be taken to HDU for 24 hours.

Summary

In this case, the patient had an uneventful Caesarean under epidural top-up. It is important to ensure that the epidural is functioning well, and, if there is any doubt about this, then it should be re-sited. However, if she had had no epidural and a *de novo* spinal was required for operative delivery, a CSE technique has advantages. The epidural needle acts as a long introducer, and a smaller dose of spinal can be used to avoid a high block, and epidural top-ups then used if the spinal block is too low. Finally, as surgery is likely to be prolonged, due to the technical difficulties caused by her obesity, the anaesthetic can be prolonged with epidural top-ups. In some cases, the epidural can be maintained for post-operative analgesia if the patient is deemed at high risk of chest complications. Post-partum education on weight loss is essential, as it is well known that the weight gained during pregnancy is often not lost in obese women whose problems are therefore compounded in the next pregnancy.

Further reading

National Institute for Health and Clinical Excellence (2008). *Diabetes in pregnancy: management of diabetes and its complications from pre-conception to the postnatal period. Clinical guidelines, CG63*. Available at: <http://www.nice.org.uk/CG063>.

Peripartum cardiomyopathy

Background

Peripartum cardiomyopathy is associated with the onset of cardiac failure in the last month of pregnancy up to 5 months post-partum, with no identifiable cause and in the absence of pre-existing heart disease. It was responsible for 11 deaths in the last CEMACH report (2006–08), with one of these deaths being a late death. It has an incidence of 1:1200–4000 live births, with most cases occurring post-partum. The aetiology of this condition is poorly understood but may be an exaggerated immune response to pregnancy or due to viral, autoimmune, or toxic factors. It is associated with older maternal age, greater parity, black race, and multiple gestations. Women may present with fatigue, dyspnoea, oedema, orthopnoea, paroxysmal nocturnal dyspnoea, chest pain, and nocturnal cough. The diagnosis can be missed, as the symptoms may be attributed to those of pregnancy. On examination, there may be an elevated JVP, hepatomegaly, a new regurgitant murmur, and bibasal crepitations.

Learning outcomes

1 Acknowledge the differential diagnoses of a parturient presenting with cardiac failure

2 Appreciate the benefits of shared care with the obstetric and cardiology services for patients with peripartum cardiomyopathy

3 Optimally plan the anaesthetic input to delivery with regards to appropriate analgesia and cardiovascular monitoring.

CPD matrix matches

2B05; 2B06

Case history

Your patient is 37 years old, of parity 2 + 1, with two previous normal deliveries at term. She is now 37 + 6 weeks pregnant and presents to the obstetric triage with increasing fatigue, worsening ankle oedema, and shortness of breath on exertion. On further questioning, her breathlessness has been deteriorating over the past couple of weeks, and she finds herself short of breath mobilizing within the house and has been unable to get out of the house in the past week. She has been waking up at night, coughing and out of breath, and is sleeping with four pillows to prop herself up. She has had occasional episodes of chest pain lasting up to 45 minutes at a time. She has no significant past medical history, is not on any medication, and has no allergies. She smokes ten cigarettes a day.

On examination, the patient has just returned from the toilet and appears dyspnoeic, and her face looks a little puffy. She has a regular pulse of 110 bpm, BP 100/65 mmHg, oxygen saturations 93% on air; her JVP is elevated at 6 cm. She has bilateral coarse crackles on chest examination and an audible 3rd heart sound. Abdominal examination is unremarkable, with a fundal height of 38 cm. Her CTG is reassuring with a baseline of 130 bpm, with good variability and accelerations. There is no uterine activity noted.

Her bloods show Hb 110 g/L, WCC 13.4×10^9/L, Plt 237×10^9/L, urea 4.5 mmol/L, Na^+ 131 mmol/L, K^+ 3.6 mmol/L, Cr 58 mmol/L, urate 0.4 mmol/L. Her blood group is A positive, and a group and save has been performed.

What is the differential diagnosis?

- Peripartum cardiomyopathy
- Other cardiomyopathy
- Sepsis
- Lower respiratory tract infection (LRTI)
- Pre-eclampsia
- Ischaemic heart disease with possible MI
- PE.

What other investigations should be performed?

- CXR: shows upper lobe diversion with some fluid in the horizontal fissure, suggestive of LV failure
- ECG: shows sinus tachycardia, with occasional ventricular ectopics. There is left axis deviation and inverted T waves inferiorly. Sinus tachycardia is a frequent finding in pregnant women, as is the left axis deviation that occurs, due to the displacement of the heart by the gravid uterus. Non-specific T wave changes are also not uncommon
- Echocardiography: shows an ejection fraction of <25%, with LV shortening of around 10% (normal is >30%) and end-diastolic dimension of 6 cm. This is severe LV dysfunction.

What is the most likely diagnosis?

In view of an absent past history of any cardiac condition, this is likely to be peripartum cardiomyopathy.

Which individuals should be involved in her care?

A multidisciplinary approach is required. The consultant obstetrician, anaesthetist, and cardiologist should be involved.

How would you manage her symptoms?

All patients are likely to be commenced on diuretics, oxygen, digoxin, and vasodilators, e.g. nitrates or amlodipine. She should also be commenced on LMWH, in view of her ejection fraction of <35% which predisposes her to a mural thrombus. Angiotensin-converting enzyme (ACE) inhibitors and angiotensin-2 antagonists are contraindicated in the pregnant state, as they may cause neonatal kidney malformations.

Case update

Your patient's condition deteriorates over the next 48 hours, with increasing oxygen requirements. She is dyspnoeic at rest and unable to lie flat. She now has crackles to her midzones despite treatment. CTG remains reassuring. A speculum examination shows a parous os, and the cervix is 2 cm long and 2 cm thick.

How should she be managed?

Delivery needs to be expedited. The mode of delivery needs to be discussed with the patient and the obstetricians. This lady is decompensating. Because the pregnancy is near term, there is no great benefit to the fetus in delaying delivery. She should be managed in a tertiary referral centre.

Your patient is keen for a vaginal delivery. What would be the benefits of this? How should this be managed by the anaesthetic team?

The benefits of a vaginal delivery include reduced blood loss, greater haemodynamic stability, avoidance of surgical stress, and reduced post-operative infections and pulmonary complications. The anaesthetic management of this course of action should include:

- A planned induction so that anticoagulants can be appropriately omitted
- She would benefit from arterial and central line monitoring during labour, and she requires careful fluid management, oxygen therapy, and diuretics, in view of her LV failure

◆ Early epidural for labour to reduce cardiovascular stress and also is beneficial in reducing afterload

◆ A shortened second stage to reduce cardiac work. Elective forceps with Syntocinon® infusion 10 IU in 100 mL of saline over 30 min.

Case update

This patient is induced, but her CTG is unreassuring, and it is decided that she requires a Caesarean section. She now has 6-pillow orthopnoea. She has not had any anticoagulant for >12 hours.

What should be your management of this situation?

Operative delivery of this patient should involve a consultant anaesthetist, and ideally a cardiac anaesthetist should be available. A regional technique, such as an epidural or a CSE, are feasible options, but, in view of the severity of her dyspnoea, this lady will be unable to lie flat for surgery, and, as a consequence, she will require a general anaesthetic. The anaesthetic planning should include:

◆ Antacid prophylaxis with ranitidine and sodium citrate prior to induction

◆ Large-bore IV access and arterial line sited prior to induction

◆ Minimize pressor response to laryngoscopy with an opiate (alfentanil or remifentanil)

◆ Thiopentone and suxamethonium for RSI with cricoid pressure

◆ Vasopressors prepared: phenylephrine to offset the vasodilation caused by general anaesthesia. Also have prepared noradrenaline, dobutamine, or adrenaline for infusion

◆ Once anaesthetized and delivered, it may be of benefit to insert a CVC or pulmonary artery catheter to optimize the post-operative cardiac management

◆ Ventilate with increased PEEP to help LV failure

◆ Restrict fluid intake to losses plus 80 mL/hour, and insert a urinary catheter to guide subsequent fluid therapies

◆ Syntocinon® 10 IU in 100 mL over 30 min following cord clamping

◆ Give a dose of furosemide after delivery, ensuring there is no hypotension following the Syntocinon® dose.

What should be her post-operative management?

She should be cared for in an ICU/HDU/coronary care unit (CCU) setting with cardiology input. She should be commenced on an ACE inhibitor. If she is keen to breastfeed, then enalapril and captopril are felt to be the safest. She requires thromboprophylaxis, due to the risk of intracardiac and pelvic thrombi.

What is her long-term prognosis?

About 50% of patients recover to a normal ejection fraction. This is more likely if the ejection fraction at diagnosis was >30%. Recovery should occur within 6 months. If there is no improvement by 6 months, then the 5-year mortality is 85%. The cardiac transplant rate is 14%.

Your patient is keen for more children. What should she be advised?

There is a high recurrence rate for peripartum cardiomyopathy, so she should have contraceptive advice and be warned against any further pregnancies.

Summary

When managing the patient with peripartum cardiomyopathy, a standard vaginal delivery is optimal in the majority of cases, once the woman is stabilized. The advantages of this mode of delivery are the reduction in haemorrhage, greater haemodynamic stability, avoidance of surgical stress, and reduced post-operative infections and respiratory complications.

Further reading

Adamson DL, Dhanjal MK, and Nelson-Piercy C (2011). Cardiomyopathies. In: Adamson DL, Dhanjal MK, and Nelson-Piercy C, eds. *Heart disease in pregnancy*, pp. 137–50. Oxford University Press, Oxford.

Royal College of Obstetricians and Gynaecologists (2011). *Cardiac disease and pregnancy (Good practice No. 13)*. Available at: <http://www.rcog.org.uk/cardiac-disease-and-pregnancy-good-practice-no-13>.

Sliwa K, Hilfiker-Kleiner D, Petrie MC, *et al.* (2010). Current state of knowledge on aetiology, diagnosis, management, and therapy of peripartum cardiomyopathy: a position statement from the Heart Failure Association of the European Society of Cardiology Working Group on peripartum cardiomyopathy. *European Journal of Heart Failure*, **12**, 767–78.

Case 5.5

Severe sepsis in pregnancy

Background

Sepsis is now the leading cause of direct maternal deaths in the UK, with a rate of 1.13 deaths per 100 000 maternities. There was a dramatic rise in this from the previous triennium (2003–2005) where it accounted for 0.85 deaths per 100 000 maternities. This is the first time that sepsis has been the leading cause of direct maternal death since reporting started in 1952. In the 2006–2008 CMACE report, sepsis accounted for a total of 29 deaths—26 direct and three late deaths. Group A β-haemolytic *Streptococcus* (GAS) was responsible for 13 of the deaths, *Escherichia coli* for five, and *Staphylococcus aureus* for three. GAS commonly causes sore throats and upper respiratory tract infections (URTIs).

The commonest sites of infection during pregnancy are the genital tract, urinary tract, breast, lung and skin and soft tissue. Many of the patients who died from GAS had reported a sore throat or had been in contact with children who had a throat infection. The diagnosis of sepsis in pregnancy may be difficult, as the signs and symptoms may be less distinctive. Important signs of sepsis that may be missed are diarrhoea and vomiting, constant abdominal pain, hypothermia, and leucopenia. Evidence of fetal distress or an absent fetal heart without placental abruption are also indicators of sepsis. This is because the uteroplacental circulation is not autoregulated, and thus fetal oxygenation is reliant on maternal oxygenation and cardiovascular stability.

Learning outcomes

1 Recognize the presenting features of sepsis in the parturient at term
2 Commence appropriate antimicrobial therapy
3 Recognize and manage DIC as a complication of sepsis in pregnancy.

CPD matrix matches

2B05; 2B06

Case history

A 38-year-old lady from Ghana, parity 1 + 2, presents in the early hours of the morning at 36 + 3 weeks gestation with possible spontaneous rupture of membranes. She had a previous normal delivery in Ghana 12 years previously. This pregnancy has been uncomplicated. The patient has no other medical history, takes no regular medication, and has no allergies. She has no anaesthetic history and is a non-smoker.

The obstetricians perform a speculum examination of this lady and can see clear liquor draining from the cervix which is posterior. A high vaginal swab is taken. Fetal monitoring is reassuring with a reactive trace. However, there is no uterine activity on the CTG. She is allowed to go home with the advice to return the following day for induction if she fails to go into labour.

She re-attends, as advised, 24 hours later and is given a pessary to induce labour. She begins to contract, and, 12 hours later, she is 2–3 cm dilated. She is admitted to the labour ward, and baseline observations are performed. Her observations include: HR 105 bpm, BP 126/74 mmHg, temperature 38.4°C, RR 21 breaths/min, and oxygen saturations 97% on air.

Comment on these observations. What is the diagnosis?

She is tachycardic, pyrexial, and tachypnoeic. There is evidence of sepsis, as she has three features of the SIRS, and the cause of this is likely to be secondary to infection from prolonged rupture of membranes.

What investigations should be performed?

Blood cultures, high vaginal swab, urine sample for microscopy and culture, FBC, U&E, coagulation, and blood group typing and saving of sample. An ABG analysis would also be appropriate, paying particular note to lactate and the base excess.

What treatment should be given?

This lady requires broad-spectrum antibiotics. CMACE recommends IV co-amoxiclav or a third-generation cephalosporin, in addition to IV metronidazole.

She should be commenced on IV fluid therapy and catheterized, with hourly urine output monitoring. Paracetamol can be administered for its analgesic and antipyretic properties.

Case update

This lady is re-examined 4 hours later, and her cervix is now 4 cm dilated, with meconium-stained fluid discharge. The CTG shows a fetal tachycardia at 165 bpm.

The maternal observations are: HR 110/min, BP 120/70 mmHg, temperature 38.0°C, and RR of 24 breaths/min. The obstetricians decide to commence a Syntocinon® infusion to augment the labour and plan to re-examine after 2 hours.

An hour later, there are signs of fetal distress on the CTG with late decelerations. The mother is re-examined, and her cervix is 6 cm dilated. Her tachycardia, tachypnoea, and pyrexia are worsening. Her blood results demonstrate a neutrophilia with a WCC of 25×10^9/mL. In view of the fetal distress, it is decided to perform a Caesarean section.

What would be your choice of anaesthetic for this patient?

As this patient is septic, regional anaesthesia is relatively contraindicated, due to the risk of spinal abscess formation. This lady requires a general anaesthetic which proceeds with an uneventful induction. During the operative delivery, the obstetricians comment that there appears to be foul-smelling residue within the uterus.

What is the likely diagnosis?

Chorioamnionitis.

What are the risk factors for peripartum sepsis?

See Table 5.1.

Table 5.1 Obstetric and patient risk factors for peripartum sepsis

Obstetric factors	Patient factors
Prolonged spontaneous rupture of membranes	Increased BMI
Retained products of conception	Diabetes/impaired glucose tolerance
Amniocentesis	Black
Cervical cerclage	Anaemia
Prolonged labour with >5 vaginal examinations	Vaginal discharge
	Impaired immunity
	History of pelvic infection
	History of GAS infections
	Poor socio-economic background

What are the likely organisms?

Sepsis in pregnant women is often caused by more than one organism. The commonest pathogens are GAS (*Streptococcus pyogenes*) and *Escherichia coli*.

Following delivery in theatre, the patient's heart rate increases to 150 bpm and blood pressure is 82/40 mmHg. What is the likely differential diagnosis of this altered physiology?

- Sepsis
- Secondary to Syntocinon® bolus
- Haemorrhage
- Embolus: either thromboembolic or amniotic fluid embolism
- Supraventricular tachycardia.

What treatment would you give in the first instance?

- Fluid resuscitation: the Surviving Sepsis campaign recommends 20 mL/kg fluid bolus of crystalloid or colloid
- Antimicrobials: as sepsis is the most likely cause, then consideration of broadening the antibiotic cover with piperacillin/tazobactam, meropenem, or ciprofloxacin and gentamicin. Clindamycin would be an option to cover GAS, as it is better for inhibiting exotoxin production by this organism, and metronidazole should be prescribed in all cases, if not already commenced for anaerobic cover. Teicoplanin or linezolid are recommended if methicillin-resistant *Staphylococcus aureus* (MRSA) is considered.

Case update

She remains hypotensive intraoperatively, with a BP of 75/30 mmHg and a tachycardia of 136 bpm. The patient had been catheterized at the start of the operation and had a residual of 50 mL. Her urine output during the past 30 min is 12 mL.

How would you define her condition?

This patient has septic shock, as she is hypotensive.

How would you manage this patient?

- Senior help: if not already present, the consultant anaesthetist should be informed of the deterioration. She should be referred to intensive care for post-operative placement due to the potential for renal failure and progressive septic shock

- ◆ ABC management: the patient should remain intubated and further IV fluid boluses cautiously titrated against the response in BP, provided there is no evidence of pulmonary oedema. Boluses of vasopressors may be required, e.g. metaraminol which can be used safely as she is post-delivery
- ◆ An arterial line should be sited for BP monitoring and sampling. ABGs should be analysed for acidosis and to check oxygenation, lactate, and Hb. All bloods should be resampled, including coagulation, due to the risk of DIC developing. A CVC to monitor fluids and as the administration of vasopressors, e.g. noradrenaline, is likely to be required.

Case update

The Caesarean section is ongoing, and the estimated blood loss is at 1400 mL. The obstetricians comment that the patient is 'oozy'. The midwife checks up the blood results taken prior to the start of surgery: Hb 82 g/L, WCC 27.5 × 10^9/L, Plt 53 × 10^9/L, APTT 66 s, APTT ratio 2.1, PT 30 s, INR 2.5, fibrinogen 0.3 g/L.

Comment on these results. Why is the patient 'oozy'?

The patient is anaemic, and the Hb is likely to have dropped in view of the intra-operative blood loss. The WCC is elevated, and the patient has thrombocytopenia. The coagulation screen suggests the patient has developed DIC, resulting in increased blood loss at the surgical interface.

How would you manage this situation?

If not already present, the consultant anaesthetist should be in attendance. Senior obstetric support should be requested to ensure the optimal surgical techniques are being employed.

Blood products should be requested from the transfusion laboratory. An initial request of 2–4 U of red cells, 4 U of FFP, and a pool of platelets is an appropriate starting point. Cryoprecipitate may be given for the low fibrinogen level, although this may respond to FFP alone. The administration of further clotting factors should be guided ideally with frequent near-patient coagulation testing, if available, e.g. thromboelastography.

As a component of DIC, the patient is also likely to have hyperfibrinolysis which can be treated with IV tranexamic acid, usually 1 g as a loading dose, and then 0.5 g/hour as an infusion or a further 1 g 8 hours later.

The surgery is completed with a total of 3.5 L blood lost. What would be your post-operative plan for this patient?

This patient has septic shock, requiring vasopressors, which has been complicated by DIC and major obstetric haemorrhage. She should be kept intubated at this time to allow for a period of stability before considering extubation, and she should be transferred to the ICU for further care.

Summary

The RCOG guidelines recommend the need for a multidisciplinary approach to the management of sepsis and the use of early warning scoring systems. It advocated adhering to the Surviving Sepsis campaign guidelines of administration of broad-spectrum antibiotics within the first hour of recognition of sepsis after appropriate blood cultures, swabs, and samples have been taken. However, antibiotic administration should not be delayed if it is not feasible for these to be performed in a timely manner. As well as routine bloods, the measurement of serum lactate provides invaluable evidence of tissue perfusion and should be measured in cases where severe sepsis is suspected.

Further reading

Lucas DN, Robinson PN, and Nel MR (2012). Sepsis in obstetrics and the role of the anaesthetist. *International Journal of Obstetric Anesthesia*, **21**, 56 67.

Chapter 6

Paediatric anaesthesia

Dr Karen McGrath
Dr Euan McGregor

Prematurity

Background

The WHO defines prematurity as childbirth occurring at <37 completed weeks of gestation, irrespective of birthweight. It is divided as: extremely preterm (<28 weeks), very preterm (28–32 weeks), and moderate to late preterm (32–37 weeks). Prematurity is generally associated with an increased rate of neonatal and infant morbidity. Risks increase from low birthweight (LBW) newborns (<2.5 kg) to very low birthweight (VLBW) newborns (<1.5 kg).

Learning outcomes

1 Outline the anatomical and physiological differences in the premature infant presenting for surgery

2 Be aware of the potential difficulties related to chronic lung disease

3 Discuss an analgesic plan for elective surgery in the ex-premature infant.

CPD matrix matches

2D01; 2D02

Case history

Baby J was born at 28 weeks' gestation, with a birthweight of 1.2 kg. He was admitted to the special care baby unit (SCBU) where he required CPAP and supplemental oxygen, nasogastric feeding, monitoring of blood sugars, and provision of glucose. He is now 37 weeks corrected gestational age (CGA), has been successfully weaned from his CPAP and oxygen therapy, and has been established on oral feeding. He is ready for discharge home but has previously been noted to have an inguinal hernia. Plans are made for him to attend his local paediatric hospital for repair of his hernia. He has an appointment to attend in 4 weeks' time; by then, he will be 41 weeks CGA.

Using a systems-based approach, outline the problems relating to prematurity

Respiratory

◆ Anatomical factors: neonates are obligate nasal breathers until 4–6 months of life; this is thought to be because of a relatively large tongue in a small oral cavity and an epiglottis that can reach the uvula. This leaves little in the way of an air space to breathe through. If there is nasal congestion, this can dramatically increase the work of breathing through the narrow nasal passages. The differences between the paediatric and adult airways are magnified due to the size of the premature neonate. The larynx is anterior, and the epiglottis is large and floppy; therefore, many anaesthetists would use a straight-bladed laryngoscope to facilitate endotracheal intubation. The cricoid cartilage is the narrowest part of the airway, and the trachea is short, around 4 cm at term; therefore, precision with tube placement is paramount

◆ Physiological factors: the premature neonate's diaphragm fatigues easily due to a reduced level of type 1 muscle fibres. Their chest wall is highly compliant, and their accessory muscles of respiration are inefficient. Pathology, such as URTIs, can cause a significant increase in the work of breathing which can result in respiratory distress or apnoeic spells. Neonates have a higher metabolic rate and therefore consume a greater volume of oxygen per kilogram per minute. They also have a very small functional residual capacity (FRC). These two factors combined can lead to extremely rapid rates of oxygen desaturation during periods of apnoea, e.g. during induction of anaesthesia or secondary to illness and exhaustion. The immature CNS and the respiratory centre, in particular, do not respond to hypoxia and hypercarbia in a predictable manner. Hypoxia and hypercarbia can cause respiratory depression and apnoea, as opposed to causing a stimulus to respiratory activity in the older child and adult

◆ Ventilatory support: the premature neonate may require respiratory support by way of both invasive and non-invasive ventilation or supplemental oxygen. Neonates requiring prolonged oxygen support (>28 days) are said to be oxygen-dependent, and some may be discharged on home oxygen. Prolonged ventilation may result in pneumonia, barotrauma, hyaline membrane disease, and residual chronic lung damage.

Cardiovascular

In utero, the PVR is greater than the SVR due to the presence of fluid within the alveoli, causing hypoxic pulmonary vasoconstriction. As a result, the muscle of the LV is not well developed and is therefore unable to significantly increase the force of ejection brought about by the increased preload with a resultant fixed stroke volume. The major determinant of cardiac output is the HR. The sympathetic nervous system is relatively immature, compared with the more dominant parasympathetic nervous system. This is why hypoxia can result in bradycardia and lead to a significant reduction in cardiac output.

Neurological

Premature infants have a higher risk of intraventricular haemorrhage with subsequent long-term neurological defects. The risk increases with increasing prematurity, LBW, respiratory distress syndrome, coagulopathy, hypoxia, and acidosis. There is poor autoregulatory control of cerebral blood flow, and fluctuations in the BP may increase the risk of intraventricular haemorrhage. Both overtransfusion and anaemia should be avoided.

Retinopathy of prematurity is related to the gestational age and duration of oxygen therapy. $PaCO_2$ and pH levels also have an affect. Lower levels of oxygen saturation (around 90%) are acceptable in this age group. In neonates born before 32 weeks' gestation, early low oxygen saturation levels and late high oxygen saturation levels have been found in a meta-analysis to reduce the risk of retinopathy of prematurity.

Thermoregulation

Preterm infants have a large surface area to body weight ratio. This leads to an increased rate of heat loss. This is compounded with less 'insulation' in the form of subcutaneous fat. They are reliant on brown fat stores for non-shivering thermogenesis, but, under anaesthesia, especially with volatile agents, this process is inhibited. Before the age of 3 months, shivering does not occur.

Glycaemic control

In children <1 month old, there is a real risk of hypoglycaemia due to reduced glycogen storage. They require a source of glucose in their IV fluids if feeding is not established.

Fluid and electrolyte balance

Total body water is expressed as a percentage of the body weight. It is higher for a term neonate than it is for an adult, with a term newborn being 75% water (40% extracellular fluid, ECF; 35% intracellular fluid, ICF) and an adult being 60% water (20% ECF; 40% ICF). During the first 6 months of life, there is a gradual decrease of body water as percentage of the body weight to 60%. Infants normally lose weight during the first week after birth. Term newborns usually lose 5–10% of their weight, almost all of which is water loss. This weight loss is greater in preterm than term infants and is associated with a diuresis. The post-natal diuresis is approximately 1–3 mL/kg/hour in term infants and is greater in preterm infants. Preterm neonates have proportionally more water (>80%), and they may lose 10–15% of their weight in the first week of life. Small-for-gestational-age preterm infants may also have a particularly high body water content. Estimated circulating blood volume is 90–100 mL/kg in a premature neonate, 85 mL/kg in a full-term neonate, 80 mL/kg in a child, and 70 mL/kg in an adult.

Neonates have a decreased capacity to concentrate or dilute urine in response to changes in the intravascular volume status and are at risk of dehydration or fluid overload. This is more pronounced in preterm infants. The normal maturation of renal function increases with increasing gestational age.

Haematological

Poor red blood cell production from immature bone marrow results in anaemia. Thrombocytopenia may occur, and sepsis should be actively excluded. All newborns should receive vitamin K at delivery, as a very small number of newborns (1 in 10 000) may have vitamin K deficiency bleeding.

Sepsis

Reduced cellular and tissue immunity increases the risk of sepsis.

Gastrointestinal

Hepatic enzyme function is immature. There may be difficulty establishing feeding as a consequence of a poor suck reflex. This reflex does not begin until about the 32nd week of pregnancy and is not fully developed until about 36 weeks. Premature infants with LBW are at risk of necrotizing enterocolitis. The exact cause of necrotizing enterocolitis is unknown, and it is not known whether some underlying pathology contributes to premature birth and LBW.

If baby J had chronic lung disease and an ongoing oxygen requirement, how might you modify your anaesthetic technique?

Patients with bronchopulmonary dysplasia require higher peak ventilation pressures and inspired oxygen to achieve an acceptable SpO_2. Post-operative nasal CPAP or ventilation may be required.

The risks of post-operative apnoeic episodes increase after general anaesthesia, even in babies born at term. For those born with a gestational age of 32 weeks, the risk of apnoea is <1% after 56 weeks post-conceptual age. With a gestational age of 34 weeks, the risk of occurrence of apnoea is <1% at 54 weeks post-conceptual age.

Spinal anaesthesia is indicated in patients such as this case or where there are significant risks of administering general anaesthesia, e.g. a difficult airway.

Performing spinal anaesthesia in this patient group is technically very challenging, and a good understanding of the anatomical landmarks and their correlation to spinal cord levels is required. There are significant differences in where Tuffier's line crosses the spinal axis in neonates, compared with older children and adults. The top of the iliac crests is thought to be at the L5–S1 level in neonates and infants, up to the age of 1 year. The spinal cord ends at L3 level at birth, compared to L1/L2 in older children and adults.

The procedure is performed with the patient awake, and it must be borne in mind that the duration of action of a subarachnoid block is much shorter than in an adult. Therefore, an experienced surgeon should be scrubbed and ready to commence the surgical procedure, whilst spinal anaesthesia is performed. When there are bilateral procedures required, prioritization of the most severely affected or highest risk side should take place first.

What measures can be taken to maintain normothermia perioperatively?

- Raise the ambient room temperature
- Minimize heat losses by limiting exposure for procedures, e.g. IV cannulation
- Cover the head with a bonnet
- Active warming measures, e.g. heating mattress and forced air warmers
- Warm and humidify anaesthetic gases.

What are the analgesic options?

- Simple analgesia, e.g. paracetamol
- Local anaesthetic by subcutaneous infiltration, nerve block (ilioinguinal), or neuraxial blockade (caudal)
- Avoid NSAIDs in <44 weeks' gestation
- Aim to minimize opioid use.

You decide to perform a caudal. How do you explain this to baby J's parents?

Before performing any nerve block or central neuraxial procedure, the parent/guardian should be given sufficient information in a way they can understand to give informed consent. This should include both the benefits and reasonable risks. A patient information leaflet could be used to support this.

What is a caudal?

A caudal is a procedure allowing access to the epidural space to deliver local anaesthesia. It is most commonly used alongside general anaesthesia to provide post-operative analgesia for procedures performed below the umbilicus.

How is a caudal epidural block performed?

A good understanding of the anatomy of the sacrum is required, and an awareness of the levels of the spinal cord and dural sac termination is essential. In children, the procedure is most commonly performed under general anaesthesia, in the lateral position with hips and knees flexed. There should be a trained assistant present, a working IV cannula sited, and resuscitation equipment easily accessible.

This is an aseptic technique, performed with similar sterile precautions as when performing an epidural. The sacral hiatus should be identified with the sacral cornuae laterally. A 22G needle/cannula should be inserted at around 45°, and, when the sacrococcygeal ligament is punctured, the angle should be flattened off, and the needle/cannula advanced by a few millimetres. It is important to take care not to advance too far, as this can cause a dural puncture.

Time should be taken to allow for the CSF or blood to flow freely from the inserted needle/cannula if inadvertent placement has occurred. The needle/cannula should be aspirated, prior to the administration of local anaesthetic.

The dose of local anaesthetic administered should be predetermined and should not breach recommendations on the maximal safe dosing of the chosen local anaesthetic.

Who will perform this procedure?

This is a simple technique with a low complication rate when appropriate care is taken. Therefore, a competent anaesthetist could perform this procedure, with supervision if required.

What are the advantages and disadvantages of caudal anaesthesia?

Advantages

- ◆ Provides good post-operative analgesia
- ◆ Minimizes opioid requirement.

Disadvantages

- ◆ Failure/technical difficulty
- ◆ Risks of intravascular injection
- ◆ Risks of dural puncture

- Rectal perforation
- Subcutaneous injection
- Urinary retention
- Leg weakness
- Nerve damage.

Is this patient suitable for day case admission?

No. He should be admitted for apnoea monitoring post-operatively. General anaesthesia can increase apnoea risk for 12–24 hours post-operatively. Apnoeic episodes are common in preterm infants, with risk factors for apnoeas, including:

- Gestation age <45 weeks
- Preterm <34 weeks
- History of apnoeas
- Anaemia
- Chronic lung disease.

His operation proceeds uneventfully and he is comfortable, following the caudal. In addition to apnoea and oxygen saturation monitoring, what additional post-operative instructions would you give?

- Post-operative analgesia
- Glucose-containing IV fluids and blood glucose monitoring until feeding re-established
- Oxygen therapy, if required, to achieve an acceptable SpO_2 level.

Summary

Delivering safe and effective anaesthesia and analgesia to an ex-premature infant requires meticulous attention to detail of the basic principles of anaesthesia. Airway and ventilatory management must take account of the fact that many ex-premature infants may have significant chronic lung disease, causing difficult oxygenation throughout the perioperative period, and may be prone to apnoeas in the post-operative period. Fluid management should account for their basal maintenance requirements of fluid, electrolytes, and glucose. Hypothermia is common and may delay recovery, so efforts to minimize heat losses and maintain normothermia should be made at all times. Employing effective regional analgesic techniques, ideally avoiding systemic opioids where possible, should optimize the post-operative recovery.

Further reading

Chen ML, Guo L, Smith LE, Dammann CE, and Dammann O (2010). High or low oxygen saturation and severe retinopathy of prematurity: a meta-analysis. *Pediatrics*, **125**, e1483–92.

Doyle E and McCormack J (2012). Sacral epidural (caudal) block. In: McLeod G, McCartney C, and Wildsmith T, eds. *Principles and practice of regional anaesthesia*, pp. 153–7. Oxford University Press, Oxford.

Intravenous fluid for children

Background

Recent guidance from the NPSA has emphasized the importance of accurate fluid management in paediatric patients across the perioperative period. This resulted from the analysis of a series of children who died from hyponatraemic coma. Recommendations on the types of fluid and monitoring of fluid balance and electrolytes have been widely employed throughout paediatric services.

Learning outcomes

1 Prepare appropriate fasting guidelines for elective paediatric surgery
2 Assess fluid dehydration in a child presenting for emergency surgery
3 Appreciate the risks associated with hyponatraemia in the perioperative period.

CPD matrix matches

2D02; 2D04

Case history 1

A 3-year-old boy who weighs 15 kg is scheduled for major elective orthopaedic surgery for an open reduction of a dysplastic hip. You are performing a preoperative assessment on the day prior to surgery.

What fasting instructions would you give his parents?

+ Clear fluids: 2 hours
+ Breast milk: 4 hours
+ Solids and formula milk: 6 hours.

Case update

You review him briefly at 11 a.m. for surgery on the afternoon list. His mother tells you that he did not have any breakfast and last ate and drank at 7.30 p.m. the previous night. He is upset, because he is hungry.

Is this the optimal fasting regimen for this patient?

The ideal fluid management in paediatric practice varies between those patients on a morning list and those on an afternoon list. For a patient on a morning list, it is assumed that an otherwise healthy child scheduled for a morning list is adequately hydrated up until going to bed the previous night. Ideally, the child would have been given a 200 mL clear fluid drink before 7.00 a.m. For a patient on the afternoon list, they should have been given breakfast by 7.30 a.m. and ideally a clear fluid drink before 11.30 a.m.

However, even a prolonged fast, as in this case, as opposed to a 2-hour fast for clear fluids, is unlikely to be physiologically significant in terms of the cardiovascular status of the normally well child. It is likely, however, to result in a very unhappy and uncooperative child.

Your patient is the only case on the afternoon list starting at 1.30 p.m. It is now 11.15 a.m. How would you proceed with his fasting status and fluid management?

Explain to the parents regarding fasting for theatre and that it is not possible for their son to have anything to eat, as his surgery is planned for 1.30 p.m. He can have a clear fluid drink to be finished at 11.30 a.m. Sugar-containing fluids would be preferable, given his prolonged fasting period.

Perioperative hypoglycaemia is rare in most children, and the majority of normal, healthy children over 1 month of age will maintain a normal blood glucose. Children at risk of hypoglycaemia should be commenced on isotonic glucose-containing IV fluids preoperatively.

Your patient is taken to theatre at 1.30 p.m. His surgery will take approximately 3.5 hours, and he has an epidural sited for analgesia. Calculate his maintenance fluid requirements.

This is traditionally calculated in paediatric practice using the 4–2–1 formula, as described by Holliday and Segar in 1957. Hence, for this 15 kg patient:

First 10 kg (A): 4 mL/kg/hour (i.e. 40 mL/hour)

Second 10 kg (B): 2 mL/kg/day (i.e. 10 mL/hour)

For each kg over 20 kg (C): 1 mL/kg/day (i.e. 0 mL/hour)

Maintenance total (D) (which is $D = A + B + C$): 50 mL/hour.

In any case of prolonged fasting, it is also important to consider any fluid deficit.

What type of maintenance fluid would you use?

An isotonic fluid such as 0.9% NaCl, Hartmann's solution, or Plasma-Lyte®. Your patient is having prolonged surgery (>3 hours) and regional anaesthesia;

he should be given dextrose during surgery and should have his blood glucose level measured regularly.

What is this patient's fluid deficit?

He has been fasting for 18 hours, with a 200 mL drink 2 hours previously. His hourly maintenance fluid requirement is 50 mL/kg. Therefore, his deficit is:

$$(18 \times 50) - 200 = 700 \text{ mL}$$

Ideally, if he had been given breakfast at 7.30 a.m., with a clear fluid drink at 11.30 a.m., his fluid deficit would have been:

$$(6 \times 50) - 200 = 100 \text{ mL}$$

An IV fluid bolus of 10–20 mL/kg of isotonic fluid should be given during surgery, and the remaining deficit replaced over 24 hours, in addition to maintenance fluid requirements.

You give your patient a 300 mL (20 mL/kg) bolus of fluid at the start of surgery. His remaining fluid deficit is 400 mL which should be replaced over 24 hours at 16 mL/hour, in addition to his maintenance fluids of 50 mL/hour; hence, his total fluid infusion rate should be 66 mL/hour, until full oral intake has been re-established. A single isotonic fluid should be used for both maintenance and correction of fluids.

What fluids would you use in the post-operative period?

Continue isotonic fluid with dextrose, until his oral intake is satisfactory. As per NPSA guidelines, any patient having prolonged IV fluid infusion should have electrolytes and blood glucose checked at least every 24 hours, more frequently if there is an abnormal result.

Case history 2

A 6-year-old girl (19 kg) presents with a 2-day history of abdominal pain, vomiting, and poor oral intake. Clinically, she has acute appendicitis and is moderately dehydrated (5%), but her vital signs are stable.

How would you assess her dehydration preoperatively?

She should have an IV cannula inserted and bloods for U&E and blood glucose. The assessment of dehydration includes the consideration of:

• Fluid deficit (to replace the fluid lost from dehydration):

A child's water deficit in mL can be calculated following an estimation of the degree of dehydration expressed as % of body weight:

$$\text{Deficit (mL)} = \% \text{ dehydration} \times \text{weight (kg)} \times 10$$

The clinical assessment of hydration is difficult and often inaccurate. The gold standard of assessment is acute weight loss, but this is often difficult due to the lack of pre-illness weight. In this case, the fluid deficit is $5 \times 19 \times 10 = 950$ mL. This should be replaced over 24 hours with isotonic fluid such as NaCl 0.9%, Hartmann's solution, or Plasma-Lyte®.

- Maintenance fluid requirements:

First 10 kg (A): 4 mL/kg/hour (i.e. 40 mL/hour)

Second 10 kg (B): 2 mL/kg/hour (i.e. 18 mL/hour)

For each kg over 20 kg (C): 1 mL/kg/hour (i.e. 0 mL/hour)

Maintenance total (D) (where D = A + B + C): 58 mL/hour.

Both fluid deficit and maintenance fluids requirements should be managed by giving a single isotonic fluid.

- Ongoing losses:

Where possible, ongoing losses, e.g. through vomiting, should be measured every 4 hours and additionally replaced with an isotonic fluid such as 0.9% NaCl, Hartmann's, or Plasma-Lyte®.

If her vital signs were unstable at presentation (e.g. tachycardic, tachypnoeic, with a prolonged CRT), how would this have altered your management?

- Call for senior help
- IV or intraosseus access: obtain urgent U&E and glucose
- Fluid bolus of 20 mL/kg of 0.9% NaCl (i.e. 380 mL)
- Reassess the clinical condition, and repeat fluid bolus, as required
- Consider the need for blood if Hb is low or if >40 mL/kg of fluid is required.

Case history 3

A 7-year-old boy is admitted for observation, following a head injury, and continues to have frequent vomiting. You are asked to prescribe IV fluids for him.

What is the appropriate fluid for this child?

In some circumstances, including head injuries, children should only ever be administered isotonic fluids such as 0.9% NaCl (with or without glucose), Hartmann's solution, or Plasma-Lyte® (with or without glucose). Hypotonic fluids must be avoided.

Some children, including those with head injuries and those in the postoperative period, may develop hyponatraemia due to increased antidiuretic hormone (ADH) secretion. In these situations, fluid restriction to 60–70% of normal maintenance rate requirements may be beneficial. Senior and specialist advice should be sought where there is uncertainty about the best course of action.

Summary

The calculation of accurate fluid and electrolyte requirements is integral to the optimal perioperative management of a paediatric patient. Consideration must be given to potential deficits and ongoing losses and the awareness of the risks of hyponatraemia, and, as such, there is little place for hypotonic fluid use in general paediatric practice. Clinicians must be mindful of the incidence of hyponatraemia and must monitor electrolytes regularly in children receiving prolonged crystalloid fluid infusions.

Further reading

Association of Paediatric Anaesthetists of Great Britain and Ireland (2007). *APA consensus guideline on perioperative fluid management in children.* Available at: <http://www.apagbi.org.uk/sites/default/files/Perioperative_Fluid_Management_2007.pdf>.

Holliday MA and Segar WE (1957). The maintenance need for water in parenteral fluid therapy. *Pediatrics*, **19**, 823–32.

McGrath KL and Davis A (2008). Peri-operative fluid management in infants and children—what's new? *Care of the Critically Ill*, **24**, 102–5.

Moritz ML and Ayus JC (2007). Hospital acquired hyponatraemia—why are hypotonic parenteral fluids still being used? *Nature Clinical Practice*, **3**, 374–82.

National Patient Safety Agency (2007). *Patient safety alert 22. Reducing the risk of hyponatraemia when administering intravenous infusions to children.* Available at: <http://www.nrls.npsa.nhs.uk/EasySiteWeb/getresource.axd?AssetID=60073&>.

Royal Children's Hospital Melbourne. *Clinical practice guidelines: intravenous fluids.* Available at: <http://www.rch.org.au/clinicalguide/guideline_index/Intravenous_Fluids/>.

Royal Children's Hospital Melbourne. *Clinical practice guidelines: dehydration.* Available at: <http://www.rch.org.au/clinicalguide/guideline_index/Dehydration/>.

The uncooperative child

Background

Children can present to hospital out of hours and as acute emergencies, and therefore it is not always possible to prepare an anxious or uncooperative child for theatre. On the other hand, in the elective setting, fantastic work can be carried out by play specialists to prepare children preoperatively. As for any clinical interaction, the anaesthetist needs to judge the level of understanding the patient has and communicate with them at an appropriate level to gain trust and cooperation. Interactions with children may be particularly challenging due to fear, pain, previous experiences, and a lack of comprehension or explanation.

Learning outcomes

1 Understand the various non-pharmacological approaches to managing the anxious or uncooperative child
2 Consider different oral premedicants in paediatric anaesthesia.

CPD matrix matching

2D02; 2D06

Case history 1

A 4-year-old girl is admitted as a day case for multiple dental extractions. This is her first general anaesthetic, and she is otherwise well. She has no known allergies and is appropriately fasted. She has not long arrived on the ward, and the nurse looking after her tells you she is very withdrawn and clinging to her mother.

How do you proceed?

Introduce yourself to the child and her parents; try to engage with them and build a rapport. Undertake your standard preoperative anaesthetic assessment, and ask specifically about recent illnesses, including cough or cold symptoms, as this can increase the risk of anaesthetic problems due to a reactive and irritable airway.

Explain the available options for the induction of anaesthesia, specifically discussing IV or inhalational induction. Use age-appropriate and non-threatening descriptions of both techniques, e.g. the use of 'magic cream' to allow the placement of a small plastic straw/tube or 'sleepy wind' via a face mask. Involve the parents in ascertaining what they believe to be most acceptable to the child, but, if the child has been under anaesthesia before or is of an appropriate age, let them make the decision how they wish to proceed with their anaesthetic. If there is a play specialist available, inform the parents of their role in supporting the child and the parents.

Consider premedication in circumstances where the child appears to be distressed, uncooperative, has had a previous bad experience, or where the child has behavioural or learning difficulties limiting their understanding and compliance. An appropriate premedicant should be prescribed, taking into account the onset time, duration of effect, and side effects, so that the parents or carers can be appropriately informed.

Case update

The parents are happy with your explanation of the procedure and would like to try an IV induction. You convey this to her named nurse and the play specialist who starts to prepare the child.

What techniques can be used by the play specialist?

- Play to build rapport and trust
- An illustrated storybook about a child's journey in hospital
- Props such as face masks, choosing a pleasant smell for inside the face mask, stickers/drawings on 'magic cream' dressing, and blowing up balloons
- 'Carrot and stick': find out what the child's interests are, and suggest reading a book about it later, i.e. in the anaesthetic room
- Distraction techniques in anaesthetic room: books, toys, talking, etc.

It is important to make realistic promises and fulfil them to maintain trust.

Case update

The nurse calls you back to the ward to consider premedication for your patient. She cooperated well with the play specialist but will not allow her name bands or topical anaesthetic cream to be put on. It has not been possible to obtain baseline observations. You are in agreement with her nurse, and return to speak to the parents about the premedication.

What premedication would you prescribe?

There are a number of options, but possible choices for oral premedication are:

◆ Midazolam 0.5 mg/kg, up to a maximum of 20 mg: quick onset of around 30 min and offset. It is important to note that benzodiazepines can cause paradoxical agitation in children with autistic spectrum disorder, in which case ketamine may be a better choice

◆ Clonidine 1–4 micrograms/kg: peak onset 60–90 min

◆ Combination of midazolam and clonidine, particularly if either alone has been unsuccessful previously

◆ Ketamine 5 mg/kg: quick onset, with longer duration than midazolam.

Children with attention deficit hyperactivity disorder (ADHD) may require larger doses of benzodiazepines, and the response may be paradoxical agitation. Ketamine may have an unpredictable effect, and the side effects of nausea and vomiting may be accentuated. Clonidine may be a more effective premedicant in this group of patients.

Case update

The patient is brought to the anaesthetic room with her parents approximately 30 min following premedication with midazolam. She is settled and looking a little drowsy but reading the book the play specialist had promised. As she had refused Emla® cream, the play specialist had shown her a face mask and practised blowing up balloons. You put a strawberry smell in the mask at her request, and proceed with a successful inhalational induction.

This was your patient's first visit to hospital. Is there any other way she could have been prepared?

◆ Parents: being truthful and explaining where they are going, why, and what to expect. Patient information leaflets may be helpful

◆ Preoperative visit with the play specialist: ideally about a week beforehand. These visits are usually done in groups, and the child can meet other children undergoing a similar experience. However, visits can be performed on a one–to-one basis, if required, e.g. a very anxious child or one with special needs:

  • Show slides
  • Use puppets to illustrate 'magic cream' and face masks, and mimic the patient journey
  • Tour of hospital
  • Meet staff who will be looking after them.

Case history 2

On the same dental list is a 9-year-old boy also for dental extractions. He is ASA 2 with mild asthma and takes a salbutamol inhaler infrequently when playing sport. He has no known drug allergies. He had a previous general anaesthetic in another hospital for a grommet insertion 3 years ago. There is no family history of problems with anaesthesia.

He admits to being nervous when you go to see him on the day case unit. Mum tells you that he was very upset when he went off to sleep last time. He had an IV induction last time and does not want the needle again. He did not have any premedication on that occasion.

What do you tell this patient and his mother?

Explore his fears, and reassure him that he can go to sleep another way, by breathing some 'sleepy wind'. Discuss the face mask, and offer a nice smell of his choosing to put inside the face mask. Explain that it is similar to using his inhaler with the spacer device, as he did when he was younger, and he can practise with the play specialist beforehand. He and his mum seem reassured, and they have no further questions.

They are seen by the play specialist and prepared for theatre. The nurse, play specialist, and yourself agree he appears more settled and decide against premedication.

However, on arrival in the anaesthetic room, he appears wary. You offer him a choice of smells for the mask and ask him if he would like to hold it himself. He places his hands over his face and refuses to use the mask. He becomes very upset and says, 'I don't want to do this' and 'you can't make me'.

How do you proceed?

Explore his fears, and try to encourage him to proceed. The play specialist and yourself talk to him about the agreed plan, but he is adamant that he will not proceed and buries his face into the bed, crying. He is becoming more upset, with no progress within 10 minutes and mum is asking if you can hold him down.

What do you do now?

Explain to mum that physical restraint is not appropriate. Give the patient and his mum the option of sending him back to the ward for premedication to calm him down so that hopefully he can be brought back later in the list to proceed with his cooperation.

Mum is keen to get the procedure done today and agrees to premedication. He is more settled after the premedication, and you perform a successful inhalational induction on the subsequent attempt.

What would you do if this boy refused to take the premedication?

Cancel the procedure, explaining to mum that it is not an emergency procedure and can be done at a later date. Arrange for this child to come on a preoperative visit prior to rescheduling. Document on his anaesthetic form that you recommend premedication on the next attempt at anaesthesia.

What differences are there in preparing an older child for theatre, compared to a younger child?

- More involved in their treatment
- Increased awareness and knowledge
- Can communicate their fears and discuss them
- May have specific requests, e.g. inhalational induction
- Require a more detailed explanation of events
- Communication is very important
- Distraction is less useful, as many want to know what is happening and why.

What if you need to perform a rapid sequence induction in an uncooperative child?

This is a very difficult situation. It is important to make a balanced decision, based on all risks, in this case, a delay in surgery *versus* an unprotected airway and a possible risk of aspiration. Ideally, these cases should be discussed with a consultant anaesthetist, as they can be particularly challenging to manage. As previously, honest descriptions of the intended sequence of events should be communicated to the child and their parents during the preoperative assessment. Potential options include:

- Proceed with attempts to cannulate the child with the parent's consent and restraint: this would generally be considered an unsatisfactory option, as this may result in physical or psychological harm to the child
- Perform an inhalational induction in head-down and left lateral position: this is a challenging technique to deliver safely in the unfasted child, and it is likely to end in a suboptimal airway management during induction
- Send to the ward, and give oral anxiolysis, e.g. midazolam 0.5 mg/kg, and wait for 20 min; then prepare to deliver an IV RSI. The risks of the short delay to surgery are likely to be considerably offset by the benefits of a smoother induction with optimal and safe airway control.

Summary

Considerable skill is required in overcoming the fears of an anxious and uncooperative child in both the emergency and elective surgical situation. Engaging the child and parents in honest conversations about the antici-pated course of events, along with support from play therapists, will over-come the vast majority of anxieties. In a small number of patients, oral premedication will be effective and facilitate either an IV or inhalational induction. It is vitally important to maintain trust with the child and par-ents, and, as such, physical restraint must never be used.

Further reading

Cote CJ (2008). Round and round we go: sedation—what is it, who does it, and have we made things safer for children? *Pediatric Anesthesia*, **18**, 3–8.

Krauss B and Green SM (2006). Procedural sedation and analgesia in children. *Lancet*, **367**, 766–80.

POEMS for children. Available at: <http://www.poemsforchildren.co.uk>.

Sinha M, Christopher NC, Fenn R, and Reeves L (2006). Evaluation of nonpharmacologic methods of pain and anxiety management for laceration repair in the pediatric emer-gency department. *Pediatrics*, **117**, 1162–8.

Sury MR and Smith JH (2008). Deep sedation and minimal anesthesia. *Pediatric Anesthesia*, **18**, 18–24.

Pyloric stenosis

Background

Congenital hypertrophic pyloric stenosis is thickening of the smooth muscle of the pylorus, which obstructs gastric outflow. It occurs in one in 300–400 children. There is a male predominance of 4:1. The condition has a polygenic mode of inheritance. The incidence is higher in the offspring of affected parents and is more common in autumn and spring. Caucasians are more likely to develop pyloric stenosis than Afro-Caribbean or Asian infants.

Learning outcomes

1 Understand the common presenting features of congenital pyloric stenosis
2 Ensure metabolic correction prior to surgery
3 Discuss an appropriate anaesthetic technique for a neonate with pyloric stenosis.

CPD matrix matches

2D02; 2D04

Case history

Baby M was born at 39 weeks' gestation by spontaneous vaginal delivery following an uneventful pregnancy. There were no maternal risk factors for sepsis. He was the first born child, both parents being in good health with no significant past medical history. His birthweight was 3.2 kg, and the early neonatal period was uneventful.

On the 23rd day of life, baby M presented with a 1-day history of vomiting with feeds, mostly effortless, but occasionally forceful. He was still passing stool and urine, although his wet nappies had decreased in frequency. He had been feeding well (160 mL/kg/day) and was gaining weight. His current weight was 4.45 kg (50th centile). No close contacts had been unwell.

He was unsettled, but otherwise clinical examination was unremarkable.

What are the differential diagnoses?

+ Gastro-oesophageal reflux
+ Pyloric stenosis
+ Viral illness
+ Urinary tract infection (UTI).

What is your initial management plan?

+ Admit for observation of feeds
+ IV access and bloods: FBC, U&E, LFTs, CRP, capillary blood gas (CBG)
+ Urinalysis
+ If temperature >38°C: full septic screen.

Comment on the initial results

+ Hb 14.2 g/L, WCC 14.3, Neutr 3.86, Lymph 9.58, Plt 376
+ Na$^+$ 140, K$^+$ 5.2, urea 2.9
+ Bil 21, ALT 20, ALP 219, γGT 44, Alb 44
+ CRP <2
+ pH 7.39, pCO$_2$ 6.72 kPa, BE 6 mmol/L, HCO$_3^-$ 30.6
+ Urinalysis: negative.

These results are essentially within normal limits.

Case update

The following day, this child appeared more settled. Overnight, a small posset was noted post-feeds. He was otherwise well, and there were no concerns regarding sepsis. Given that he was thriving and the short duration of symptoms, he was discharged with no further follow-up.

However, 5 days post-discharge, baby M was readmitted with a 3-day history of worsening vomiting, up to 1 hour following feeds. It was milky, non-bilious, and occasionally forceful. He had become increasingly agitated, and his wet nappies had decreased in frequency. He was constipated, and his weight had fallen to 3.96 kg. He remained apyrexic and had mildly sunken fontanelle but was well perfused. Clinical examination revealed a palpable mass to the right of his umbilicus, following a test feed.

What is the likely diagnosis?

+ Congenital hypertrophic pyloric stenosis.

What is the initial management of this condition?

+ Obtain IV access and baseline bloods, including CBG
+ Nil by mouth (NBM); commence IV fluids
+ Pass an NG tube
+ USS to confirm the diagnosis.

Case update

The USS confirmed pyloric stenosis, and his initial CBG results were:

+ pH 7.46, pCO$_2$ 6.27 kPa, BE 8 mmol/L, HCO$_3^-$ 31 mmol/L, Cl$^-$ 94 mmol/L, K$^+$ 3.3 mmol/L, Na$^+$ 138 mmol/L.

Comment on this CBG

There is a hypochloraemic, hypokalaemic metabolic alkalosis.

What IV fluid regime would you prescribe?

+ Maintenance fluids with potassium chloride (150 mL/kg/day)
+ NG losses: 0.9% normal saline (mL for mL).

Outline the ongoing management for your patient

+ NBM
+ Regular NG aspiration and replacement with 0.9% saline
+ Continue maintenance fluids, guided by repeated CBGs
+ Surgical pyloromyotomy only when the infant is adequately rehydrated and metabolic abnormalities corrected. This may take 24–28 hours or more.

Case update

A repeat CBG was taken 5 hours later, showing: pH 7.47, pCO$_2$ 5.9 kPa, BE 7.4 mmol/L, HCO$_3^-$ 30.5 mmol/L, Cl$^-$ 96 mmol/L, K$^+$ 3.9 mmol/L, Na$^+$ 133 mmol/L.

How would you interpret this CBG? Would you change the management plan?

+ There is a persistent hypochloraemic metabolic alkalosis, with no improvement since commencing IV fluids
+ Increase maintenance fluids to 180 mL/kg/day, then repeat CBG.

Case update

A repeat CBG 3 hours later shows: pH 7.48, pCO_2 5.51 kPa, BE 6.6 mmol/L, HCO_3^- 29.9 mmol/L, Cl^- 94 mmol/L, K^+ 4 mmol/L, Na^+ 137 mmol/L. This demonstrates a persisting hypochloraemic metabolic alkalosis, some improvement in BE and HCO_3^-. However, full correction would not be expected in such a short time period, so the recommendation would be to continue at the current rate, and then to repeat CBG.

The CBG 12 hours later shows: pH 7.36, pCO_2 5.69 kPa, BE –1.6 mmol/L, HCO_3^- 22.9 mmol/L, Cl^- 105.6 mmol/L, K^+ 5.4 mmol/L, Na^+ 141 mmol/L.

What is your interpretation of these results?

◆ Normal CBG.

It is now appropriate to proceed with surgical pyloromyotomy.

Describe the anaesthetic management of surgical pyloromyotomy

◆ Generally these infants have an IV cannula *in situ* and IV fluids running

◆ Aspirate the NG tube in left, right, lateral, and head-down positions. IV and inhalational induction are both safe techniques, following an NG aspiration

◆ Options for induction:
  • RSI: thiopentone (5–7 mg/kg) and suxamethonium (2 mg/kg)
  • IV induction and a non-depolarizing muscle relaxant
  • Inhalational induction and a non-depolarizing muscle relaxant
  • Inhalational induction, followed by intubation under deep volatile anaesthesia

◆ Intubate with an appropriately sized ETT (either uncuffed or microcuffed). Have a smaller sized ETT available.

◆ Pressure-controlled IPPV is the normal practice

◆ Maintenance is with volatile in oxygen and air

◆ The surgeon may ask for the stomach to be distended with 40–60 mL of air, injected through the NG tube, to check for mucosal perforation. The air is aspirated prior to wound closure

◆ Reverse the non-depolarizing muscle relaxants with neostigmine (50 micrograms/kg) and glycopyrrolate (10 micrograms/kg)

◆ Aspirate the NG tube at the end of surgery, and extubate the infant awake.

How would you control post-operative pain?

* Regular paracetamol
* Local anaesthetic infiltrated to the incision or laparoscopic port sites by the surgeon
* Bilateral rectus sheath blocks can be used for periumbilical incisions.

What post-operative instructions would you give?

* NBM
* Reintroduce feeds as per surgeon's instructions (clear fluids initially, followed by milk, if tolerated)
* Continue maintenance fluids until feeding is re-established
* Overnight SpO_2 and apnoea monitoring.

Discussion

Infants generally present aged <12 weeks, commonly between the 3rd and 5th weeks of life. It usually affects full-term infants; only a small number of cases are premature infants. The infant presents with progressive non-bilious vomiting, following a feed, which may become projectile. Concurrent constipation is common. There may be mild jaundice, attributable to glucuronyl transferase deficiency which develops as a consequence of starvation.

Associated abnormalities are found in 6–20% of infants, including oesophageal atresia, congenital cardiac anomalies, Hirschsprung's disease, intestinal malformation, anorectal anomalies, minor renal anomalies, and inguinal hernias. There is loss of weight or failure to thrive, and the infant is ravenously hungry. On clinical examination, varying degrees of dehydration and apathy may be present.

What are the clinical signs of dehydration in infants?

The diagnosis is made on history and examination. The upper abdomen may be distended, with visible gastric peristaltic waves moving from left to right during feeding. An olive-sized mass may be palpated to the right of the umbilicus, more apparent after vomiting. USS shows hypertrophy of the pylorus wall (thickness >4 mm or length >16 mm).

Gastric outlet obstruction initially produces regurgitation and eventually vomiting. Vomiting causes loss of fluid, H^+, Cl^-, and a variable amount of Na^+ and K^+ Secondary hyperaldosteronism develops as a result of hypovolaemia. This causes the kidneys to avidly retain Na^+ (to correct for intravascular volume depletion) and excrete increased amounts of K^+ into the urine, thereby

Table 6.1 Definitions and grading of dehydration in children, and associated clinical signs

Severity	Mild	Moderate	Severe
Fluid loss (% body weight)	5	10	15
Anterior fontanelle	Normal	Sunken	Moderately depressed
Skin turgor	Normal	Decreased	Greatly decreased
Mucous membranes	Moist	Dry	Very dry
Eyes	Normal	Sunken	Markedly sunken
Pulse	Normal	Increased	Increased and feeble
Respiration	Normal	Tachypnoea	Rapid and deep
Urine output (mL/kg/hour)	<2	<1	<0.5

Data from Duggan C et al., 'The management of acute diarrhea in children: oral rehydration, maintenance, and nutritional therapy', *MMWR*, 1992, 41, RR-16, pp. 1–20.

retaining Na^+ and K^+ ions. Infants may be dehydrated, with a hypochloraemic, hypokalaemic, hyponatraemic metabolic alkalosis. Increasingly, medical care is sought quickly, and many infants only have a mild metabolic derangement or none at all.

Prior to theatre, infants should be adequately rehydrated, with a urine output of >1 mL/kg/hour. Laboratory and CBG results should be monitored and the following targets achieved before surgery:

◆ Serum Cl^- >100 mmol/L

◆ Serum Na^+ >135 mmol/L

◆ Serum HCO_3^- <26 mmol/L.

Summary

Pyloric stenosis is not a surgical emergency. Dehydration and metabolic abnormalities should be corrected prior to theatre. A 20 mL/kg bolus of 0.9% saline may be given for resuscitation, if necessary. Generally, infants receive maintenance fluids with added potassium chloride as 150% of their calculated maintenance requirements. An NG tube is passed, and losses are replaced, mL for mL, with 0.9% normal saline until volume and metabolic normality are achieved.

Further reading

Fell D and Chelliah S (2001). Infantile pyloric stenosis. *British Journal of Anaesthesia CEPD Reviews*, **1**, 85–8.

Habre W, Schwab C, Gollow I, and Johnson C (1999). An audit of postoperative analgesia after pyloromyotomy. *Pediatric Anesthesia*, **9**, 253–6.

Pappano D (2011). Alkalosis-induced respiratory depression from infantile hypertrophic pyloric stenosis. *Pediatric Emergency Care*, **27**, 124.

Wilkinson DJ, Chapman RA, Owen A, and Marven SS (2011). Hypertrophic pyloric stenosis: predicting the resolution of biochemical abnormalities. *Pediatric Surgery International*, **27**, 695–8.

Chapter 7

Neuroanaesthesia

Dr Keith Kelly
Dr Ivan Marples
Mr Peter Bodkin

Case 7.1

Principles of neuroanaesthesia

CPD matrix matches

2A03, 2F01

Principles of neuroanaesthesia

Many of the principles (though not all) regarding head injury transfer hold true for neuroanaesthesia. Techniques should optimize cerebral metabolism (cerebral metabolic rate of oxygen, $CMRO_2$) and the cerebral blood flow and should not cause rises in ICP. Generally accepted principles are:

- To prevent rises in ICP
- To maintain an adequate cerebral perfusion pressure (CPP)
- To use techniques with minimal interference with cerebral autoregulation
- To affect rapid and smooth awakening at the end of the procedure. Slow emergence from anaesthesia may be a sign of an expanding haematoma, and techniques should be used to minimize the confounding effects of anaesthesia.

The importance of an optimal patient positioning in neurosurgery cannot be overemphasized. Cases can be long and complex, with multiple pieces of equipment to negotiate. A good operating theatre set-up will have staff members, familiar with the positioning requirements for a variety of neurosurgical procedures, working together within specified roles.

What are the specific considerations in patient positioning in neuroanaesthesia?

- Provision of optimal venous drainage to prevent excessive intraoperative bleeding
- Avoidance of prolonged, excessive pressure on the skin and nerve bundles, for example
- Special thought will be required for patients with unstable spines, ankylosing spondylitis, scoliosis, spasticity, gross obesity, or indeed cachexia, in consideration of pressure areas, chest excursion, and operative exposure

♦ Use of gravity to optimize the opening of soft tissue planes, thus avoiding or minimizing the requirement for retraction, especially on the brain

♦ The recognition of scenarios that have a risk of air embolism and the provision of appropriate methods of reducing this risk or being able to treat it if it occurs

♦ The increasing use of ancillary equipment poses special problems and may create a crowded operating room:

- A frameless neuronavigation requires an unobstructed line of site between the infrared beam source and the reference star and pointer (newer electromagnetic equipment is beginning to be used that avoids this problem)

- The microscope placement is important for both the operating surgeon and assistant

- Allowing optimal X-ray penetrance from image intensifiers (i.e. ensuring the arms are pulled down so that the shoulders are not obstructing the view when operating on the lower cervical spine)

- Ultrasound guidance equipment is optimally used when a pool of saline may be maintained over the area of interest; therefore, the operative area should be kept horizontal

- Endoscopy generally requires a set-up where two surgeons can comfortably work opposite each other with a good view of a monitor

- The use of the Budde halo (ring for attaching retractors) will require some thought as to how the position will affect its placement and draping. Similar principles may be said of the Mayfield clamps (see Figure 7.1a)

- The introduction of intraoperative MRI in some units will also bring new problems with patient positioning

♦ Awake craniotomies require an extra level of attention to detail. Patients must be comfortable on the operating table, have appropriate screening, but maintain access to theatre personnel. Their neurological functions (speech, limb movement) also need to be assessable.

What is the anaesthetist's role in preventing a raised intracranial pressure when managing the airway?

The anaesthetist may help by using tape to secure ETTs, not ties which act like a 'neck tourniquet'. All should be done to optimize venous drainage from the head. Our practice is to use armoured ETTs to minimize kinking and flexing of the neck. Patients are generally positioned head up.

Positioning is critical in neurosurgery.

Proper positioning will provide an optimal venous drainage away from the surgical field. Appropriate positioning will also allow gravity to expose tissue plains and minimize the requirement for surgical retraction of the brain (thus reducing post-operative brain swelling).

There are a number of commonly adopted positions on the operating table (see Figures 7.1b–f):

- The supine position (e.g. used for anterior and middle cranial fossae and anterior cervical work) (see Figures 7.1b–c)
- The lateral position (e.g. used for posterior fossa, occipital regions, and lumbar peritoneal shunts)) (see Figure 7.1d)
- The prone position (an alternative for posterior fossa, craniocervical junction, posterior spine) (see Figure 7.1e).

The sitting position

This position had been popular as an approach to the posterior fossa and posterior approaches for high cervical work (see Figure 7.1f). The perceived advantages (access to the operative field, drainage of fluid away from the surgical field under gravity, decreased blood loss, and historically, if the patient had been allowed to breathe spontaneously, localization due to changes in the respiratory

(a)

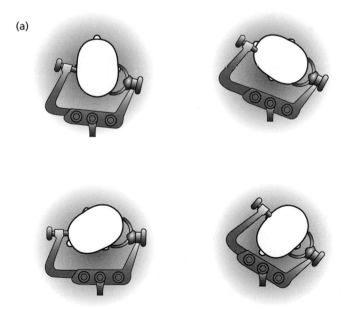

Fig. 7.1 (a) Various positions of Mayfield clamps.

(b)

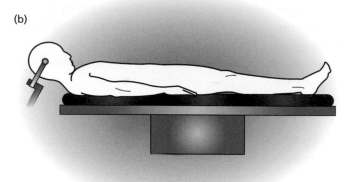

Fig. 7.1 (b) Variation on supine positioning; head in Mayfield pins on a non-slip mattress.

(c)

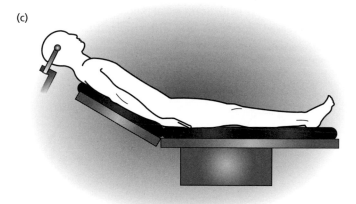

Fig. 7.1 (c) Further variation on the supine position.

pattern when operating on the brainstem) are now largely thought by many to be outweighed by the disadvantages.

These disadvantages include:

1 Hypotension (causing stroke, particularly quadriplegia). One of the reasons for the advantage of reduced blood loss was due to the reduced perfusion pressure of the site of surgery being higher than that of the heart. It may result in cardiovascular instability

(d)

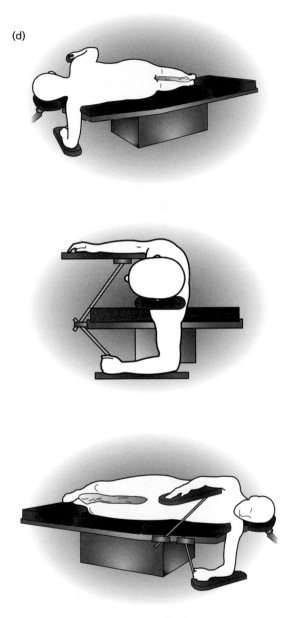

Fig. 7.1 (d) Variations on the lateral/park bench position.

(e)

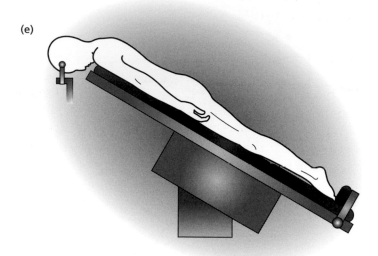

Fig. 7.1 (e) One version of prone positioning. In addition to being on a non-slip mattress, the patient should have footguard to prevent the body weight from 'hanging' from Mayfield pins. Ankles should be kept in a neutral position, e.g. rolled towel under the ankles (not shown).

(f)

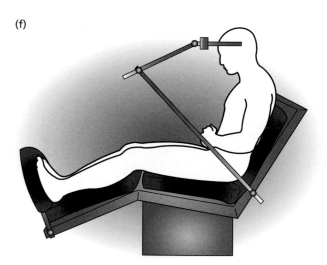

Fig. 7.1 (f) Version of the sitting position.

2 Air embolus, particularly if the patient were breathing spontaneously

3 Macroglossia caused by tongue swelling

4 Pressure sores.

Consequently, the use of the sitting position in neurosurgery has been on the wane in recent years in the UK and other countries. A survey of neurosurgical units in the British Isles in 1991 showed that only 8 (20%) of the UK centres still used this position for posterior fossa surgery, in comparison to 19 (53%) 10 years prior to that. There are still advocates for its retention as a 2002 editorial on the subject notes. However, as centres abandon its use, the number of staff familiar with its use will diminish.

Cases will tend to be longer than in other subspecialties, so due care must be taken over pressure areas to prevent neuropathies.

We acknowledge that a large caseload in neurosurgical units encompasses neck and other spinal surgery. However, given that we are restricted to a small number of cases in each chapter of this book, we have illustrated the teaching points by describing cases with intracranial pathology. This chapter concentrates on the intracranial aspects of neurosurgery.

Further reading

Greenberg MS (2010). *Handbook of neurosurgery*, 7th edn. Thieme, New York.

Leonard IE and Cunningham AJ (2002). The sitting position in neurosurgery-not yet obsolete! *British Journal of Anaesthesia*, **88**, 1–3.

Mishra LD, Rajkumar N, and Hancock SM (2006). Current controversies in neuroanaesthesia, head injury management and neurocritical care. *Continuing Education in Anaesthesia, Critical Care & Pain*, **6**, 83–5.

Rhoton AL (2008). *Cranial anatomy and surgical approaches*. Lippincott Williams and Wilkins, Philadelphia.

St-Arnaud D and Paquin M-J (2008). Safe positioning for neurosurgical patients. *AORN Journal*, **87**, 1156–68.

Acute subdural haematoma

Learning outcomes

1 Management of subdural haematoma, including appropriate timing of operation, and technique.

CPD matrix matches

2F01

Case history

A 70-year-old, 85 kg, and 1.83 m tall man presented to hospital with a 5-day history of frontal headache. Previous medical history included well-controlled AF, migraines, gastro-oesophageal reflux disease, and osteoarthritis. He did not recall any history of trauma. Neurosurgical services in the hospital were contacted.

His medication included: warfarin, digoxin 125 micrograms/day, diltiazem 300 mg/day, pantoprazole 20 mg/day, Seretide® and salbutmol inhalers.

On admission, examination findings were: BP 160/100, pulse ventricular rate 81, no heart murmurs, chest clear. GCS 15. No focal deficits.

Initial investigations were:

- Na$^+$ 136 mmol/L, K$^+$ 4.9 mmol/L, urea 6.4 mmol/L, Cr 63 micromoles/L, estimated glomerular filtration rate (eGFR) >60 mL/min
- Hb 143 g/L, WCC 13.9 × 10^9/L, Plt 142 × 10^9/L
- Clotting: APTT 29 s (ratio 1.0), INR 2.7, fibrinogen 3.9 g/L
- Brain CT scan: 11 mm left-sided subdural haematoma (see Figure 7.2).

What is the likely cause of the patient's subdural haematoma? What should be the initial management of this patient?

The generally accepted anatomical source of bleeding in subdural haemorrhage is from the bridging veins passing from the cortical surface to the large venous

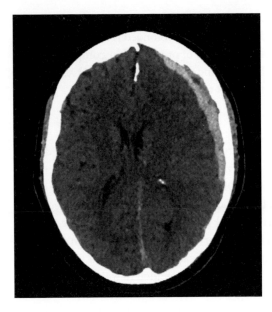

Fig. 7.2 Admission axial non-contrasted CT scan showing an acute left subdural haematoma, 11 mm in depth with a 4 mm midline shift.

sinuses, most particularly the superior sagittal sinus. These haemorrhages are rather more common in the elderly. This is because, as one gets older, the brain shrinks and the bridging veins have longer to travel and are therefore more liable to being torn by trauma. This can be quite trivial and not remembered by the patient. Often the patient is asymptomatic for some time, but, as blood products break down, the haematoma tends to enlarge and cause more mass effect. In this case, the patient's risk of an intracranial haemorrhage is increased by him being on warfarin therapy. This is quite a frequent scenario in neurosurgery and requires careful management from anaesthetics, neurosurgery, and the haematology service.

In general, an acute intracranial haemorrhage will always require normalization of the INR. The length of time off anticoagulants is a trade-off between the risks of a rebleed and thrombosis, which will have to be judged on an individual basis.

Consideration has to be given as to why a patient was on warfarin, and, if an additional specialty were to have started warfarin (such as cardiac surgery, cardiology, or neurology), then they should be included in this discussion. The patient may be taking warfarin for a recently diagnosed thrombotic event or because they have a metallic heart valve. Particularly in patients who have metallic heart valves, there is a fine balance to be struck between the safe reversal of their clotting and a thrombotic event.

In this patient's case, it was to reduce the chance of thrombotic events secondary to AF. The decision was made to reverse the prolonged INR with 5 mg of IV vitamin K and 2000 U of Beriplex® (a form of prothrombin complex concentrate (PCC), a combination of blood clotting factors II, VII, IX, and X, as well as protein C and S). This corrected the INR to 1.1.

Case update

The patient was admitted to the neurosurgical ward. It was considered most appropriate to keep him under observation and defer surgery. The evacuation of an acute subdural haematoma (ASDH) (when the appearance is white on CT scan) requires a craniotomy, as the blood is thick and firm. Over 1–2 weeks, the subdural blood will liquefy (turning black on CT) and may be evacuated via one or two small burr holes (14 mm in diameter). This is much less traumatic for the patient. Given that his only symptom was headache, he had no focal deficits, and he remained fully alert and oriented, it was decided to wait.

As the haematoma will go through various phases (from liquid to solid to liquid again), it was felt best to observe the patient until the haematoma had liquefied, then to evacuate, unless his condition deteriorated. He was noticed to be rather sleepy and slightly confused on the eighth day after admission, reducing his GCS from 15 to 14. A repeat CT scan was performed, showing a new midline shift of >1 cm (see Figure 7.3).

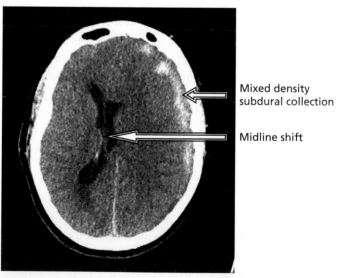

Mixed density subdural collection

Midline shift

Fig. 7.3 Axial non-contrasted CT scan showing a left mixed-density subdural haematoma, now with a 13 mm midline shift and effacement of the left lateral ventricle, prior to surgery.

Given the deterioration in GCS and the worsening appearance on CT scan, the decision was made to evacuate the haematoma now. The appearance of the subdural on CT was still dense (white) and so was not yet amenable to surgery via burr hole; therefore, he was prepared for a craniotomy.

How may a subdural haematoma be differentiated from an extradural haematoma?

Classically, a subdural haematoma occurs due to venous bleeding, and an extradural haematoma (referred to as an epidural haematoma in North American literature) from arterial bleeding (see Table 7.1 and compare Figures 7.2 and 7.4 which contrasts the patient's initial CT head scan with another CT scan of a patient demonstrating an extradural haematoma).

Discuss which anaesthetic techniques could broadly be used for this patient. What are the relative advantages and disadvantages?

Local anaesthesia is sometimes adopted for burr hole surgery if the patient is compliant. It is also sometimes used when resecting tumours in eloquent areas.

Table 7.1 A comparison of common features of subdural and extradural haematomas

	Subdural haematoma	**Extradural haematoma**
Source	Bridging veins	Middle meningeal artery, commonly from fracture of the overlying squamous temporal bone (can be caused by any meningeal artery), or from ooze from the bone at any fracture site
Shape	Crescentic	Lentiform
Relationship to skull suture lines	Will spread over the whole hemisphere	Classically does not cross sutures due to adherence of periostium
Acute/chronic	Can be either	Almost always acute
Urgency of treatment	If chronic and causing minimal symptoms, may be managed expectantly. If acute, especially in the young, and with mass effect, should be treated as per extradural haematoma	Generally, this is a lifesaving emergency of the highest urgency
Age of patient	Often older, although acute subdural haematoma in a young person indicates a very significant injury	Usually younger

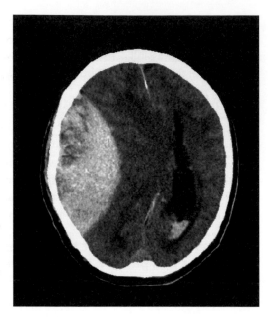

Fig. 7.4 Example of an extradural haematoma. Note the lentiform shape (convex), compared to the concave subdural haematomas. Also note the marked midline shift.

For trauma craniotomies, however, there is no rationale to favour awake surgery, as the urgency of the situation, as well as the need for surgical control, dictates the requirement for general anaesthesia.

We stress that this decision should be made before embarking on the procedure. We do not think it is good practice to start under local anaesthesia and to then convert to a general anaesthetic mid-procedure (potentially with the head open).

There are two broad categories of technique used for an asleep technique in neuroanaesthesia: TIVA and a volatile-based technique.

Total intravenous anaesthesia with propofol

Propofol theoretically has fewer deleterious effects on autoregulation, reduces $CMRO_2$, and thus optimizes the cerebral blood flow, and consequently the ICP. Propofol has an antiemetic profile, reducing the likelihood of PONV. In the presence of a critically elevated ICP, arguably it is the technique of choice.

However, due to its accumulation in adipose tissue, propofol may lead to prolonged wakening. As end-tidal propofol concentrations cannot be routinely measured, a depth of anaesthesia monitor is advisable. One may wish to continue a propofol infusion when receiving an intubated head injury transfer (particularly as they are most likely to have been established on a propofol infusion for the transfer).

Volatile technique

All volatile agents reduce cerebral autoregulation to a varying degree. Sevoflurane starts to affect autoregulation at 1.5 MAC; isoflurane starts to effect autoregulation at 1.0 MAC, and desflurane at only 0.5 MAC.

The counter argument is that, when the cranium is actually open, the ICP is at atmospheric pressure anyway, so does this matter as much? The co-administration of an agent, such as remifentanil, reduces this deleterious effect.

There are surprisingly few direct comparisons between sevoflurane and desflurane on longer-duration intracranial cases. One of the few studies, which directly compares sevoflurane against desflurane, found no difference in emergence time (12.2 ± 4.9 min with sevoflurane; 10.8 ± 7.2 min with desflurane), but a marginally quicker time to extubation (15.2 ± 3.0 min for sevoflurane; 11.3 ± 3.9 min for desflurane; p <0.001) and recovery (18.2 ± 2.3 for sevoflurance; 12.4 ± 7.7 for desflurance; p <0.001). Results shown are means with standard deviations.

The short orientation memory concentration test (SOMCT) score, as a test for the return of mental capacity, was marginally better with desflurane; however, the scores with sevoflurane were still within the normal range.

Worries about desflurane's effect on autoregulation may be more theoretical than real. A pragmatic use may be when there is a definite advantage such as an elevated BMI.

Case update (anaesthetic technique used)

A 20 g left radial arterial line and BIS depth of anaesthesia monitor were placed prior to induction. Anaesthesia was induced with propofol 150 mg and rocuronium 80 mg, and the hypertensive response to intubation obtunded with a remifentanil infusion, supplemented with a bolus of remifentanil 70 micrograms. The trachea was intubated with an 8.0 mm internal diameter armoured ETT. The maintenance of anaesthesia was with an oxygen/air/sevoflurane technique, with continuation of the remifentanil infusion (basic rate 0.1 micrograms/kg/min), and the target for the BIS monitor was 40–45. A urinary catheter was sited after induction. Intermittent metaraminol boluses were used to maintain an adequate CPP. The patient was ventilated to maintain $ETCO_2$ in the low normocapnia range.

Analgesia was with IV paracetamol and fentanyl 50 micrograms administered towards the end of the operation, to supplement the 20 mL 50/50 mix of 1% lidocaine with 1/200 000 adrenaline/0.5% bupivacaine infiltrated by the surgeon. Granisetron was administered as an antiemetic.

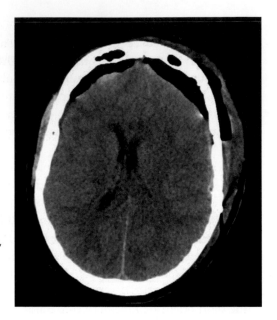

Fig. 7.5 Post-operative scan showing an almost complete removal of a subdural collection, some expected post-operative intracranial air (pneumocephalus), and resolution of the midline shift.

The patient woke up with a GCS of 14 (due to confusion). Post-operative analgesia was with regular paracetamol, supplemented with PCA morphine and dihydrocodeine, as required.

On the day after the procedure, his GCS fell from 13 (E3 V4 M6) to 11 (E4 V2 M5), and he appeared vacant. He then had two episodes of facial twitching, lasting for 2 and then 3 min. A CT scan of the head performed post-operatively is shown in Figure 7.5.

He was given a loading dose of 1 g phenytoin, followed by supplementary levetiracetam.

His seizure activity ceased. However, his INR, which had originally been corrected to within the normal range, was prolonged 3 days later to 1.8 and then 2.1.

What do you think may have caused this increase of the INR? How may you treat this?

A drug interaction between the newly commenced anticonvulsant and any residual warfarin still in the body (by displacement of protein binding) was considered. This would have been problematic, as the anticonvulsant was required to stop seizure activity.

However, on discussion with haematology colleagues, it was felt that the prolonged INR was due to a deficiency of vitamin K. Supplements of vitamin K were administered, and the INR returned to normal.

Case update

There were no further seizures. After a few more days on the ward, the patient was discharged home with an appropriate support package. GCS on discharge was 15, and activities of daily living had returned to normal. He was scheduled for follow-up in the outpatient clinic.

Summary

The evacuation of a subdural haematoma represents a significant caseload in emergency neurosurgery. There are differences between subdural and extradural haematomas. Of note, subdural haematomas may go through various stages of maturation, and the timing of any intervention may take this into account, as well as any correction of clotting abnormality. As patients may have other comorbidities, there may be discussions with other specialties, especially if the patient has been commenced on anticoagulants by these colleagues.

Further reading

Magni G, La Rosa I, Melillo G, Savio A, and Rosa G (2009). A comparison between sevoflurane and desflurane anesthesia in patients undergoing craniotomy for supratentorial intracranial surgery. *Anesthesia & Analgesia*, **109**, 567–71.

Endovascular treatment of subarachnoid haemorrhage due to ruptured berry aneurysm

Learning outcome

1 Current anaesthetic management of subarachnoid haemorrhage

2 Anaesthesia for interventional neuroradiology

3 Management of acute rupture of aneurysm.

CPD matrix match

2A06, 2A07, 2F03

Case history

A 46-year-old right-handed man presented to his local district general hospital with a history of sudden-onset headache whist exercising in the gym. A CT brain showed subarachnoid blood. His past medical history includes type II diabetes mellitus, treated with metformin, and a smoking habit of 50 cigarettes per day. Despite this, his usual exercise tolerance was more than a mile. He was referred to the regional neurosurgical unit for operative intervention with a GCS of 15. BP ranged from 127/72 to 147/75; pulse was 82 bpm and regular.

A subsequent diagnostic angiogram under local anaesthetic demonstrated that the likely source of the subarachnoid blood was from a ruptured berry aneurysm of the anterior communicating artery.

What is the aetiology and incidence of subarachnoid haemorrhage (SAH)?

The background incidence of spontaneous SAH in the UK is approximately 1 per 10 000 population per annum. Nearly twice as many females as males are affected, and there can be a familial association in some cases. The peak age for aneurysmal SAH is 45–55 years.

Rupture of berry aneurysms accounts for about 80% of cases, with arterio-venous malformations accounting for a further 5%. The remaining 10% is made up of other vascular malformations, non-aneurysmal perimesencephalic bleeds, and vasculitides.

What are the independent risk factors for an aneurysmal subarachnoid haemorrhage?

These include: hypertension, smoking, binge drinking, drugs (cocaine/amphetamines), substantial positive family history (two or more first-degree relatives affected), autosomal dominant polycystic kidney disease, and certain rare inherited collagen vascular disorders.

Independent predictors of poor outcome after an aneurysmal subarachnoid haemorrhage

- Reduced GCS on admission (reflected in the World Federation of Neurosurgeons grade)
- Increasing age
- High-volume blood load on CT scan.

Non-independent predictors

- Larger aneurysm size and posterior circulation aneurysms.

What is the usual current intervention for this disease?

Since the 2002 publication of the International Subarachnoid Aneurysm Trial (ISAT), endovascular coiling has become the mainstay of intervention, replacing clipping in the majority of cases where it is technically feasible. ISAT recruited 2143 patients (mean age 52 years) with a diagnosis of SAH secondary to rupture of a berry aneurysm, between 1994 and 2002, and randomized patients to either endovascular coiling or standard clipping. Measured outcomes were the risk of death or dependency at 1 year and were reported as coiling (24%) vs clipping (31%). This represented an absolute risk reduction of 7.4% and a relative risk reduction of 24%.

The follow-up, reported in 2009, recorded 24 rebleeds after 1 year:

- Thirteen from target aneurysm (10/13 in the coil arm), p 0.06.

The 5-year mortality was 11% for the coiled group and 14% for the clipped group (p 0.03). The proportion of independent survivors was the same. If the study were reviewed again, as the technology is improving constantly one could argue that follow-up results now would be even better if more advanced coils had been available in 2002.

In the light of ISAT, are there still indications for the clipping of aneurysms? If so, what are they?

There will still be a requirement for the clipping of aneurysms. The major indications for clipping include:

1 No endovascular services available in the region (and transfer to another centre not feasible)

2 The anatomy of the aneurysm precludes coiling (e.g. branch vessels arising off the aneurysm sac; the neck of the aneurysm is too wide, so a coil will not stay *in situ*; or impossible to position the coil)

3 A simultaneous urgent surgical procedure also required (such as the evacuation of haematoma).

What are the problems associated with a subarachnoid haemorrhage, and what may be done to lessen them?

Hydrocephalus

Ten to 30% of patients will have significantly impaired consciousness, due to an obstructive hydrocephalus. This may require CSF drainage.

Haematoma

After a bleed from an aneurysm, a haematoma may form around the bleeding point. There may be subsequent swelling, causing significant ICP rises. This may necessitate surgical evacuation. There is a theoretical risk of aneurysmal rupture on opening the dura and evacuating the clot. This could reduce the ICP and therefore remove the tamponade effect of the haematoma, thus encouraging a rebleed. Two broad approaches may be considered:

1 The surgeon evacuating the haematoma must be prepared to clip the aneurysm if further bleeding occurs

2 If it can be arranged in time, the aneurysm is protected by coiling, prior to the haematoma evacuation. Obviously, the ICP pressure problems may preclude the time taken to do this.

Vasospasm

Vasospasm (also referred to as delayed ischaemic neurological deficit, DIND) can be clinical or radiological. Clinical vasospasm is the development of neurological deficits, deterioration in the conscious level, or worsening headache. Radiologically, one may see narrowed arteries on angiography. The two entities do not necessarily coincide, and spasm may be acting at a microcirculation level.

Breakdown products from the haemorrhage may cause vasospasm. Classi-cally, the highest incidence for this was between the 4th and 12th day after the bleed, though there was a large degree of interpatient variation. The traditional management was the 'triple H' therapy (hydration, haemodilution, hyperten-sion). The rationale was that an adequate fluid load and driving pressure were required to drive blood through the vasospastic vessels. A haematocrit at 0.3 was said to be the optimum compromise between decreased viscosity and good oxygen-carrying capacity.

However, there are caveats with this. Patients may have neurogenic pulmo-nary oedema or cardiac impairment, precluding an aggressive fluid manage-ment. The aneurysm may not be fully protected, or there may be other aneurysms which do not justify treatment but should not be subjected to hypertension.

In practice, many units strive towards the aims of the triple H therapy, but without slavishly adhering to the original protocols, principally by adequate hydration. Good hydration may maintain an adequate perfusion pressure and dilute the haematocrit, but without using an inotrope or respectively requiring venesection. If a patient with delayed cerebral ischaemia secondary to vasos-pasm fails to respond to the triple H treatment, then balloon angioplasty under general anaesthesia may be considered. Although anecdotal reports indicate a 15–20% absolute benefit from this technique, robust data on its efficacy are lacking (no RCTs), and there is a 2–5% morbidity/mortality rate associated with the procedure.

What are the anaesthetic issues regarding anaesthetizing for endovascular coiling of a subarachnoid haemorrhage?

The procedure itself is not particularly painful or stimulating to the patient. The major indication for general anaesthesia is to guarantee that the patient will not move during the procedure and to enable control of the HR and BP, as required.

The procedure takes place in an IR suite. An example of such a suite is shown in Figure 7.6. There is restricted access to the patient. There are critical points in the procedure where movement would be not just embarrassing to the profes-sional pride of the anaesthetists, but also life-threatening to the patient. These times are:

1 When the microcatheter is being inserted into the aneurysm under digital fluoroscopic control ('roadmap')

2 When coils are being deployed in the aneurysm.

The roadmap involves taking an X-ray at one particular point, subtracting all extraneous details from it, and superimposing the real-time image of the guide

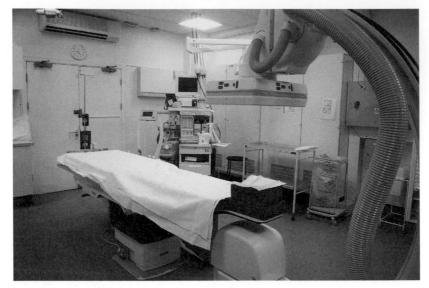

Fig. 7.6 Photograph of a typical interventional radiology suite.

catheter upon this. It is done to reduce the dose of radiation administered to the patient. However, if the patient moves after the roadmap image has been taken, the catheter will not actually be where it appears on screen and may be advanced inadvertently through the wall of the vessel or aneurysm. That the patient should not move whist the coil is being deployed is intuitively obvious.

The anaesthetist must not move the table, so care should be taken to avoid resting on it. A free-standing drip pole should be used near, though not directly attached to, the table so that fluid bags or infusions can be changed with minimal disturbance. Similarly, a means of administering bolus drugs without touching the table should be made ('remote injector').

Either TIVA, based on propofol and remifentanil, or a gaseous technique, using oxygen/air/sevoflurane, are common. The use of infusions of muscle relaxants is controversial; the author's preference is to use them.

A depth of anaesthetic monitor has proved useful, especially the recent development of the dual hemisphere BIS. In addition to allowing the measurement of the depth of anaesthesia, this development may allow the activity between the hemispheres to be compared.

Case update

After siting a 20 g left radial arterial line under local anaesthetic and after the administration of 2 mg IV midazolam, the patient was anaesthetized with propofol, remifentanil (bolus and infusion), and atracurium (bolus and infusion). In addition to standard monitoring, a bihemisphere BIS monitor was sited, and a urine catheter was placed after induction. BP was stable at 110/60; pulse was 55, and BIS at 40–45.

About 1 hour into the procedure, at the siting of the second coil, the BP rose suddenly to 200/120, pulse to 80, and BIS fell to 6. The anaesthetic chart is shown in Figure 7.7.

What do you think has happened, and how should this patient be managed?

The most likely event is an acute rupture of the aneurysm. Several actions must be taken quickly. There is usually a hypertensive response to the rupture as in this case. This must be obtunded. Optimize oxygenation. Reverse any administered heparin (in our unit, with protamine). This event, particularly if surgery is required, is the only time protamine use would currently be considered in our unit. The interventional neuroradiologist may wish to rapidly continue packing the aneurysm with as many coils as practicable to occlude the re-ruptured aneurysm. Our usual practice is to obtain an urgent CT head scan to confirm the diagnosis and to assess the extent of the bleed and damage and also if there are any treatable complications such as an obstructive hydrocephalus which may require drainage.

If an external ventricular drain (EVD) is indicated, then the next step is to take the patient to theatre urgently.

Which problems may present around the time of the procedure? How should these problems be managed?

+ Rupture of the aneurysm on the table: as discussed previously
+ Delayed return of consciousness: exclude a pharmacological reason
+ Consider a thromboembolic event: consider Reopro® or other potent anti-platelet agents
+ Consider vasospasm: consider glyceryl trinitrate (GTN) or nimodipine intra-arterially (not a licensed use) ± angioplasty
+ A further management point: at the preoperative assessment stage, it is worthwhile stressing to the patient that their headache will not instantaneously disappear on wakening from their general anaesthetic.

Case update

The patient had an urgent CT scan of head whist under the same general anaesthetic. To facilitate transfer to the CT scanner, then to theatre, and ultimately to

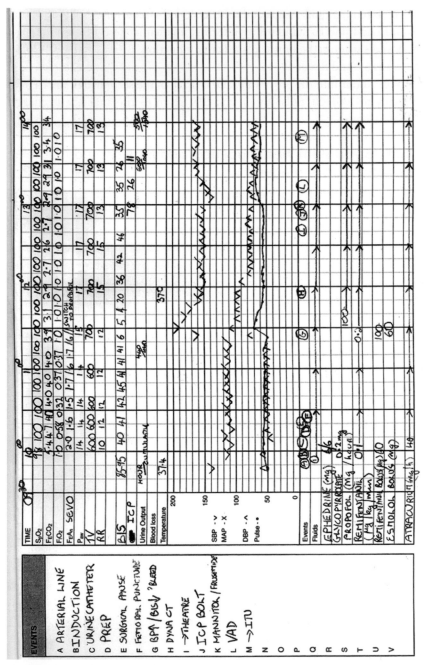

Fig. 7.7 The anaesthetic record of the interventional neuroradiology case that is described in the text.

ICU, a propofol infusion was substituted for sevoflurane, although the remifentanil and atracurium infusions were continued. The patient was taken to theatre, and an intracranial bolt for pressure monitoring reasons was inserted. The initial ICP was 75 mmHg. A ventricular access device was inserted, and the ICP fell to 6 mmHg almost immediately. The patient was then taken to intensive care for sedation and ventilation.

Sedation was lightened 24 hours later, and he was subsequently extubated, although reintubated 72 hours later for a further 5 days. Four days after the final extubation, he was discharged from the ICU to the neuro HDU, with a GCS of 13 (E4 V3 M6).

After a further 2 weeks on the regional neurosurgical ward, he was discharged to the referring district general hospital for continuing rehabilitation. GCS on discharge was 14, due to confusion. He was scheduled for follow-up in the neurovascular clinic at 6 months.

Summary

The management of subarachnoid treatment has been revolutionized in recent years since the widespread introduction of endovascular treatment. This has taken the management out of the operating theatre and into the radiology suite. Although the procedure is less invasive, the anaesthetic technique should be no less vigilant, as the patient must not move. The anaesthetic technique should allow the administration of drugs and fluids without causing movement of the X-ray table or patient. This may involve mounting infusion pumps and fluids on a free-standing pole and having a remote injection set for bolus drugs.

Although the large majority of subarachnoid haemorrhages (SAHs) are now managed by an endovascular technique, there will still be a requirement for clipping of aneurysms.

Further reading

Dorairaj IL and Hancock SM (2008). Anaesthesia for interventional neuroradiology. *Continuing Education in Anaesthesia, Critical Care & Pain*, **8**, 86–9.

Molyneux A, Kerr RSC, Birks J, *et al.* (2009). Risk of recurrent subarachnoid haemorrhage, death or dependence and standardised mortality ratios after clipping or coiling of an intracranial aneurysm in the International Subarachnoid Aneurysm Trial (ISAT): long-term follow-up. *Lancet Neurology*, **8**, 427–33.

Molyneux A, Kerr R, Stratton I, *et al.* (2002). International Subarachnoid Aneurysm Trial (ISAT) of neurosurgical clipping versus endovascular coiling in 2143 patients with ruptured intracranial aneurysms: a randomised trial. *Lancet*, **360**, 1267–74.

Clipping of aneurysm

Learning outcomes

1 General management of a major craniotomy

2 Anaesthesia for clipping of aneurysm

3 The concept of neuroprotection.

CPD matrix matches

2A03, 2F01

Case history

As mentioned in Case 7.3, there will still continue to be a need for clipping of aneurysms. A 44-year-old female right-handed lecturer was admitted following a spontaneous grade I SAH. She had been standing in her classroom and developed sudden onset of severe headache and collapsed to the ground. After a brief loss of consciousness, she awoke surrounded by colleagues. She did not have any focal weakness but noticed her speech slurred.

Imaging confirmed a diffuse SAH. Urgent cerebral angiography showed two aneurysms. A middle cerebral artery (MCA) aneurysm was successfully coiled the day after admission, but a complex aneurysm of the anterior communicating artery (ACOM) was found to be uncoilable. It was thought that the MCA aneurysm was an incidental finding, and the ACOM aneurysm had bled. Following coiling, she was transferred to the neurosurgical HDU, pending surgical clipping of the ACOM aneurysm. The patient was taken to theatre for this procedure the next day.

The patient arrived in the anaesthetic room (GCS 15), with a left radial arterial line, a large-bore cannula in the left cephalic vein, and a urinary catheter *in situ*. She was induced with remifentanil TCI 4 ng/mL (weight 68 kg, height 1.67 m, BP before induction 124/78, pulse 68), propofol 150 mg, and vecuronium 10 mg. Anaesthesia was maintained with remifentanil TCI and desflurane in an oxygen/air mix, FiO$_2$ 0.4. She was ventilated to maintain an ETCO$_2$ of 4%. She was positioned semi-recumbent, a gel pad behind the left shoulder and the head tilted to the right and held in Mayfield tongs. Surgery proceeded via a pterional craniotomy.

Prior to the definitive clipping of the ACOM aneurysm, the surgeon applied a temporary clip to the feeding artery to improve access to the neck of the aneurysm. In order to protect the brain from a period of anoxia, due to an interrupted blood flow, thiopentone 375 mg was delivered IV. The temporary clip was applied for 3 min; a permanent 10 mm clip was applied to the neck of the ACOM aneurysm, and the temporary clip removed. The time taken for surgery was 2 hours and 15 min. Five 0.5 mg increments of metaraminol were delivered IV during surgery to maintain a CPP of 60 mmHg. The patient received ondansetron 4 mg and cyclizine 50 mg plus morphine 6 mg prior to emergence.

After dressings were applied to the wound, and the Mayfield tongs removed, the patient was allowed to waken. She was extubated on return of airway reflexes and adequate respiratory effort. Over a period of 1 hour in the recovery suite, the highest recorded GCS was 9. She maintained adequate respiratory parameters and blood oxygenation throughout, and blood gases revealed PaO_2 20.5 kPa (oxygen 4L/min via Hudson mask), $PaCO_2$ 5.5 kPa, H^+ 45 nmol/L, HCO_3^- 23 mmol/L, and BE −0.9 mmol/L. Post-operative CT brain showed a small pneumocranium, consistent with surgery, no increase in subarachnoid blood load, and no subdural collection of blood or fluid.

Due to a persisting low GCS, the patient was intubated prior to transfer to intensive care, with an ICP monitor sited and a plan to treat a raised ICP, if and when it occurred, and to sedate overnight and re-evaluate the next day. The ICP fluctuated but did not rise sufficiently to require treatment. She was extubated the morning after admission to the ICU. Thereafter, she was E3–4 M6 V1–4 (i.e. GCS quite variable although always obeying commands). She developed a high-volume, low-osmolarity urine flow, which was treated with desmopressin for 24 hours.

It became apparent that she had a left 6th nerve palsy, with an accompanying left-sided proptosis, as well as a conjunctival infection. Despite, on paper, GCS being 15, she did have marked neuropsychological issues which required inpatient rehabilitation. The rehabilitation issues were as follows:

1 Mood and cognition: she had cognitive impairments across a broad spectrum of domains, with frontal lobe functions, in particular, being affected, with mild executive impairments, impaired judgement and insight, and also with reduced spatial awareness. Forgetfulness and impairments of short-term memory were also problematic. In addition, she was quite tearful

2 Communication: she scored well on formal tests, including the Galveston Orientation and Amnesia Test (GOAT) 100/100 and Frenchay Aphasia Screening Test (FAST) 27/30. She was easily distracted. She was able to touch-type, but not as efficiently as previously

3 Cranial nerves: lateral rectus palsy is gradually improving and is expected to recover fully

4 Upper and lower limb function: peripheral neural examination was broadly normal, although she did have reduced sensation, with sensory inattention on the left. This is gradually improving

5 Long-term prognosis: she is continuing to improve; now that her aneurysms have been successfully treated, hopefully there should be no recurrence.

What are the principles behind the use of temporary clips? How may the anaesthetist facilitate this technique?

When access to the aneurysm may be difficult, the surgeon may wish to apply a temporary clip. This stops the blood flow in a small portion of the cerebral circulation. Obviously, this may cause ischaemia. If the $CMRO_2$ can be reduced, then the period of ischaemia can be prolonged.

Which other methods of neuroprotection have been tried?

Many methods have been tried. None has been an undisputed success.

Hypothermia has been intermittently in and out of fashion. The Intraoperative Hypothermia for Aneurysm Surgery Trial (IHAST) of 1001 patients found mild hypothermia (33°C vs 36.5°C) did not improve the neurological outcome after clipping, as judged by comparing GCS at 90 days post-operatively. This study also noted the following:

◆ Post-operative bacteraemia was commoner in the hypothermic group (5% vs 3%)

◆ 25% of the hypothermic group were still intubated 2 hours post-operatively. That said, so were 13% of the normothermic group.

Summary

As mentioned in Case 7.3, although the majority of SAHs caused by berry aneurysms can now be treated with an endovascular procedure, there will still be a need to treat some aneurysms with the older clipping technique for the foreseeable future. This may require the placement of a temporary clip to allow better access to the aneurysm. This will be applied for as short a time as possible, but this period can be prolonged if the $CMRO_2$ is reduced, necessitating neuroprotection. Methods of affecting this are controversial.

The rehabilitation of a patient after an SAH is an important component of management.

Further reading

Todd MM, Hindman BJ, Clarke WR, and Torner JC; Intraoperative Hypothermia for Aneurysm Surgery Trial (IHAST) Investigators (2005). Mild intraoperative hypothermia during surgery for intracranial aneurysm. *New England Journal of Medicine*, **352**, 135–45.

Posterior fossa craniectomy

Learning outcomes

1 Anaesthetic management of major craniectomy/craniotomy

2 Problems particularly associated with posterior fossa procedures

3 Analgesia after a craniotomy.

CPD matrix matches

2E01, 2F01

Case history

A 39-year-old man (83 kg, 1.84 m tall) presented with a 3-week history of headache and ataxia. An MRI demonstrated a cystic lesion in the right cerebellar hemisphere. There was a working diagnosis of a cerebellar haemangioblastoma.

What are the major features of an intracranial haemangioblastoma? How should this patient be worked up for theatre?

Cerebellar haemangioblastomas may be sporadic or present as part of a syndrome such as von Hippel–Lindau disease (vHLD) (in 20%). They are benign and may be solid or cystic, and the intracranial lesion is almost always in the posterior fossa. There is an association with polycythaemia.

vHLD may be associated with retinal angiomas, haemangioblastomas of the spinal cord or brain, renal cell carcinoma, and, in 10% of cases, phaeochromocytoma. Thus, screening for phaeochromocytoma may be undertaken. vHLD is an autosomal dominant inherited condition, with a 90% penetrance and an incidence of 1 in 36 000 live births. In appropriate cases, genetic counselling will be offered. Typical presenting complaints are similar to those in the patient (headache, nausea and vomiting, cerebellar signs).

Case update

The patient had an unremarkable previous medical and family history. Screening for phaeochromocytoma was negative.

- Preoperative medication included: paracetamol, omeprazole, dexamethasone (recently commenced to reduce swelling around the lesion)
- BP 110/74–135/70; pulse 75 regular.

Preoperative investigations included:

- Initial investigations: Na$^+$ 141 mmol/L, K$^+$ 4.3 mmol/L, urea 5.5 mmol/L, Cr 61 micromoles/L, eGFR >60 mL/min
- Hb 145 g/L, WCC 10.4 × 10^9/L, Plt 270 × 10^9/L
- Clotting: APTT ratio 1.0, INR 1.0, fibrinogen 2.7 g/L
- ECG: sinus rhythm.

What are the problems especially associated with posterior fossa procedures?

- Positioning which may include the prone position
- Vital structures in the posterior fossa
- Generally perceived as more painful than other approaches, as greater dissection through more muscle (trapezius) and more bone
- A high incidence of PONV.

How may a patient be kept comfortable after a craniotomy? What are the salient points for this?

Analgesic regimens between neurosurgical units are highly variable. This allows requirements to be tailored to those of the unit, but is not necessarily evidence-based. Patients must be kept comfortable, but without causing an altered consciousness or a respiratory depression (and hence a raised PaCO$_2$ and all that means for ICP). Also the analgesic must not affect clotting, specifically the platelet function, and must not reduce the seizure threshold.

The means we use in our own unit are as follows:

- Regular paracetamol, starting with an IV administration perioperatively. That said, we review the requirement for regular paracetamol on a daily basis, changing to 'as required' use or discontinuing the paracetamol completely when a regular use is no longer deemed necessary
- Should the patient be sufficiently conscious to use a PCA, we give it, usually with morphine. As an intermediate between paracetamol and morphine, we usually prescribe dihydrocodeine, usually on an 'as required' basis
- We avoid tramadol, because it lowers the seizure threshold
- The use of NSAIDs after a craniotomy is highly contentious. Opinions range from the perioperative administration of drugs, such as parecoxib, after a

dural closure, through the administration of NSAIDs after a period of between 6 and 24 hours, to an absolute abstention in a patient who has undergone an intracranial procedure. Our unit very rarely administers NSAIDs after a craniotomy, always after discussion with our neurosurgeons, and never within the first 24 hours. On the rare occasion when NSAIDS are used, it is when pain control has been problematic with other means

- We have been recently impressed by the use of clonidine IV (variable; slow IV bolus dose; when used, 30 micrograms is commonly the dose) as an adjunct to analgesia in patients who have difficulty in managing pain. Although mildly sedating, we find the patients easy to rouse and no appreciable effect on respiration. As the patients are usually catheterized, we find no problems with urinary retention

- A mixture of lidocaine and bupivacaine containing 1/400 000 adrenaline is usually administered by neurosurgical colleagues at the start of the procedure. We do not administer a local anaesthetic at the end of the procedure, as the dura has been opened, and there is a danger that the local anaesthetic may track beneath the dura. The bupivacaine may exert an effect for some hours after the procedure.

Some units use scalp blocks for craniotomies.

The old-fashioned prejudice was that the only safe opiate to give after intracranial surgery was codeine. This has been challenged. Now some colleagues prescribe morphine. Discuss this point.

Codeine is a prodrug, which is demethylated (to morphine) in the liver to its most active form. Some patients lack the enzyme to do this, and the intrinsic analgesic property of unaltered codeine is poor.

In doses used clinically, morphine was no more likely to cause side effects of respiratory depression and sedation than codeine. Morphine did, however, provide more predictable and persistent analgesia, as reported by Goldsack and colleagues.

Codeine is still used in many units, despite 50% of anaesthetists thinking it is poor analgesic, as described by Stoneham and Walters. Codeine should not be administered IV.

Case update

After 1 mg of IV midazolam, an arterial line was sited, followed by induction with propofol, remifentanil, and atracurium. Maintenance of anaesthesia was with a combination of oxygen/air/sevofluanne and an infusion of remifentanil and atracurium. A right internal jugular central line was sited, prior to preparation and prone positioning. Surgery, conducted under Brainlab® (neuronavigation) guidance, was uneventful, as was the post-operative course.

The patient was comfortable with the post-operative analgesia regimen of morphine PCA and regular paracetamol.

The patient went home 5 days post-operatively (GCS 15) and was doing well at the post-operative outpatient follow-up.

Summary

Posterior fossa procedures are especially challenging for a number of reasons, including positioning on the operating table and the close proximity of vital intracranial structures. They also tend to be more painful and to have a relatively high incidence of PONV. Analgesia regimens vary between units, and some of the agents used are highly controversial.

Some conditions associated with posterior fossa lesions (e.g. von Hippel–Lindau syndrome) may require screening for further associated medical conditions such as phaeochromocytoma or cysts.

Further reading

Greenberg MS (2006). Cerebellar haemangioblastoma. In: *Handbook of neurosurgery*, 6th edn, pp. 459–61. Thieme, New York.

NSAIDS and neurosurgery

Jones SJ, Cormack J, Murphy MA, and Scott DA (2009). Parecoxib for analgesia after craniotomy. *British Journal of Anaesthesia*, **102**, 76–9.

Kelly KP, Janssens MC, Ross J, and Horn EH (2011). Controversy of non-steroidal anti-inflammatory drugs and intracranial surgery: et ne nos inducas in tentationem? *British Journal of Anaesthesia*, **107**, 302–5.

Sebastian J and Hunt K (2006). United Kingdom and Ireland survey of the use of non-steroidal anti-inflammatory drugs after intracranial surgery. *Journal of Neurosurgical Anesthesiology*, **18**, 267.

Shafer AI (1995). Effects of nonsteroidal antiinflammatory drugs on platelet function and systemic hemostasis. *Journal of Clinical Pharmacology*, **35**, 209–19.

Umamaheswara Rao GS and Gelb AW (2009). To use or not to use: the dilemma of NSAIDs and craniotomy. *European Journal of Anaesthesiology*, **26**, 625–6.

Haematoma after intracranial surgery

Palmer JD, Sparrow OC, and Iannotti F (1994). Postoperative hematoma: a 5-year survey and identification of avoidable risk factors. *Neurosurgery*, **35**, 1061–4; discussion 64–5.

Taylor WAS, Thomas NW, Wellings JA, and Bell BA (1995). Timing of postoperative intracranial hematoma development and implications for the best use of neurosurgical intensive care. *Journal of Neurosurgery*, **82**, 48–50.

Attitudes to pain control after neurosurgery

De Benedittis G, Lorenzetti A, Migliore M, Spagnoli D, Tiberio F, and Villani R (1996). Postoperative pain in neurosurgery: a pilot study in brain surgery. *Neurosurgery*, **38**, 466–70.

Goldsack C, Scuplak SM, and Smith M (1996). A double-blind comparison of codeine and morphine for postoperative analgesia following intracranial surgery. *Anaesthesia*, **51**, 1029–32.

Hockey B, Leslie K, and Williams D (2009). Dexamethasone for intracranial neurosurgery and anaesthesia. *Journal of Clinical Neuroscience*, **16**, 1389–93.

Kahn LH, Alderfer RJ, and Graham DJ (1997). Seizures reported with tramadol. *Journal of the American Medical Association*, **278**, 1661.

Kotak D, Cheserem B, and Solth A (2009). A survey of post-craniotomy analgesia in British neurosurgical centres: time for perceptions and prescribing to change? *British Journal of Neurosurgery*, **23**, 538–42.

Oscier C and Milner Q (2009). Peri-operative use of paracetamol. *Anaesthesia*, **64**, 65–72.

Stoneham MD and Walters FJM (1995). Post-operative analgesia for craniotomy patients: current attitudes among neuroanaesthetists. *European Journal of Anaesthesiology*, **12**, 571–5.

Tramer MR (2000). Systematic reviews in PONV therapy. In: Tramer MR, ed. *Evidence-based resource in anaesthesia and analgesia*, pp. 157–78. BMJ Books, London.

Awake craniotomy

Learning outcomes

1 Indications for awake craniotomy

2 Techniques for awake craniotomy.

CPD matrix matches

2A03, 2A07

Case history

A 55-year-old, right-handed male architect had presented with a 5-week history of dizziness, disorientation, visuospatial changes ('walking into objects, unaware that they were there'), and right arm weakness. He was otherwise well and had no other medical history, except for an uneventful appendicectomy in his teens. He was a lifelong non-smoker who seldom drank alcohol.

An MRI scan of his head showed a left-sided enhancing parieto-occipital mass, approximately 40 x 70 mm in dimension. He took no medication prior to diagnosis and had been commenced on a course of dexamethasone (with omeprazole) 2 weeks prior to admission, which led to some resolution of his symptoms.

Due to the position of the tumour, it was intended to perform this procedure as an 'awake' technique, with which the patient was in full agreement.

What are the major indications for an awake craniotomy?

1 A tumour in an eloquent part of the brain, described previously (i.e. in order to damage as little of the normal brain tissue as possible)

2 Movement disorders (including benign intention tremor, Parkinson's disease, and secondary to multiple sclerosis)

3 Epilepsy with a particularly circumscribed focus of electrical activity.

Less established indications are obesity and obsessive–compulsive disorder.

Case update

◆ On examination:
  • BP 122/73, pulse 82, weight 99 kg, height 1.92 m
  • GCS 15. No obvious focal deficits after 2 weeks on steroids
◆ Blood results:
  • Na$^+$ 135 mmol/L, K$^+$ 4.7 mmol/L, urea 5.8 mmol/L, Cr 63 micromoles/L, eGFR >60 mL/min
  • Hb 159 g/L, WCC 18.3 × 10^9/L (on dexamethasone), Plt 232 × 10^9/L
  • Clotting screen: normal
◆ ECG: sinus rhythm.

What are the goals of the anaesthetic technique used for an awake craniotomy? Which anaesthetic techniques may be used for an awake craniotomy?

There are a number of tenets for an awake craniotomy. First and foremost, it must be a technique acceptable to the patient. The patient must be comfortable and crucially not move during the critical parts of the procedure. They must waken up quickly.

The broad categories may be classified as follows:

◆ **Local anaesthetic for the entire procedure**: some advocate scalp blocks. However, scalp blocks to both sides of the head, incorporating all the nerves which have to be blocked, may approach the maximum recommended dose for that local anaesthetic.

The patient must be exceptionally compliant. Obviously, this lengthens the time for which the patient is awake, and many patients will find this intolerable. Hence, the so-called:

◆ **Asleep/awake/(asleep) technique**: in this technique, the patient has a general anaesthetic for the initial part of the procedure, during which potentially uncomfortable parts of the procedure are performed (siting the stereotactic frame, skin incision, and the initial part of the craniotomy). The patient is then woken up, and the rest of the operation is performed (the awake phase).

The patient may then be put back off to sleep. However, this is often not necessary and may require instrumentation of the patient's airway from the front, with the head held rigidly in Mayfield pins. As such, many anaesthetists do not re-sedate the patient after they have been woken up.

Whichever technique is used, the patients must be carefully selected and informed of the likely format of the case. Performing the entire procedure under local anaesthetic may be unacceptable to a significant number of patients (and surgeons)!

The technique used most recently in our centre is an asleep/awake technique. For the preparatory parts of the procedure perceived as being the most uncomfortable, the patient is asleep. That said, the administration of a longer-acting local anaesthetic is used (bupivacaine), particularly to the Mayfield pins.

Several recent developments have revolutionized this procedure. These include:

- The LMA, which may be the reinforced model. The LMA (as opposed to formal intubation) has greatly facilitated a smooth awakening. The administration of the non-sedative antisialogogue glycopyrrolate about 1.5 hours prior to the anticipated removal of the LMA may reduce coughing caused by secretions

- Propofol infusion, guided by a depth of anaesthesia monitor (such as BIS), allows an appropriate depth of anaesthesia with minimal agent. That said, many colleagues prefer to use a volatile-based technique with an agent such as sevoflurane

- Remifentanil IV infusion allows the suppression of spontaneous ventilation (and hence the ability to ventilate through the LMA. This stops an inappropriately high $PaCO_2$). It also allows rapid offset and has minimal sedative properties

- The depth of anaesthesia monitoring (such as BIS) allows the minimal required amount of sedative to be given which facilitates a rapid awakening.

Dexmedetomidine by infusion has been used as a sedative with analgesic properties in several countries. It has the advantage of a rapid recovery. However, it was not widely available in the UK at the time the case discussed here took place and was initially being introduced with the licensed indication intended for ICU administration. Subsequently, other centres have used it in theatre to good effect.

The less selective α2-agonist clonidine has been used by some anaesthetists, based on experience gained on ICU (to ease the withdrawal from alcohol dependency). However, the use of clonidine infusions in theatre and in ICU is currently unlicensed in the UK.

Case update

Technique

A 20G left radial arterial line was placed after induction with propofol TCI, with a remifentanil infusion at 0.1 micrograms/kg/min to suppress attempts to breath, and supplemented with an 80 microgram bolus to facilitate LMA placement. An armoured size 4 disposable laryngeal mask was used to maintain the airway. Once asleep, glycopyrrolate 0.3 mg was administered as an antisialogogue in anticipation of the removal of the LMA. The patient was kept asleep with a TIVA technique, based on the propofol/remifentanil regimen and ventilated through the LMA with oxygen and air. Clonidine (30 micrograms/hour) was commenced after induction and ran until about 20 min prior to the anticipated awakening.

The depth of anaesthesia was monitored, using bihemisphere BIS. A transcutaneous carbon dioxide monitor was sited on the right earlobe as a means of continuously monitoring the arterial carbon dioxide, prior to removal of the LMA. This was checked against intermittent ABGs and found to give close concurrence. As $ETCO_2$ monitoring is lost when the LMA is removed and ABG is intermittent, the transcutaneous carbon dioxide monitor maintained continuous information on the carbon dioxide levels. A urinary catheter was placed asleep.

Mayfield pins were placed and the head positioned. The scalp was infiltrated with 0.375% bupivacaine with 1/200 000 adrenaline. This was done by blocking the left-sided auriculotemporal, zygomaticotemporal, supraorbital, supratrochlear, and greater and lesser occipital nerves with a few mL infiltrated around the three Mayfield pins. A total of 40 mL of this solution was used.

When the surgeons had gained adequate access, the request to lighten the anaesthesia was made; the propofol was switched off, along with the remifentanil infusion. The anaesthetic chart is shown in Figure 7.8.

The rest of the resection was performed with attention paid to any changes in motor function or speech. BP increased from 115/60, immediately prior to awakening, to 150/80. In order to prevent an overshot, a test bolus of esmolol was administered (to no detriment). Remifentanil was recommenced at 0.02 micrograms/kg/min, and propofol TCI at 0.7 micrograms/mL, leaving the patient calm and easily rousable. Mannitol 20% 100mL was administered twice to reduce brain swelling. Morphine 2 mg was administered towards the end of the case. The patient remained comfortable throughout and did not require to be put back off to sleep.

Post-operative course

The patient was GCS 15 immediately post-operatively. Post-operative analgesia was achieved with regular paracetamol and morphine PCA. Pathology samples had shown a high-grade glioma, and he was referred for chemo- and radiotherapy with adjuvant temozolomide. He was discharged 72 hours after the procedure, with follow-up in clinic. He remained well 6 months post-surgery.

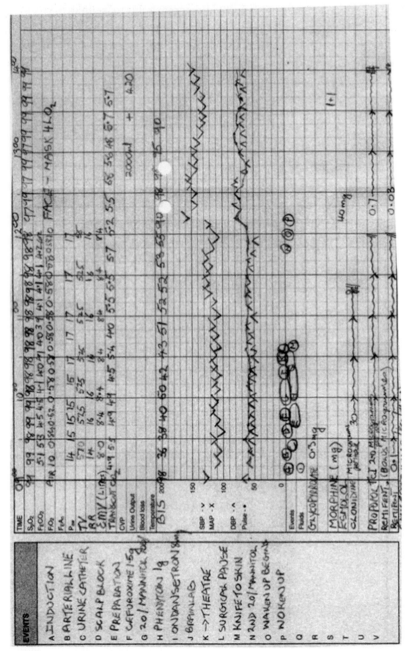

Fig. 7.8 An anaesthetic chart for the awake craniotomy case described in the text.

Summary

There are a number of indications for awake craniotomy, including a tumour in eloquent areas of the brain, epilepsy surgery, and movement disorders. Patients should be carefully selected, and a patient who does not wish to have an awake craniotomy is an absolute contraindication to this technique.

There is no undisputed technique, and each variation has its advocates. A common variation is to have the patient asleep for the potentially uncomfortable initial phase of the operation, then awake, and, if necessary, re-sedated ('asleep/awake/asleep'). The asleep phase is achieved with propofol infusion or a volatile technique. Dexmedetomidine has been available in some countries as part of the technique for awake craniotomies.

The laryngeal mask and depth of anaesthesia monitoring have greatly facilitated this procedure.

Further reading

Bilotta F and Rosa G (2009). Anesthesia for awake neurosurgery. *Current Opinion in Anaesthesiology*, **22**, 560–5.

Burnand C and Sebastian J (2014). Anaesthesia for awake craniotomy. *Continuing Education in Anaesthesia, Critical Care & Pain*, **14**, 6–11.

Costello TG and Cormack JR (2004). Anaesthesia for awake craniotomy: a modern approach. *Journal of Clinical Neuroscience*, **11**, 16–19.

Jones H and Smith M (2004). Awake craniotomies. *Continuing Education in Anaesthesia, Critical Care & Pain*, **4**, 189–92.

Chapter 8

Ear, nose, and throat anaesthesia

Dr Anil Patel

Bleeding tonsils

Background

Tonsillectomy is the commonest operation performed in the UK, and, each year, >50 000 tonsillectomies are carried out. In 2005, the National Prospective Tonsillectomy Audit published data on 33 921 patients who underwent a tonsillectomy between July 2003 and September 2004. Children aged <5 years accounted for 23%, children aged 5–16 years for 49%, and 16 years or over for 28% of all tonsillectomy procedures. The aim of the audit was to investigate the occurrence of haemorrhage and other complications in the first 28 days after tonsillectomy.

The National Prospective Tonsillectomy Audit is the largest audit undertaken for tonsillectomy and described the primary and secondary tonsillar haemorrhage rates. Primary complications occurred during the initial stay and delayed discharge, and required a return to theatre or a blood transfusion. Secondary complications required readmission to hospital within 28 days of the initial surgery.

In 33 921 patients, 95% recovered uneventfully, whilst 0.9% required a return trip to theatre. The remainder suffered less severe complications such as mild bleeding, pain, or vomiting. There were 1197 (3.5%) complications involving either a primary or secondary tonsillar haemorrhage, and 318 (0.9%) patients required a return to theatre within 28 days of their initial operation. Of these, 150 (0.4%) patients were returned to theatre during their initial hospital stay, whilst 176 (0.5%) patients were returned to theatre during a readmission.

Adults had higher haemorrhage rates than children. The highest haemorrhage rates were seen in patients with quinsy (5.4%). Patients with a pharyngeal obstruction had a lower rate of haemorrhage than patients with recurrent acute tonsillitis (the most common indication for surgery).

Learning outcomes

1 Recognize the signs and symptoms of post-tonsillectomy haemorrhage

2 Deliver appropriate resuscitation prior to surgical intervention

3 Discuss anaesthetic techniques for emergency operative management of a patient with bleeding tonsils.

CPD matrix matches

2A07; 2D01; 2D02; 2D04

Case history

A healthy 7-year-old child was scheduled for a routine tonsillectomy for recurrent acute tonsillitis on an elective ear, nose, and throat (ENT) morning operating list. The child had a previous general anaesthetic for dental clearance of damaged teeth 1 year ago, with no complications and an uneventful recovery at home. The tonsillectomy procedure had been postponed on two previous occasions because of an active acute tonsillitis.

On this occasion, the child had finished a course of antibiotics prescribed by the GP 2 days prior to admission. Preoperative assessment revealed a fit and healthy 7-year-old boy with large tonsils. Preoperative oral paracetamol and diclofenac were given 1 hour before surgery. Following IV induction with fentanyl and propofol, flexible LMA insertion, and spontaneous ventilation, general anaesthesia had been uneventful. Large tonsillar tissues were resected, and <10 mL of blood had been lost intraoperatively, and IV fluids were continued into the post-operative period. Recovery was uneventful, and observations were normal, following which the child was returned to the ward.

Five hours later, the nursing staff on the ward have asked for an ENT and anaesthestic review of the child. There has been no obvious blood loss from the mouth, but the child has vomited once, is occasionally spitting out blood, and is not eating, and the nursing staff are concerned, because he looks very tired.

Is the child bleeding?

Although there is no obvious blood loss from the mouth, significant blood can still be lost and swallowed over several hours following a tonsillectomy. The child has vomited on one occasion, and this was reported as containing blood. This child is not eating and complains of feeling sick, and the parents have noticed that he seems to be constantly swallowing which suggests there may be significant bleeding and swallowing of blood. Oxygen should be administered but may not be tolerated.

When and where is the bleeding?

Primary haemorrhage is usually within the first 6 hours post-operatively but can present immediately in the recovery area. The bleeding is usually as a result of venous or capillary oozing from the tonsillar bed. Secondary haemorrhage is within 28 days of the initial surgery and can be as a result of vessel ties coming loose, sloughing, or infection of the tissue overlying the tonsillar bed.

How much has the child bled?

It is not possible to identify the amount of blood lost, because much of it is swallowed, and therefore hypovolaemic assessment and resuscitation are clinical.

Early indicators of significant bleeding and hypovolaemia are:

◆ Tachycardia: an increased HR is the principal physiological response to hypovolaemia

◆ CRT (>2 s): hypovolaemia resulting in reduced skin perfusion

◆ Mottling, pallor, and peripheral cyanosis: hypovolaemia resulting in reduced skin perfusion

◆ Temperature: a difference of >2°C between the core temperature and skin temperature

◆ Tachypnoea: in response to metabolic tissue acidosis secondary to tissue hypoperfusion

◆ Urine output: reduced urine output secondary to hypovolaemia and renal hypoperfusion.

Late indicators of significant bleeding and hypovolaemia include:

◆ BP: hypotension is a late sign

◆ Reduced conscious level/GCS: altered consciousness level is a late sign.

Severe indicators of massive blood loss and hypovolaemia include:

◆ Bradycardia: a reduced HR in the presence of severe hypovolaemia is a pre-terminal sign requiring immediate treatment.

Case update

On examination, the child has a HR of 145, CRT of 3 s, RR of 28 breaths/min, and BP of 83/38 mmHg; he looks pale and has cool peripheries and periods of agitation and sleeping.

Significant bleeding has occurred; the child is hypovolaemic and requires immediate resuscitation and then transfer to theatre.

How much and what type of fluid for resuscitation?

Resuscitation is usually with isotonic crystalloid or colloid in the first instance, because blood is usually not immediately available. Hypotonic fluids should not be used. Hartmann's solution or 0.9% saline are suitable crystalloid solutions. Blood is given as soon as it is available. The response to an initial bolus dose of 20 mL/kg is assessed clinically by various indicators of hypovolaemia: HR, CRT, skin perfusion, temperature, and tachypnoea.

More fluid may be required and is administered after repeated assessment of the clinical signs. General anaesthesia should follow resuscitation, avoiding the potential catastrophic cardiovascular complications after induction of general anaesthesia in a hypovolaemic child.

Case update

After 35 mL/kg of fluid, the child has a HR of 95, CRT of 2 s, RR of 21 breaths/min, and BP of 84/43 mmHg; he looks pale. Blood has been taken for coagulation screening and cross-matching, and blood is now available. Coagulation screening results are not yet available. A decision is made to take the child to the operating theatre.

Who should be involved with a second general anaesthetic on a resuscitated child?

Although the general anaesthetic 5 hours previously was uneventful, a second general anaesthetic on a resuscitated child will be more challenging, requiring an experienced anaesthetist. Senior anaesthetic and surgical help should be sought and may well be needed.

What are the specific anaesthetic concerns for a bleeding child?

- ◆ Full stomach: this may be because the child has eaten and drunk fluids after the operation on the ward before bleeding has been recognized or, more commonly, as a result of swallowed blood

- ◆ Difficult intubation: any child with a bleeding tonsil should be treated as a patient with a full stomach and will require tracheal intubation. The original procedure may have been performed with a tracheal tube or with a flexible LMA. If the child had been intubated, a record of the ease of direct laryngoscopy and tracheal intubation will be present. Irrespective of the ease of the previous laryngoscopy and tracheal intubation, all children have the potential to convert from an easy laryngoscopy and intubation to a difficult intubation. It can often surprise the novice how quickly a normal airway can convert to a difficult airway in the presence of blood, clots, and bleeding, and as a result of the swelling and oedema secondary to surgical and anaesthetic instrumentation. Precautions for a potential difficult intubation should be taken

- ◆ Parental anxiety: both parents and child will be anxious. Expectations of a routine day case procedure will have transformed to a bleeding child, requiring resuscitation and an emergency operation.

What anaesthetic equipment is required?

In addition to all standard equipment for an emergency, preparations for a potentially difficult intubation should be made. This might include a selection of direct laryngoscope blades, video laryngoscopes, and tracheal tubes of various sizes. Typically, a smaller tracheal tube may be required because of associated swelling and oedema, and, on initial placement, this may become blocked with clots and blood. A second tracheal tube of a similar size may be needed.

Following placement of a tracheal tube, swallowed blood should be suctioned from the stomach after the insertion of wide-bore orogastric tubes. Standard orogastric feeding-type tubes are not suitable for suctioning large amounts of blood from the stomach, because they are easily blocked. At the end of the operation, the stomach should be suctioned again before extubation.

What induction technique should be employed—a rapid sequence induction or an inhalational induction?

Either technique can be used, and the final decision will depend on the experience of the anaesthetist. The chosen technique is the one they are most experienced in and feel comfortable with. The surgeon should be scrubbed and prepared in case of difficulty with the tracheal intubation.

- RSI: this involves a rapid sequence intubation with cricoid pressure, as appropriate. Preoxygenation is attempted but may not be tolerated by an anxious bleeding child, and gentle ventilation may be necessary after the administration of muscle relaxants and before tracheal intubation. This technique allows laryngoscopy in a more familiar supine position under optimal intubating conditions with muscle relaxation

- Inhalational induction: this, in a child with a bleeding airway, is challenging. It can be a slow process and may lead to a deep plane of anaesthesia with cardiovascular instability. The left lateral position allows blood, clots, and secretions to drain away from the airway but makes laryngoscopy and tracheal intubation more difficult, because most anaesthetists are unfamiliar with laryngoscopy and tracheal intubation in a lateral position. To optimize laryngoscopy and tracheal intubation, some anaesthetists will turn the child into a supine position and may administer muscle relaxants.

What are the intraoperative considerations?

Further fluid resuscitation, careful monitoring, and the administration of blood products may be necessary, guided by Hb assessment.

Standard surgery monitoring should include temperature measurement, active warming with blankets and fluid, eye protection, and peripheral nerve monitoring. At the end of the procedure, residual neuromuscular blockade is reversed, and the child extubated awake in a left lateral head-down position or in the 'tonsil' position, which places a pillow under the child's lateral chest, which allows any residual blood or secretions to drain away from the airway.

What are the appropriate post-operative care instructions?

Following extubation, careful observations should be continued in the recovery area. Further bleeding may still occur, and the repeat tracheal intubation and surgery may result in further swelling and oedema. Careful observations of the airway, cardiovascular and respiratory status, and Hb level should be made. Once the child appears stable, they can be transferred to a high dependency area on the ward where careful observations must be continued overnight.

Summary

More than 50 000 tonsillectomies are performed each year in the UK, with a tonsillar haemorrhage rate of 3.5%. Of these, 0.4% required a return to theatre during their initial hospital stay, and 0.5% returned to theatre during a readmission. Principles in the management of bleeding tonsils include the recognition of the signs and symptoms of post-tonsillectomy haemorrhage, appropriate resuscitation prior to surgical intervention, recognition of a full stomach, and the potential for a difficult intubation. Following the placement of a tracheal tube, swallowed blood should be suctioned from the stomach after the insertion of wide-bore orogastric tubes, and, following surgery, careful observations of the airway, cardiovascular and respiratory status, and Hb level should be made.

Further reading

Gobindram A and Patel A (2008). ENT emergencies. *Anaesthesia and Intensive Care Medicine*, **9**, 277–328.

Case 8.2

Acute epiglottitis

Background

Acute epiglottitis is an acute inflammatory condition of the epiglottis, arytenoids, and aryepiglottic folds, with gross swelling and oedema of the structures at the laryngeal inlet, resulting in an acute upper airway obstruction. The onset and progression of symptoms are rapid and can lead to complete upper airway occlusion, hypoxaemia, and death. Acute epiglottitis is a medical emergency and requires prompt recognition and management.

The anatomy of the paediatric airway is different to adults. The tongue and arytenoid structures are relatively large, and the infant nares are small. The larynx and epiglottis have a higher position in the infant which descends with age. The epiglottis shape is longer, softer, and omega-shaped and changes to a more adult configuration as the larynx descends. These differences mean any reduction in the calibre of the airway has a greater effect on airflow than in adults.

Acute epiglottitis is caused by infectious agents, including *Haemophilus influenzae* type B, group A *Streptococcus pneumoniae*, *Haemophilus parainfluenzae*, *Staphylococcus aureus*, and β-haemolytic streptococci. The principal agent was *Haemophilus influenzae* type B, but, since the introduction of the *H. influenzae* B (HiB) vaccine in 1992, the incidence of acute epiglottitis has fallen dramatically, and many trainees may never have seen a case.

Learning outcomes

1 Recognize the signs and symptoms of life-threatening airway pathology

2 Discuss appropriate preoperative interventions

3 Plan a safe induction technique for a child with upper airway compromise.

CPD matrix matches

1C01; 2A01

Case history 1

A healthy 2-year-old boy has developed a cough, sore throat, and rhinorrhoea, with a low-grade temperature over the last 5 days. This morning, the child's temperature was 37.4°C, and a barking cough with a loud inspiratory stridor was noticed. The parents were concerned with this new noise, and they presented with the child to the ED. The child is swallowing fluids and is able to lie down but has suprasternal retractions, nasal flaring, oxygen saturations of 93% on air, and a RR of 26 breaths/min.

Case history 2

A healthy 3-year-old girl was entirely well until the last 12 hours when she developed a high temperature of 38.9°C, and severe throat pain, and she is now unable to swallow. The parents have brought the child to the ED. She is distressed, sitting upright, with inspiratory and expiratory stridor. Oxygen saturations are 88% on air, and there is significant nasal flaring and suprasternal and intercostal retractions, with a RR of 38 breaths/min.

What is the diagnosis?

In children, acute epiglottitis typically occurs at age 2–5 years old. The main differential diagnosis is croup, which occurs in younger children aged 6 months to 3 years, has a more gradual onset over a number of days, and rarely appears toxic.

The 2-year-old boy has croup (laryngotracheobronchitis). Croup is an acute viral URTI, in which there is inflammation, with swelling and oedema in the larynx and trachea, reducing airflow and producing the characteristic barking cough. There is a gradual onset of symptoms with low-grade fever, sore throat, and URTI over a number of days preceding to a loud barking cough, hoarseness, and inspiratory stridor. Swallowing is normal with no drooling, and children are usually able to lie down. Treatment depends on the severity of the respiratory distress at presentation. Initial therapy in early cases involves humidification therapy to limit airway drying, steroids therapy to reduce inflammation, and nebulized adrenaline to reduce mucosal oedema quickly. Occasionally, children with croup can present with severe respiratory distress and need urgent intubation.

The 3-year-old girl has acute epiglottitis with its typical presentation of sudden onset in a previously well child. A sore throat, abrupt onset of fever, dysphagia, drooling, open mouth, muffled voice, inspiratory and expiratory stridor, and severe respiratory distress are characteristic. The child will often assume the tripod position, sitting upright with their hands outstretched and still, with the neck extended and head held forward in an attempt to improve the mechanical advantage of the respiratory muscles. These children are toxic, distressed, and anxious. Prompt diagnosis and urgent intervention is required.

What is the severity of respiratory distress?

An assessment of the severity of the respiratory distress guides the diagnosis and future management in children with upper airway obstruction. Inspiratory stridor is classically a sign of supraglottic upper airway obstruction, and expiratory stridor is a feature of intrathoracic airway obstruction. With severe upper airway obstruction, both inspiratory and expiratory stridor can be present. The presence of stridor is always a worrying sign, but its absence or reduction in volume may suggest the child is becoming tired and may soon be unable to maintain the airway.

The RR, body position, chest wall and abdominal movements, retractions with the use of accessory muscles, air entry, and cyanosis all indicate the severity of respiratory distress. The level of consciousness will be affected with a normal child becoming anxious, restless, and eventually lethargic with a depressed level of consciousness. With reduced air entry, hypoxaemia and cyanosis develop, with hypercarbia and resultant cardiovascular system compromise and tachycardia. With exhaustion, the RR can fall, and air entry diminishes dramatically.

Case 1 has mild/moderate respiratory distress, with retractions, nasal flaring, oxygen saturations of 93% on air, and a RR of 26 breaths/min. Simple humidification may be the only treatment required, with careful assessment of the respiratory distress and the addition of steroids and nebulized adrenaline

Case 2 describes a child with severe respiratory distress, sitting upright with inspiratory and expiratory stridor. Oxygen saturations are 88% on air, and there is significant nasal flaring and suprasternal and intercostal retractions, with a RR of 38 breaths/min. Immediate intervention is required.

Discuss the management of acute epiglottitis

The diagnosis is made on the history and examination, with the least possible disturbance of the child. Keep the child in whatever position she feels is most comfortable, with the examination working around this position. The child may prefer to stay in the parent's arms. Very gentle examination without disturbing the child will provide information on the degree of respiratory distress, and a gently placed pulse oximeter will provide information on oxygen saturation readings. The child may tolerate a gently placed oxygen mask held near to the face by the parents; if this appears to be unsettling the child, it should be moved further away or removed.

Both the child and parents should be kept calm and an explanation of the proposed management given to the parents. Preparation for a difficult intubation and an emergency tracheostomy should be made.

In this example, indirect laryngoscopy, placement of IV lines, oropharyngeal examination, IM injections, and lateral neck radiographs should not be undertaken, because further distress may precipitate a complete airway obstruction.

In a cooperative adult with acute epiglottitis, very careful flexible fibreoptic laryngoscopy, IV lines, and a careful oropharyngeal examination by experienced personnel can be performed.

Which team members should be involved?

Senior experienced anaesthetic and surgical staff should be involved as early as possible, and intubation should be delayed until they arrive. Operating room staff should be informed early and equipment assembled and prepared. Equipment for an emergency surgical airway, emergency cricothyrotomy, jet ventilation, various sizes of oral and nasal tracheal tubes, a flexible fibrescope, and a rigid bronchoscope may be needed. The child should be transferred with the parents and emergency equipment to the operating room, with minimal disruption and distress, accompanied by senior staff.

Discuss the options for induction and intubation

In the operating room, an inhalational induction with sevoflurane or halothane in oxygen is commenced, with the child usually sitting or in the preferred position. Nitrous oxide is not used. An experienced surgeon able to perform a tracheostomy should be scrubbed and ready.

Inhalational induction with sevoflurane 8% in oxygen can be a long process, taking between 5 and 10 min, because alveolar ventilation is very slow with acute airway obstruction.

Further monitoring and IV access are established as anaesthesia deepens. IV fluids and atropine may be administered to reduce the likelihood of bradycardia associated with intubation. The child may be positioned into a supine position to aid laryngoscopy and the parents asked to leave. On laryngoscopy, the epiglottis and aryepiglottic folds are swollen, and the classic 'cherry-red' epiglottis may be seen. Often, the glottic opening is not seen, and the only clue may be a small mucous bubble during spontaneous ventilation or by gentle pressure on the child's chest.

A tracheal tube, usually 1–3 mm smaller than normal, is placed. Initially, this is an oral tube, and, once the child is stable, this is replaced to a nasal tube which is less likely to become dislodged during the subsequent ventilation on a paediatric ICU. Great care must be taken to prevent dislodgement of the nasal tracheal tube.

In adults with a compromised airway, inhalational induction is often unfamiliar, difficult, and slow, and the depth of anaesthesia can be hard to assess. The patient may become more hypoxic and hypercarbic with long periods of instability, arrhythmias, and apnoea. The traditional view is that the technique is safe, because, if the patient obstructs, the volatile agent will no longer be taken up and the patient will lighten and wake up. This frequently does not happen, and the technique is often not reliable. Some centres therefore use an IV induction technique in adults with epiglottitis, with a backup plan of a surgical airway, and, in some cooperative patients, the surgical airway may be placed before induction under local anaesthetic.

What are the appropriate post-intubation care instructions?

A post-intubation CXR should be taken to ensure optimal tube placement and to assess for LRTIs. Throat and blood cultures are taken, antibiotic therapy (usually a third- or fourth-generation cephalosporin) commenced, and the child transferred to a paediatric ICU, with the appropriate sedation and muscle relaxation to allow controlled ventilation. Extubation is normally possible within 48 hours, with rapidly resolving swelling and oedema of the epiglottis.

Summary

Acute epiglottitis is a medical emergency with a rapid onset and progression of symptoms which can lead to complete upper airway obstruction and death. In children, the main differential diagnosis is croup which occurs in younger children, has a more gradual onset over a number of days, and rarely appears toxic. The diagnosis of acute epiglottitis is made on the history and examination with a sudden onset in a previously well child of sore throat, fever, dysphagia, drooling, open mouth, muffled voice, inspiratory and expiratory stridor, and severe respiratory distress. Senior experienced anaesthetic and surgical staff should be involved as early as possible, and intubation should be delayed until they arrive. Equipment for difficult airway management and emergency surgical airway must be immediately available.

Further reading

Gobindram A and Patel A (2008). ENT emergencies. *Anaesthesia and Intensive Care Medicine*, **9**, 277–328.

Patel A (2011). What is epiglottitis and how is it managed? In: Calder I and Pearce A, eds. *Core topics in airway management*, 2nd edn, p. 303. Cambridge University Press, Cambridge.

Case 8.3

Inhaled foreign body

Background

Adults and children can present following the inhalation of a foreign body, but, in young children, this is the commonest indication for a bronchoscopy and one of the leading causes of death. Adults can usually recall the event and the diagnosis is more confident, whereas, in children, this is more difficult, often relying on history, symptoms, and suspicion.

Typically, between the ages of 1 and 4 years old, children are crawling and starting to walk and often put objects in their mouth, nose, and ears. Distress or exercise may result in an uncoordinated inhalation of a foreign body in the mouth, bypassing the usual epiglottic, vocal cord, and laryngeal apparatus protective mechanisms.

What happens next depends on the size and nature of the material inhaled and where it stops. If the foreign body is large and causes complete obstruction of the glottis or trachea, unless immediate action is taken, the child will die from asphyxia at home. Partial airway obstruction presents with various degrees of compromise and urgency, depending on the size of the foreign body, its material, and where the object has stopped. It is this group of children that requires very careful assessment, investigation, and optimal communication and cooperation between the surgeon taking out the foreign body from the airway and the anaesthetist managing this shared airway.

Learning outcomes

1 Recognize the signs and symptoms of aspirated foreign bodies
2 Instigate appropriate planning for surgical intervention for the removal of a foreign body in the airway
3 Be aware of the difficulties of delivering anaesthesia for rigid bronchoscopy and the hazards of a shared airway.

CPD matrix matches

1C01; 2A01; 2D02

Case history 1

A healthy boy, aged 6 years old, has seen the GP for the second time in the last week. He had been diagnosed with a chest infection 5 days earlier and been started on oral antibiotics. Over the last 5 days, he had developed a wheeze, continued to cough intermittently, and remained pyrexial. The boy has mentioned to the parents that the coughing had started 10 days ago after he had been eating some peanuts.

Case history 2

A healthy girl, aged 3 years and 10 months, has had a persistent cough for the last 24 hours and has presented to the casualty department. A wheeze is present, particularly over the right side of the chest. The parents mention that she started intermittently coughing after a children's party the previous day and that this has got worse overnight. She is apyrexial; her RR is 26 breaths/min; oxygen saturations are 97% on air, and she looks otherwise well.

Case history 3

A 2-year-old boy presents to the casualty department with a 1 hour history of severe coughing. The coughing had started following a choking episode during a meal which the child had been unable to finish. The parents had initially thought the coughing would settle, but, over the last hour, it had got worse. In between periods of coughing, the child was crying and obviously distressed. He was short of breath, with a RR of 38 breaths/min and oxygen saturation of 93% on air, and was beginning to develop intercostal and sternal recession. There was no stridor, cyanosis, or aphonia, and he was apyrexial.

Is there evidence of an inhaled foreign body in these cases?

These three cases highlight the variation in presentation following the inhalation of a foreign body. Foreign bodies within the larynx and trachea can present with acute dyspnoea, stridor, coughing, cyanosis, and aphonia, suggesting an obstruction at a laryngeal level. At the other end of the spectrum of presentations, the child may look well, with no symptoms or signs other than a cough.

In an emergency with a foreign body in the larynx or trachea, the Heimlich manoeuvre or management according to the basic life support 'choking child' algorithms with abdominal thrusts and back blows will be necessary.

Most children presenting to hospital have partial airway obstruction as a result of a foreign body in the bronchus, and they present with a sudden onset of choking followed by coughing, wheezing, hoarseness, and shortness of breath. There may be clinically detectable reduced air entry and wheezing on the side of the obstruction.

Case 1 describes a typical history from a child with a late presentation. There may have been some coughing at the time of inhalation, but this may have settled and the child and parents been unaware of its significance. The child may present much later if the obstruction does not pose a functional problem with mucosal irritation, oedema, and pneumonitis distal to the obstruction. Subsequently, the child may have been treated for a chest infection or asthma and finally present with intractable secondary LRTIs

Case 2 describes a child who may have inhaled a foreign body, with the diagnosis requiring an awareness and a degree of suspicion. If left alone, the child may re-present with airway compromise due to obstruction and infection

Case 3 describes a child who has presented with an acute partial airway obstruction, is unwell, and will require urgent management to remove the foreign body.

What are the differential diagnoses?

The history, symptoms, and signs will help differentiate respiratory tract infections, including croup, and pneumothorax and asthma.

What are the foreign bodies, and where do they end up?

More than 90% of foreign bodies are organic material, and this is usually food, with nuts being particularly common. Most are found in one of the bronchi, with the majority inhaled into the right main bronchus because of its anatomical position.

Four types of obstruction have been described:

- Check valve: the foreign body in the lower airway/bronchus allows air to be inhaled past it but does not allow exhalation, resulting in emphysema
- Ball valve: air can be exhaled, but not inhaled, past the foreign body, resulting in collapse of the bronchopulmonary segment
- Bypass valve: the foreign body partially obstructs both inspiration and expiration
- Stop valve: there is total obstruction, causing airway collapse and consolidation.

What investigations should be performed?

The principal investigation will be a CXR. In cases 1, 2, and 3, a CXR with AP and lateral views should be undertaken, but, in most cases, the foreign body will not be seen because most foreign bodies will be organic material and therefore radiolucent. The CXRs are useful, because they provide secondary signs of partial or complete obstruction such as lobar collapse, consolidation, and atelectasis with stop valve obstruction, and emphysematous gas trapping changes with a check valve obstruction. Significant lobar collapse and gas trapping may cause a mediastinal shift. These secondary findings may not have developed or be visible within the first 24 hours, and most CXR investigations within the first 24 hours are negative. Fluoroscopy or CXRs in inhalation and exhalation may improve the sensitivity of the investigation.

Case 1: evidence of an inhaled foreign body is seen, with secondary signs of collapse and consolidation

Case 2: gives a reasonable history for inhalation, and confirmation with inspiratory and expiratory views may be useful. The child is reasonably stable, and the additional confirmation is worthwhile

Case 3: the positive history, symptoms, and signs are sufficient to justify a general anaesthetic and endoscopic procedure. The CXR showed no collapse, consolidation, or pneumothorax.

In all three cases, a decision is made to proceed with tracheobronchoscopy under general anaesthesia.

What urgency of intervention is indicated?

This will depend on the presentation and severity of respiratory distress. A child with a convincing history, severe respiratory distress, cyanosis, and obvious airway obstruction should be given 100% oxygen and transferred to the operating room in preparation for tracheobronchoscopy. Foreign bodies in the larynx or trachea will cause more distress and are associated with a higher mortality than those that are usually smaller and pass more distally into the bronchi.

Case 3 is the most urgent with significant respiratory distress and requires urgent intervention.

How should you manage the full stomach?

Ideally, all patients should be fasted for a suitable period. In reality, when a child has severe respiratory distress and requires urgent intervention to remove the foreign body, this becomes more important than strict fasting regimes. In cases 1 and 2, an optimal preparation with a suitable fasting period should be allowed. In case 3, urgent intervention with removal of the foreign body is required, and there should not be a delay for a suitable fasting period.

Which staff should be involved?

Once there is a suspicion of an inhaled foreign body, experienced staff should be involved. When a child has severe respiratory distress, senior anaesthetic and surgical staff should be directly involved in the operative management. Senior anaesthetic and surgical staff should be directly involved with all three cases in the operating room.

Which drugs should be considered?

+ Sedatives: the administration of any sedative premedication to a child with severe respiratory distress can lead to an unpredictable response with oversedation, worsening of airway obstruction, or total airway obstruction. Most anaesthetists do not give sedative premedication because of these concerns and rely on the presence of the parents to keep the children calm. Premedication was not given to cases 1, 2, or 3, because of the risk of total airway obstruction

+ Anticholinergics: in the past, these were routinely prescribed, particularly with the use of halothane, to reduce the associated vagal-mediated bradycardia, reflex bronchoconstriction, and secretions. With the more widespread use of sevoflurane, anticholinergics are not always used. Atropine 20 micrograms/kg or glycopyrrolate 10 micrograms/kg help reduce secretions and the reflex bradycardia associated with airway instrumentation

+ Steroids: although its efficacy is uncertain, dexamethasone is often administered, in an attempt to reduce post-operative swelling and laryngeal oedema following surgical instrumentation and removal of a foreign body. Dexamethasone 0.1 mg/kg was administered to cases 1, 2, and 3

+ Local anaesthetic: a topical local anaesthetic (lidocaine up to 4 mg/kg) is administered by spray to the vocal cords and trachea. A topical local anaesthetic is important in reducing the reflex responses and cardiovascular stimulation associated with the introduction of metal instruments into the trachea.

Should intravenous access be secured prior to induction of anaesthesia?

IV access should be established before any operative intervention. Topical local anaesthetics, such as Emla® or Ametop®, may be tolerated and, after a suitable time, IV access established. In an urgent situation with severe respiratory distress, there may be inadequate time for a topical local anaesthetic to work, and the child may become too distressed by attempts at IV cannulation. Under these circumstances, it will be more sensible to attempt IV cannulation after inhalational induction.

What equipment is required?

Familiarity with rigid ventilating bronchoscopes, attachments, and preoperative checks to ensure these are correct and working should be undertaken. Some bronchoscopes allow the attachment of a T-piece to a side arm on the bronchoscope, through which oxygen and volatile agent can pass directly into the distal trachea, acting in a similar manner to an uncuffed tracheal tube. Some bronchoscopes do not allow T-piece attachment. and therefore insufflation or IV anaesthetic techniques are required.

What monitoring should be applied?

Standard monitoring, including oxygen saturation, capnography, transcutaneous capnometry and neuromuscular monitoring if muscle relaxants are administered.

How should you conduct the induction of anaesthesia?

Traditionally, the general principle around induction and maintenance of anaesthesia is to maintain spontaneous ventilation, usually by an inhalational technique with sevoflurane or halothane, in the hope of reducing the chances of the foreign body being pushed distally into the airway. Dislodging an inhaled foreign body can convert a partial airway obstruction to a more severe, or even complete, obstruction. However, in practice, the maintenance of spontaneous ventilation in a critically obstructed airway can be extremely difficult to sustain, and IPPV may be needed, with some centres routinely using controlled ventilation and muscle paralysis. Recent trials have shown the efficacy of routine paralysis and PPV with better control of ventilation and little impact on dislodgement of the foreign body. Nitrous oxide is not used because of the increased risks associated with gas trapping.

Case 3: induction with sevoflurane in oxygen was started and at a deep plane of anaesthesia, as judged by movements, pupil size, respiratory rate and pattern, and cardiovascular parameters. Laryngoscopy was performed and a topical local anaesthetic administered. Because of its longer duration of action, sevoflurane was changed to isoflurane once a deep plane of anaesthesia had been achieved. Close observation and monitoring was required throughout the procedure to ensure the correct depth of anaesthesia to prevent movement, coughing, and laryngospasm. A rigid bronchoscope was introduced, and isoflurane oxygen insufflated through the T-piece on the bronchoscope. Grasping forceps were introduced through the rigid bronchoscope to remove the foreign body.

What are the potential intraoperative complications?

Complications occur because of inadequate anaesthesia, inadequate ventilation, and instrumentation of the airway. The consequences of inadequate anaesthesia include coughing, movements, dislodgement of the foreign body, pneumothorax, regurgitation and aspiration, and dysrhythmias. The consequences of inadequate ventilation are hypoxia and hypercarbia, promoting dysrhythmias. Instrumentation may traumatize any part of the airway and cause mucosal oedema, with respiratory distress.

During the removal of the foreign body, it can become fragmented, pushed further into the airway, become lodged, or caught up at the trachea or glottis. If the foreign body is lodged in the trachea, complete airway obstruction may result, and the foreign body needs to be removed immediately or pushed back down into the bronchus. Muscle relaxation at this critical time may be useful by providing a totally relaxed upper airway, from which the foreign body is extracted.

What post-operative care instructions are recommended?

Post-operative care involves a CXR, high dependency environment, humidified oxygen, and observation for airway oedema. Antibiotics in suspected cases of infection and IV steroids to reduce airway oedema may be indicated.

Summary

The presentation of inhaled foreign bodies varies from an emergency in a 'choking child' to a partial obstruction and a chronic cough. Most children presenting to hospital have partial airway obstruction as a result of the foreign body in the bronchus and present with a sudden onset of choking, followed by coughing, wheezing, hoarseness, and shortness of breath. The differential diagnosis includes respiratory tract infections, croup, pneumothorax, and asthma. Most foreign bodies are radiolucent and are not seen on a CXR, but secondary signs include lobar collapse, consolidation, atelectasis, and gas trapping. Traditionally, the general principle around the induction and maintenance of anaesthesia is to maintain spontaneous ventilation, usually by an inhalational technique with sevoflurane or halothane, in the hope of reducing the chances of the foreign body being pushed distally into the airway. In practice, the maintenance of spontaneous ventilation in a critically obstructed airway can be extremely difficult to sustain, and IPPV may be needed. Post-operative observation for airway oedema should take place in a high dependency environment.

Further reading

Gobindram A and Patel A (2008). ENT emergencies. *Anaesthesia and Intensive Care Medicine*, **9**, 277–328.

Patel A (2011). How might a child with an inhaled foreign body present? In: Calder I and Pearce A, eds. *Core topics in airway management*, 2nd edn, p. 304. Cambridge University Press, Cambridge.

Case 8.4

Airway obstruction

Background

An obstructed airway can be caused by tumours, infection, and trauma anywhere in the airway, from the nasopharynx, pharynx, and larynx through to the lower trachea and lower airways. Management strategies remain controversial, and experts frequently disagree on the best strategy. For adults, there are advocates of inducing general anaesthesia by an inhalational route and avoiding muscle relaxants, inducing general anaesthesia by the IV route and using muscle relaxants, avoiding general anaesthesia altogether and securing an airway by an awake fibreoptic intubation (AFOI) technique, tracheostomy under local anaesthesia, or insertion of a transtracheal catheter under local anaesthesia.

The recognition of a compromised or an anatomically distorted upper airway is vital in the preoperative assessment of head and neck patients. For elective patients, detailed investigations can be undertaken, but, in urgent cases, this may not be possible.

The exact technique chosen will be influenced by the urgency of the intervention required, the experience of the anaesthetist, the team around them, the location, surgical experience, and the site and extent of the airway obstruction. All plans can fail, and backup plans should have been discussed amongst the team, with the relevant equipment being available.

There are three questions that determine the management of the obstructed adult airway. First, what and where is the lesion? Second, how urgent is the intervention? Third, is the obstruction so significant that we should abandon attempts for general anaesthesia and use an awake technique?

Learning outcomes

1 Recognize the pathological causes of an airway obstruction
2 Define the level and severity of the obstruction
3 Describe the safe conduct of fibreoptic-guided airway management.

CPD matrix matches

2A01; 2A03

Case history 1

A 54-year-old woman presented with a large neck mass and a vocal cord palsy on the left side. She was unable to lie flat for prolonged periods, because of the difficulty in breathing, and preferred to sleep semi-upright on her left side. She had been unable to walk >20 yards without stopping and was now unable to climb her stairs at home. She had an RR of 16 breaths/min at rest and oxygen saturation readings of 95% on air. An urgent CT scan showed a large thyroid mass which was flattening the trachea to a minimal diameter of 8 mm, but no obvious local invasion into the trachea.

Case history 2

A 68-year-old man presented to the ED with increasing difficulty in breathing over the last week and was now unable to speak in full sentences. Past medical history included a hypopharyngeal carcinoma treated with surgical resection and radiotherapy 3 years previously. Over the last 24 hours, the breathing had become particularly difficult, and he was now unable to walk up his stairs at home. On examination, he had inspiratory stridor, tracheal tug, an RR of 26 breaths/min, and oxygen saturation readings of 86% on air. Careful experienced flexible nasendoscopy revealed an ulcerated mass on the left vocal cord which was obstructing approximately 70% of the laryngeal inlet.

What is causing the airway obstruction?

Case 1: a large neck mass suggests thyroid involvement which can extend into the mediastinum. If there is mediastinal involvement, there may be associated large vessel obstruction, and surgery may involve resection of the manubrium for access. Recurrent laryngeal nerve function may be compromised with expanding neck and thyroid masses

Case 2: this is likely to be a recurrence of the hypopharyngeal tumour or an infective process involving the area of previous surgical resection and radiotherapy.

The differential diagnosis of any upper airway obstruction varies according to age and the history of presentation. Benign or malignant tumours in any anatomical part of the upper airway or extrinsic compression from mediastinal masses can cause compression, luminal obliteration, or vocal cord palsy. Infection can be due to a retropharyngeal abscess, acute tonsillitis, Ludwig's angina, epiglottitis, laryngotracheobronchitis (croup), and diphtheria. Trauma, foreign bodies, haemorrhage, facial trauma, laryngeal stenosis, burns, laryngotracheal stenosis, angio-oedema, anaphylaxis, and vocal cord paralysis can all cause airway obstruction.

What is the level of the obstruction?

Case 1: the woman has a large thyroid mass that is causing compressive symptoms on the trachea which is resulting in difficulty of breathing. She does not need immediate intervention, and further investigations can be carried out. She will need a resection of the thyroid mass under general anaesthesia. There is compression of the trachea, and this may be worse following induction of anaesthesia. If laryngoscopy and tracheal intubation proves to be difficult or impossible, the option of an urgent surgical airway (plan B) would not be possible with a large mass overlying the neck. Under these circumstances and without the option of a surgical plan B, this patient should have an AFOI

Case 2: a recurrence of the carcinoma with extensive laryngeal obstruction is present. Urgent stabilization and intervention are required. Initial medical management with careful observation includes humidified oxygen, nebulized adrenaline, IV corticosteroids, and helium/oxygen mixtures if further deterioration in breathing occurs. Helium/oxygen is used as a temporary 'holding' measure whilst preparations are made for a definitive surgical intervention.

The level at which obstruction exists makes a significant difference as to the suitability of different techniques. For obstructing oral cavity lesions, the problems are first the ability to face mask-ventilate following induction of anaesthesia and, second, the difficult or impossible direct laryngoscopy around obstructing masses. At the glottis, the most common cause of obstructing lesions are tumours, and, as they enlarge, patients compensate until either an acute deterioration or a critical narrowing is reached. The key decision is to identify if it will be possible to pass a tracheal tube through the narrowing, and, if this is felt to be unlikely, an awake transtracheal catheter or awake local anaesthetic tracheostomy should be considered. Tracheal compression can occur as a result of lesions within the trachea or compression from thyroid and mediastinal masses. The upper airway may be normal at laryngoscopy, but it may not be possible to pass a tube beyond the obstruction or place a surgical airway beyond the obstruction.

Can you quantify the severity of the obstruction?

The differences between airway noises can help establish the level of obstruction, but, in severe obstruction, as the airflow becomes more restricted, the noise of breathing may disappear. An obstruction at a nasopharyngeal level typically produces a stertorous sound and at an oropharyngeal level a gurgling sound. Stridor is a high-pitched sound, and inspiratory and expiratory stridors represent extrathoracic and intrathoracic obstructions. In severe obstruction and with exhaustion, the noise will diminish.

Describe the appropriate anaesthesic technique

A full history and investigations to determine the site and extent of the obstruction and determine all the other factors associated with difficult airway management should be sought. Old anaesthetic records, imaging, and careful flexible nasendoscopy will provide useful information. The aim is to balance the urgency of the clinical situation but to provide anaesthesia in a planned manner. In an emergency, it may be necessary to proceed without the full clinical picture.

Case 1: an AFOI is performed, with the patient sitting up. This should be performed by an experienced endoscopist, with optimal topical local anaesthetic. A 'spray as you go' technique will be required to topicalize the trachea, because intratracheal injections will not be possible in a patient with a large neck mass overlying the trachea

Case 2: surgical intervention to debulk the tumour under general anaesthesia with a microlaryngoscopy tube was planned urgently. Experienced surgical and anaesthetic staff were involved, and all equipment was checked and plans made for emergency surgical tracheal access. The anaesthetic plan involved the introduction of an awake transtracheal catheter under local anaesthetic. After the introduction and confirmation of correct placement of the transtracheal catheter, IV induction of anaesthesia with propofol, fentanyl, and rocuronium was undertaken. Face mask ventilation using oxygen F_iO_2 1.0 was possible, and anaesthesia was maintained using sevoflurane 2–4% in oxygen. Direct laryngoscopy allowed the introduction of a size 4 laser-resistant tube. Surgery involved laser debulking of the mass, and, at the end of the case, he was extubated in a head-up position, fully awake.

Fibreoptic intubation is a complex highly skilled technique and should only be used in a critical airway by those familiar with it, as the risks of total airway obstruction and trauma are higher in inexperienced hands. In patients with severe glottic or subglottic narrowing, there is a significant risk of total airway blockage as the fibrescope is passed, and it may not be possible to railroad a tube past the obstruction. The recent National Audit Project 4 identified 14 failed intubations in 23 fibreoptic intubation attempts in patients with head and neck pathology, of which almost all required a surgical airway. AFOI is particularly useful when there may be difficulty with face mask ventilation or with direct laryngoscopy.

Anterior neck access by a transtracheal cannula, designed for tracheal access, can be inserted in elective, as well as more urgent, cases typically into the upper trachea between the tracheal rings, avoiding the cricothyroid area where there may be tumour extension. It is then possible to insufflate oxygen or use jet ventilation techniques via the cannula. The ability to oxygenate prior to the induction of general anaesthesia allows time for airway manipulations, so that difficult laryngoscopy is not rushed and is optimal with the highest success rates.

Is there a role for awake tracheostomy?

With severe airway compromise, sedation or general anaesthesia may, in some patients, cause total airway obstruction. This may not be relieved with airway manoeuvres, and direct laryngoscopy or flexible fibreoptic attempts at intubation may not be possible. Under these circumstances, any sedation, general anaesthesia, or attempts at airway intervention result in a patient in which we cannot ventilate or intubate. Under these circumstances, an awake tracheostomy performed by an experienced surgeon is the safest method of airway management. The ideal position for a surgical tracheostomy is supine with the neck extended, but, in severe airway compromise, this is not possible. Typically, a patient for an awake tracheostomy cannot lie flat or extend the neck, and so the procedure is undertaken in a semi-recumbent or an upright position. Oxygen should be administered throughout, and there must be no sedation or anaesthesia during the awake tracheostomy. The implicit safety of an awake tracheostomy is that the patient is awake. Any sedation or anaesthesia risks total airway obstruction and conversion of a difficult, but controlled, awake surgical tracheostomy into an immediate uncontrolled surgical tracheostomy.

Summary

Management strategies for airway obstruction remain controversial, and experts frequently disagree on the best strategy. Generally, three questions determine the management of the obstructed adult airway. First, what and where is the lesion? Second, how urgent is the intervention? Third, is the obstruction so significant that we should abandon attempts for general anaesthesia and use an awake technique? Fibreoptic intubation is a complex, highly skilled technique and should only be used in a critical airway by those familiar with it, as the risks of total airway obstruction and trauma are higher in inexperienced hands. With severe airway compromise, sedation or general anaesthesia may, in some patients, cause total airway obstruction. Under these circumstances, an awake tracheostomy performed by an experienced surgeon is the safest method of airway management.

Further reading

Patel A and Pearce A (2011). Progress in management of the obstructed airway. *Anaesthesia*, **66**, 93–100.

Patel A, Pearce A, and Pracy P (2011). Head and neck pathology. In: Cook T, Woodall N, and Frerk C, eds. *4th national audit project of the Royal College of Anaesthetists and the Difficult Airway Society: major complications of airway management in the United Kingdom*, pp. 143–54. Royal College of Anaesthetists, London.

Chapter 9

Vascular anaesthesia

Dr Alastair J Thomson
Dr Matthew T Royds

Ruptured abdominal aortic aneurysm

Background

Around two-thirds of patients with a ruptured abdominal aortic aneurysm (AAA) do not reach hospital alive. In-hospital mortality for those patients that do reach hospital is >50%. This is therefore a vascular emergency, and the patient may decompensate dramatically at any time. A number of scoring systems (e.g. Glasgow aneurysm score or the Hardmann index) have been developed to help predict the outcome of surgery following a ruptured AAA.

Learning outcomes

1 Describe the preoperative preparation and immediate anaesthetic management of a patient with a ruptured abdominal aortic aneurysm

2 Interpret point-of-care coagulation testing, and manage clotting dysfunction appropriately

3 Anticipate and manage perioperative myocardial ischaemia in the high-risk vascular patient.

CPD matrix matches

2A05; 2A07

Case history

A 70-year-old retired engineer presents to accident and emergency (A&E) with abdominal pain and a pulsatile mass in his epigastrium. Initial examination confirms that he is alert and orientated, maintaining a patent airway, and has a palpable radial pulse. His HR is 100 bpm, BP 84/60 mmHg, and SpO_2 94% on air. His previous medical history includes well-controlled hypertension and type II diabetes mellitus. He lives alone, is self-caring, and enjoys a reasonably active lifestyle, being able to walk up to 2 miles without stopping.

An urgent contrast CT scan is performed and reveals a 6.9 cm infrarenal aortic aneurysm with a large periaortic retroperitoneal haematoma. The AAA is not suitable for endovascular repair. However, given this man's relatively good health and functional status, it is very likely that he will be offered emergency open aneurysm repair.

You are the on-call anaesthetist who is called to the A&E department to help with his management. What is your initial approach?

Senior anaesthetic help is required and should be summoned immediately. A rapid ABC approach to patient assessment is taken at this stage. Whilst simultaneously stabilizing the patient, the vascular surgical and theatre teams are mobilized. Ideally, two experienced anaesthetists should be available. One anaesthetist should prepare the theatre environment and draw up the appropriate drugs, whilst the other transfers the patient to theatre.

Prior to transfer, at least two large-bore IV cannulae should be inserted; blood should be sent for basic biochemistry, FBC, and coagulation studies, and a 12-lead ECG should be performed. It is imperative that a sample of blood is also sent to the transfusion laboratory for urgent cross-matching. Depending on local hospital protocols, it may be desirable to initiate the 'major haemorrhage' protocol at this point. It is best to have red blood cells available in the operating theatre prior to the start of surgery; therefore, if there is any delay in the cross-matching process, O-negative blood should be made available. Almost invariably, FFP and platelet concentrates will be required during surgery, and this should be requested at this early stage. Ten units of red cells, 4 U of FFP, and two pools of platelets are commonly requested quantities.

Having made the diagnosis of a ruptured AAA, it is important that aggressive fluid resuscitation is avoided prior to the start of surgery and the application of an aortic cross-clamp. Unless consciousness is lost or there is evidence of myocardial ischaemia, no IV fluids should be given. This is because large volumes of IV fluids may worsen the haemorrhage by increasing the BP and causing clot disruption. In addition, they may contribute to a dilutional and hypothermic coagulopathy. This practice is referred to as hypotensive resuscitation.

Once the decision for treatment has been made, the patient should be transferred to the operating theatre, fully monitored and with resuscitation equipment available, without delay.

Describe a suitable anaesthetic induction plan for this patient

Prior to the induction of anaesthesia, invasive arterial BP monitoring is desirable. However, this should not delay the start of surgery in very unstable patients. Rapid and significant haemodynamic decompensation can occur, following the induction of anaesthesia. This is caused by a number of mechanisms, including the cardiodepressant and vasodilatory effects of anaesthetic agents, the reduction in tamponade following relaxation of the abdominal musculature, and a reduction in the sympathetic tone. Induction should therefore take place with the patient fully prepared and draped and the surgeons scrubbed and ready for incision. Large-bore IV access should be connected to a primed rapid fluid infusion/warming device. The blood and blood products should be available for immediate use.

The patient is not fasted, and so a modified RSI will be required, with the placement of a cuffed ETT. The exact choice of induction drugs is not of crucial importance. However, drugs that minimize haemodynamic disturbance may be beneficial (etomidate or ketamine). These are often supplemented by opioids (fentanyl, alfentanil, or remifentanil). A dose of suxamethonium will be required to facilitate tracheal intubation. It may be necessary to use vasopressor or inotropic drugs at this point, and a selection of drugs should be prepared in advance (e.g. ephedrine, phenylephrine, adrenaline, calcium gluconate). Anaesthesia is then maintained with either a volatile agent or propofol infusion, ideally guided by a depth of anaesthesia monitor (e.g. BIS) to reduce the likelihood of patient awareness and excessive anaesthetic depth. After the induction of anaesthesia, a CVC should be inserted.

Remember that senior experienced help is required and that good communication between the anaesthetists, surgeons, and other team members is imperative for the smooth running of the case.

The operation begins, and the surgeon manages to clamp the infrarenal aorta. However, there is still ongoing haemorrhage, and the estimated blood loss by this point is 3500 mL. Describe the management of haemorrhage in this case

In emergency aortic surgery, significant blood loss can occur very rapidly. Circulating volume must be maintained with appropriately warmed fluids (crystalloids, colloids, and blood products) administered via large-bore central or peripheral cannulae using a rapid infusion system. Fluid therapy should be guided by the clinical haemodynamic status, CVP, and, if available, cardiac output monitoring. Monitors using pulse pressure or stroke volume variation from arterial waveform analysis can provide a valuable indication of fluid responsiveness and volume status. Where skills exist, transoesophageal echocardiography (TOE) can provide extremely useful information regarding the volume status, in addition to myocardial contractility. It is imperative that the anaesthetists keeps up to date with the volumes of blood lost and fluid infused throughout the procedure.

In a major haemorrhage, a combination of colloids, crystalloids, and blood products will be required. Where available, red cell salvage should be employed, in order to reduce the requirement for allogeneic blood. The patient's Hb concentration should be monitored regularly using point-of-care monitors (e.g. HemoCue® or an ABG analyser with an inbuilt co-oximeter). This will allow anaemia to be detected rapidly and transfusion to be targeted at an appropriate Hb concentration, typically aiming to maintain above 8 g/L. Tolerance of dilutional anaemia may be associated with an increased risk of myocardial ischaemia or stroke.

It is likely that a coagulopathy will develop due to a combination of consumption (of coagulation factors and platelets) and dilution. Efforts should be made to prevent and treat hypothermia, acidaemia, and hypocalcaemia (that will worsen coagulopathy). Near-patient coagulation monitoring is now frequently used in major vascular surgery. Rotational thromboelastography (TEG®), or thromboelastometry (ROTEM®) allows the rapid diagnosis and targeted treatment of coagulopathy within minutes of a blood sample being taken.

Comment on the following ROTEM® results, and describe an appropriate management

ROTEM® is one of the commonly available forms of rotational thromboelastometry (see Figure 9.1). A citrated blood sample is added, along with reagents which activate the extrinsic (EXTEM) and intrinsic (INTEM) coagulation pathways, to a cuvette in which a pin rotates. The rotational movement of the pin is measured precisely. As clotting begins, increasing resistance to the rotational movement of the pin occurs. This is plotted against time to produce the characteristic ROTEM® trace (see Figure 9.1). A number of parameters can then be measured. In simple terms, clotting time (CT) is the time taken from the start of measurement until the first clot is detected. It represents the speed of fibrin formation and is influenced by the number of clotting factors available. It is prolonged by clotting factor deficiencies. Maximum clot firmness (MCF) is measured at the widest point of the trace. It represents stabilization of the clot by fibrin polymerization and platelet function. It is reduced by fibrinogen and platelet deficiencies.

The FIBTEM trace is produced by adding a platelet inhibitor to an EXTEM sample; thus, the contribution of platelets to the clot stabilization process is removed, and, by examining the FIBTEM MCF, it can be deduced whether the patient is deficient in platelets (a normal MCF) or fibrinogen (a low MCF) when the EXTEM or INTEM MCF is abnormal.

In the ROTEM® traces from the patient, both the CT is prolonged, and the MCF is reduced in both the EXTEM and INTEM channels, suggesting clotting factor and fibrinogen deficiencies. This diagnosis is supported by the reduced MCF in the FIBTEM. Initial treatment should be with FFP (10 mL/kg). The ROTEM® should then be repeated immediately to assess the effect of this intervention.

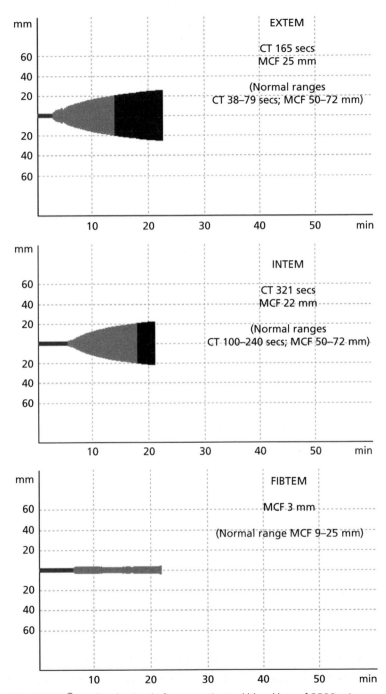

Fig. 9.1 ROTEM® results obtained after an estimated blood loss of 3500 mL.

What are the adverse effects associated with a massive transfusion?

Transfusion of large amounts of allogeneic blood products can be lifesaving, but they may also be associated with a number of adverse effects:

- Biochemical abnormalities: hyperkalaemia, hypocalcaemia
- Acidosis
- Hypothermia
- Coagulopathy
- Allergic reactions
- Transfusion-associated cardiac overload (TACO)
- Transfusion-associated acute lung injury (TRALI)
- Transfusion-associated immunomodulation (TRIM).

What are the physiological consequences of aortic cross-clamping and subsequent unclamping?

Cross-clamping of the aorta above the area of rupture is obviously a crucial step in the surgical procedure. Whilst it will dramatically reduce the rate of haemorrhage, it also increases the BP as a result of raising afterload. This abrupt increase in afterload increases the work of the LV, and this is a typical time where myocardial ischaemia can occur. There may also be a short-lived rise in preload, as the effective circulating volume is effectively reduced at this time. Tissues distal to the clamp inevitably become ischaemic during the time that the clamp is in place. Anaerobic metabolism continues in these poorly perfused tissues, with the accumulation of ischaemic metabolites and lactic acid. On release of the clamps, there is a sudden fall in afterload, as the circulation is restored to the pelvis and lower limbs. This commonly produces hypotension, resulting from a number of mechanisms—the volume of the circulation is suddenly restored, and, in addition, lactic acid and ischaemic metabolites are washed into the circulation, causing systemic vasodilatation, pulmonary vasoconstriction, and myocardial suppression. It is important to ensure an adequate preload before unclamping. However, despite this, the BP may require support with fluids and vasoconstrictors/inotropes if there is a marked hypotensive response.

How is intraoperative myocardial ischaemia detected? Suggest appropriate treatments

Myocardial ischaemia is detected by performing ST segment analysis of the ECG. Any significant depression or elevation of the ST segment can signify ischaemia. Ideally, a 5-electrode ECG should be used, with two limb leads plus one chest lead being monitored to increase the sensitivity of the test. If TOE is available, new ventricular wall motion abnormalities can indicate ischaemia.

If ischaemia is detected, efforts should be made to optimize oxygen delivery (e.g. by ensuring adequate oxyhaemoglobin saturation and correcting anaemia and hypotension). Attempting to reduce myocardial oxygen consumption may also be appropriate in some circumstances—with a β-blocker if the HR is high, or using vasodilator therapy if there is marked hypertension. Short-acting drugs, such as esmolol and GTN, are ideal in this situation.

How should this patient be cared for in the immediate post-operative period? What are the main issues following surgery for a ruptured abdominal aortic aneurysm?

All patients will require intensive care post-operatively. Careful monitoring of all organ systems is mandatory, as multiple organ dysfunction is possible. In the immediate post-operative period, efforts should be made to re-warm the patient, treat any residual coagulopathy that exists, and correct any acid–base disturbance. Ventilatory support will be required for a variable period of time (a few hours to days), whilst cardiovascular support and renal replacement therapy will be required for some patients. Intra-abdominal hypertension is common after surgery for a ruptured AAA. Ideally, the intra-abdominal pressure should be monitored to identify those patients who are developing abdominal compartment syndrome.

Summary

A ruptured AAA is a vascular surgical emergency that is associated with significant morbidity and mortality. Optimal care requires excellent communication between the different professional groups involved at each stage of the treatment process.

The anaesthetist caring for the patient with a ruptured AAA needs to be aware of the potential for profound haemodynamic instability, myocardial ischaemia, coagulopathy, and marked acid–base disturbance. It is crucial that appropriate treatments are instituted in a timely fashion to minimize the impact of these factors.

Further reading

Roberts K, Revell M, Youssef H, Bradbury AW, and Adam DJ (2006). Hypotensive resuscitation in patients with ruptured abdominal aortic aneurysm. *European Journal of Vascular and Endovascular Surgery*, **31**, 339–44.

Case 9.2

Carotid endarterectomy

Background

Carotid endarterectomy (CEA) is a preventative procedure that aims to reduce the likelihood of a major disabling stroke or death in patients who have experienced a minor stroke or a transient ischaemic attack (TIA) and who also have a significant stenosis of the ipsilateral internal carotid artery. The risk of a major stroke is highest in the period immediately following a minor stroke or TIA. Therefore, to produce the maximum reduction in risk, CEA should be performed within 2 weeks of a minor stroke or TIA.

Learning outcomes

1 Discuss the preoperative assessments and medical management prior to carotid endarterectomy

2 Appreciate the risks and benefits of regional vs general anaesthesia for carotid endarterectomy

3 Manage an acute airway compromise due to post-operative haematoma formation.

CPD matrix matches

2A03; 2A10; 2G01

Case history

A 57-year-old male accountant with a 30 pack year smoking history is scheduled for a left-sided CEA. Seven days previously, whilst in a business meeting, he experienced an episode of weakness affecting his right arm, accompanied by expressive dysphasia. His symptoms resolved completely within 20 min. Previously, he was taking no medications, but, following this event, he has been started on clopidogrel and simvastatin.

What investigative imaging would you expect this patient to have undergone prior to listing for surgery?

The patient is likely to have undergone a CT scan of the head to exclude a cerebral haemorrhage or space-occupying lesion. He will also have had bilateral carotid duplex ultrasonography performed. Clear benefits are gained by carrying out CEA in patients with symptomatic internal carotid artery stenosis of ≥70%. Some male patients (but not females) with lesser degrees of stenosis (50–69%) may benefit from CEA, but the number of patients needed to treat to prevent a stroke is higher in this group. Importantly, a duplex scan should be repeated in the hours prior to surgery to ensure that the carotid artery has not occluded completely, as there is no benefit from proceeding with surgery in this situation.

What are the important features of your preoperative assessment in this case?

A standard preoperative assessment should be made, with particular reference to the following points.

History

◆ It is essential to establish which symptoms occurred at the time of the TIA, the patient's current neurological status, and the presence of any residual deficits. The occurrence of further TIAs following the index event is also important, as patients with crescendo TIAs are at increased risk of a perioperative stroke

◆ Patients with cerebrovascular disease often have other forms of cardiovascular disease and factors which increase the risk of perioperative complications—ischaemic heart disease, hypertension, chronic kidney disease, and diabetes mellitus are common, as is a history of cigarette smoking

◆ Smokers have a higher incidence of respiratory disease, and, if surgery is planned under regional anaesthesia, the ability to lie flat and still without coughing or desaturation is important. Cognitive function and the ability to obey commands are also important if regional anaesthesia is planned.

Medications

◆ All patients should be on antiplatelet therapy. Guidelines regarding the optimal choice of drugs for secondary prevention change frequently, with either clopidogrel as a single agent or aspirin plus dipyridamole currently recommended

◆ In addition to antiplatelet drugs, statin therapy not only reduces the risk of further stroke, but also lowers the incidence of perioperative cardiac events

◆ Poorly controlled hypertension is a risk factor for perioperative stroke. Ideally, the BP should be well controlled when the patient presents for CEA, although this is often not the case. In general, antiplatelet, statin, and antihypertensive drugs should be continued throughout the perioperative period.

Investigations

◆ BP should be recorded in both arms prior to surgery, as co-existing subclavian artery stenosis (producing unequal brachial BPs) is not uncommon. In this situation, the higher reading should be used for BP measurement

◆ The results of FBC, U&E, glucose, and a 12-lead ECG should be available. A specimen should be sent to the transfusion laboratory for 'group and save'

◆ It is also important to know the result of the carotid duplex scan. Important features to note include the degree of stenosis in both the carotid artery that is to be operated on and also the contralateral carotid. A high-grade stenosis in the contralateral carotid artery increases the likelihood of an inadequate flow in the circle of Willis during the time that the carotid artery is clamped and may increase the likelihood of requiring a temporary shunt.

What are the anaesthetic options for carotid endarterectomy? What are the advantages and disadvantages of each?

CEA can be performed under either general or local anaesthesia. There is no clear-cut evidence that demonstrates the superiority of one technique over the other, although the GALA trial suggested that local anaesthesia may be better for patients in whom the contralateral carotid is occluded. Local anaesthesia is also associated with a reduced use of temporary shunts during the procedure and a reduced incidence of post-operative wound haemorrhage.

What are the common goals of anaesthesia for carotid endarterectomy?

Ideally, the patient should be pain-free, well oxygenated, and haemodynamically stable throughout the perioperative period, no matter whether local or general anaesthesia is chosen as the anaesthetic technique. Unfortunately, the BP can be labile during CEA, no matter which anaesthetic technique is chosen, and the anaesthetist must be prepared to manipulate the BP upwards or downwards at any point. A range of drugs, including esmolol, labetalol, ephedrine, and phenylephrine, should be immediately available. It has been suggested that the BP should be maintained within ± 20% of the baseline BP throughout the procedure. However, there are occasions during the period of cross-clamping where a BP in excess of this may be useful in maximizing flow in the circle of Willis and maintaining an acceptable cerebral perfusion. An arterial pressure monitoring line should be inserted prior to the start of anaesthesia.

Local anaesthesia

Superficial, intermediate, deep, or combined cervical plexus blocks, placed with or without the aid of ultrasound, have been described for CEA. Meta-analyses of a number of trials that compared the analgesic efficacy of these different types of cervical plexus blocks concluded that deep blocks do not improve the quality of analgesia, compared with superficial blocks. However, the risk of serious complications (intravascular or intrathecal injection) is significantly higher with deep blocks. Local anaesthetic techniques are often combined with IV sedation—TCIs of propofol and remifentanil (in low doses) are ideal for this purpose, as they are readily titratable and short-acting.

Advantages of local anaesthetic techniques

- Allows the assessment of neurological status throughout the case (this is the main advantage over general anaesthesia)
- Avoids the need for airway management
- Reduces the need for temporary shunt placement, hence reduces the incidence of shunt-associated complications (distal emboli and arterial dissection)
- Preserves cerebral autoregulation and blood flow to the contralateral hemisphere.

Disadvantages of local anaesthetic techniques

- Inadequate analgesia requiring supplemental local anaesthetic by the surgeon (this is almost inevitable during the dissection of the carotid sheath, as this is innervated by the glossopharyngeal nerve, not the cervical plexus)
- Oversedation (if sedative drugs are used)
- Requirement to lie flat and still
- Risks of intraoperative conversion to general anaesthesia (<2% of cases)
- Complications associated with the block (intravascular or intrathecal injection; phrenic nerve block).

General anaesthesia

CEA can also be performed under general anaesthesia. Due to the site of surgery and a difficult access to the airway, a technique that involves tracheal intubation and mechanical ventilation is most commonly used. Short-acting anaesthetic drugs that wear off quickly after surgery and allow a rapid assessment of neurology should be used. Propofol, remifentanil, and desflurane are ideal agents.

Advantages of general anaesthesia

- ◆ Immobile patient for the duration of the operation
- ◆ Control of airway and ventilation ($PaCO_2$).

Disadvantages of general anaesthesia

- ◆ No direct neurological assessment possible (with reliance on indirect monitors)
- ◆ Increased use of shunts
- ◆ Increased incidence of intraoperative hypotension.

What methods are available for monitoring cerebral perfusion during carotid endarterectomy?

Surgery performed under local anaesthesia allows regular direct clinical assessment of the conscious level, upper limb motor strength, vision, speech, and some higher cognitive functions (e.g. simple arithmetic). This is considered to be the 'gold standard' method for assessing the adequacy of cerebral perfusion and is one of the major justifications for performing CEA using local anaesthetic techniques. Obviously, this is not possible during general anaesthesia where a number of alternative indirect methods have been described to assess cerebral perfusion. These include cerebral oximetry using near-infrared spectroscopy; measurement of the cerebral blood flow in the ipsilateral middle cerebral artery using transcranial Doppler; somatosensory evoked potentials; and measurement of carotid artery stump pressures. All of these methods have significant limitations, and the decision to insert a temporary shunt, or not, is often based on somewhat arbitrary cut-off values, depending on which monitoring technique is used. Some anaesthetists and surgeons advocate the routine insertion of an elective shunt if surgery is performed under general anaesthesia.

A local anaesthesia technique is chosen. Unfortunately, the patient becomes unresponsive following cross-clamping of the internal carotid artery. Describe the subsequent management

Communication between the surgeon and anaesthetist is crucial in this situation. The anaesthetist should declare that there is likely to be an inadequate cerebral perfusion, and the surgeon should prepare to insert a temporary shunt. Meanwhile, attempts should be made to improve the cerebral perfusion by increasing the mean arterial BP to a level above the normal baseline. IV fluids, plus bolus doses of ephedrine or phenylephrine, may be required to achieve this. Any sedative agents should be discontinued. If there is no improvement in the neurological status and the patient remains unresponsive after the BP has been raised, the surgeon should proceed with the insertion of a temporary shunt which bypasses the area of the carotid artery that has been clamped. This usually results in a rapid improvement in the conscious level and neurological function. In this situation, it is appropriate to continue surgery under local anaesthesia. However, if there is airway compromise or an inadequacy of ventilation, then conversion to general anaesthesia may be required.

Prior to closure, the surgeon complains of excessive bleeding from the suture line of the arteriotomy. What are the possible causes, and how would you investigate and manage this situation?

1 Excessive heparin effect: IV heparin (in a dose 70 IU/kg) is usually administered prior to cross-clamping the carotid artery. Occasionally, an excessive heparin effect persists towards the end of surgery that makes haemostasis difficult to achieve. This can be confirmed by measuring APTT in the operating theatre, using a near-patient monitor, and protamine can then be administered, if required

2 Excessive antiplatelet effect: treatment with antiplatelet therapy, particularly when two antiplatelet drugs are used, can also lead to problems with haemostasis. Ideally, the effect of antiplatelet agents should be assessed using a near-patient platelet function analyser. If a profound antiplatelet effect is present, then platelet transfusion should be considered.

You are called to the ward by a junior doctor 2 hours following surgery, because the patient is finding it difficult to breathe. On examination, the patient is tachypnoeic and cyanosed, with a large swelling on the left side of the neck. There is audible stridor. What is the diagnosis, and what is your management?

The patient has developed a haematoma which is compressing the upper airway; this is an emergency situation that requires immediate action. Call for senior help, and administer high-flow oxygen. If the patient is *in extremis*, then insufficient time exists to return to the operating theatre. Medical staff on the ward must be prepared to remove the skin sutures (or staples) and evacuate the haematoma. Depending on the exact location of the bleeding point and how the neck has been closed, it may also be necessary to remove deeper sutures that have been used to close the cervical fascia and platysma muscle. This is an emergency, lifesaving act, following which the patient will need to return to theatre for formal exploration and haemostasis.

Summary

CEA is an effective treatment option for some patients with significant carotid artery atherosclerosis who have suffered a TIA or minor stroke. The aim of the procedure is to reduce the risk of a further stroke causing death or disability. For CEA to be of maximum value, the risks around the time of surgery need to minimized as far as possible. The combined risk of death or stroke in the perioperative period should be <3%. In order to achieve this, carotid surgery should only be performed by experienced teams of professionals who are aware of the many potential problems that the patient may experience around the time of surgery.

Further reading

GALA Trial Collaborative Group (2008). General anaesthesia versus local anaesthesia for carotid surgery (GALA): a multicentre, randomised controlled trial. *Lancet*, **372**, 2132–42.

Case 9.3

Elective aorto-femoral arterial revascularization

Background

This operation is performed to improve the arterial circulation to the lower limbs when significant occlusive disease affects the distal aorta and/or the iliac arteries. It is a major surgical procedure which involves a laparotomy and bilateral groin operations. A prosthetic graft is anastomosed to the infrarenal aorta and femoral arteries to bypass areas of arterial stenosis or occlusion.

Risks of aorto-bifemoral grafting include haemorrhage, coagulopathy, infection, major organ dysfunction (myocardial ischaemia, cerebrovascular accident, renal impairment, ARDS), limb loss, impotence, and ischaemia of the pelvic contents. The risks of an MI or death within 30 days of surgery exceed 5%.

Learning outcomes

1 Perform a detailed cardiac risk profiling prior to the proposed vascular surgery

2 Optimize medical therapies prior to elective surgery.

CPD matrix matches

2A03; 2A07

Case history

A 71-year-old retired taxi driver presents with a history of left thigh claudication that prevents him from walking >75 m. He has already been assessed by a vascular surgeon who arranged for a magnetic resonance angiogram to be performed. This revealed areas of significant stenosis in his left common iliac artery and more minor stenosis in his distal aorta. The vascular surgeon has asked you to assess his fitness for aorto-bifemoral bypass surgery.

He has type II diabetes, controlled hypertension, and a history of angina in the past. He is overweight with a BMI of 38 kg/m^2. He continues to smoke 15 cigarettes a day. Five years ago, coronary angiography was performed following a non-ST elevation MI. This demonstrated a tight stenosis in the proximal circumflex artery and 50% stenoses in the left anterior descending and right coronary arteries. The circumflex lesion was treated by the insertion of a bare metal stent. He does not currently suffer from any angina. He has no history of cerebrovascular disease.

His medications include aspirin, ramipril, and insulin. His renal function is impaired (Cr 200 micromoles/L). A 12-lead ECG shows sinus rhythm, with no evidence of ischaemic changes. Resting echocardiography shows no valvular abnormalities, and LV systolic function is within normal limits.

What alternative treatments might be considered, rather than aorto-bifemoral bypass grafting? What is the role of the anaesthetist in this decision-making process?

Aorto-bifemoral bypass grafting is a major surgical procedure that is associated with a significant risk of cardiovascular complications or death in the perioperative period. This risk is much higher in patients who have co-existing diseases.

A number of alternative lower-risk management strategies exists for this condition. The anaesthetist can play an important role in estimating the level of risk for individual patients. This information can then be used to inform decisions regarding the most appropriate choice of treatment.

Alternative management strategies that entail lower risks (which may be more appropriate for less fit patients) include conservative treatment; this would include the optimization of medical therapy by adding a statin to the current medications, smoking cessation strategies, and exercise, ideally as part of a structured exercise plan. Endovascular treatment (angioplasty and stent insertion) may be possible for short stenoses within the iliac arteries. Alternative surgical procedures that are less physiologically stressful (and associated with lower rates of perioperative complications/death) involve extra-anatomical grafts and include axillo-femoral (or axillo-bifemoral) and femoro-femoral cross-over grafts.

What is the revised cardiac risk index? How might it be used in the preoperative assessment of this patient?

The revised cardiac risk index (RCRI)* is a simple clinical risk-scoring system that was derived and validated for the prediction of major adverse cardiovascular events (MACE) after surgery. It is currently considered to be one of the best evidence-based clinical risk-scoring systems and is utilized by both European and American preoperative assessment guidelines to help predict cardiac risk in the perioperative period.

---

* Data from Lee, T. H. et al., 1999, 'Derivation and prospective validation of a simple index for prediction of cardiac risk of major noncardiac surgery', *Circulation*, 100, 10, pp. 1043–1049.

One point is allocated for:

- History of ischaemic heart disease
- History of congestive heart failure
- History of cerebrovascular disease
- Insulin therapy for diabetes mellitus
- Renal impairment (Cr >177 micromoles/L)
- High-risk surgery (intraperitoneal, intrathoracic, or suprainguinal vascular).

Rates of major cardiac events in the original validation cohort with 0, 1, 2, or ≥3 risk factors were 0.4%, 0.9%, 7%, and 11%, respectively.

How else could you quantify the perioperative risk for this patient? What further investigations might be useful?

A number of methods can be used to assess the perioperative risk, in addition to clinical risk-scoring systems.

Assessment of functional capacity

Attempts should be made to quantify exercise tolerance in terms of METs. METs are multiples of the basal metabolic requirement for oxygen (3.5 mL/kg/min). Lists of common activities and their associated METs are available. For example, carrying out light housework requires around 4 METs. This value is important, as being unable to carry out activities that require 4 METs is associated with increased risk, both in the perioperative period and longer term. If possible, it is always better to make an objective assessment of the functional capacity, rather than rely on the patient's estimates. There are a number of different ways in which this can be done; one of the simplest is to walk up stairs with the patient and observe how they manage this activity, noting any symptoms experienced and how many flights are climbed. The ability to climb two flights of stairs requires between 4 and 5.5 METs, whilst being unable to climb two flights of stairs is associated with increased risks of perioperative morbidity. Another alternative test that can be considered is the six-minute walk test. This measures the distance that can be covered in 6 min over a flat surface. The obvious limitation of any of these functional assessments is that patients with severe peripheral arterial disease will almost certainly be limited by their claudication symptoms.

Cardiopulmonary exercise testing

This is the gold standard method for objectively assessing exercise capacity. It is now commonly used by anaesthetists as part of the preoperative assessment of patients prior to major surgery. CPET (or CPX) is an integrated test of cardiorespiratory function where a period of graded exercise is performed on either a bicycle ergometer or treadmill. A number of parameters, including peak oxygen consumption (VO_2 peak), oxygen consumption at the anaerobic threshold (AT), and ventilatory equivalents for oxygen and carbon dioxide, can be determined accurately during the test. In addition, 12-lead ECG monitoring and ST segment analysis take place to detect any exercise-induced arrhythmias, or myocardial ischaemia. A low VO_2 peak, low AT, raised ventilatory equivalents for carbon dioxide, and evidence of myocardial ischaemia, in association with a low AT, have all been associated with increased risks of mortality after major surgery.

Dobutamine stress echocardiography

This involves performing conventional transthoracic echocardiography at the same time as infusing increasing doses of dobutamine intravenously. The presence and severity of any new ventricular wall motion abnormalities are noted during the period of inotropic and chronotropic stress. The number of segments of the LV that function abnormally can be correlated with the risk of perioperative cardiac complications. The test has a high negative predictive value (90–100%) for perioperative cardiac complications.

Myocardial perfusion scanning

This involves IV injection of thallium (a nuclear tracer), which is taken up by the myocardium, and dipyridamole (which induces myocardial stress by causing vasodilatation and tachycardia). Areas of the myocardium with a poor blood supply during stress can be identified by poor thallium uptake. The reversibility of ischaemia can be assessed by repeating the scan after a number of hours when the tachycardia has resolved and the thallium uptake is complete. This test has a similar high negative predictive value for perioperative cardiac complications.

Biomarkers

Elevated brain natriuretic peptide (BNP) levels have been shown to be associated with cardiac complications following major surgery. However, at present, there is no consensus regarding optimal cut-off values for use in preoperative risk stratification.

Would you recommend repeat coronary angiography?

Coronary angiography may be appropriate for selected patients being considered for major vascular surgery—if the patient is suffering from severe angina or has a strongly positive stress test or develops extensive new wall motion abnormalities during stress echocardiography. In these situations, the aim is to identify those patients with very significant coronary artery disease (left main stem or severe triple-vessel disease) whose long-term prognosis may be improved by performing coronary artery bypass grafting (CABG). However, it should be noted that CABG should not be performed routinely in patients with stable coronary artery disease prior to vascular surgery, as this approach does not improve clinical outcomes. Furthermore, it must be emphasized that percutaneous coronary intervention (PCI) with stent insertion is associated with worse outcomes, compared to optimal medical treatment of coronary artery disease, when performed immediately prior to major surgery. This is due to the high incidence of within-stent thrombosis that can occur secondary to the inflammatory and procoagulant effects of major surgery. In addition, there is a requirement for continuous dual antiplatelet therapy after stent insertion (for 3 months after a bare metal stent insertion and 12 months after a drug-eluting stent insertion)—this may have consequences for both haemostasis and regional anaesthesia.

Would you recommend any changes to medication prior to surgery?

This patient should be on long-term statin therapy for a number of reasons—to reduce the likelihood of future cardiovascular events and death, and to slow the progression of peripheral arterial disease and improve his claudication distance. In addition, when taken around the time of major vascular surgery, statin therapy reduces the risk of death or cardiac complications. These beneficial 'pleiotropic' effects of statins may result from an increased atherosclerotic plaque stability caused by reduced levels of vascular inflammation, matrix metalloproteinases, and lipid oxidation. Statins should be continued throughout the perioperative period, as the withdrawal of statin therapy may increase the likelihood of cardiovascular complications by a 'rebound' effect.

The literature concerning the role of β-blockers in reducing perioperative risk is somewhat confusing. Early studies of β-blockers in patients with, or at risk of, ischaemic heart disease demonstrated significant reductions in the risk of cardiac death or non-fatal MI after major surgery. These studies prompted the widespread use of β-blockers in patients undergoing vascular surgery. However, a number of studies have since been published that have cast doubt on the appropriateness of this approach. Most recently, the POISE study, a large randomized, placebo-controlled study of the effects of metoprolol in patients undergoing major non-cardiac surgery, has confirmed that perioperative β-blockade does reduce the incidence of MI, but this is at the expense of an increase in all-cause mortality and an excess of cerebrovascular accidents. It is postulated that the increased risk of morbidity and mortality observed in this study relates to hypotension caused by the large doses of metoprolol that were used and the timing of the start of therapy immediately prior to surgery. Notwithstanding the limitations of this study, it has raised concerns that β-blockers may not be appropriate for all patients undergoing vascular surgery. Currently, β-blockers are recommended for patients at the highest risk around the time of vascular surgery (these are patients with evidence of myocardial ischaemia on preoperative stress testing) or for those with multiple (≥3) clinical risk factors. It is also strongly recommended that chronic β-blocker therapy should be continued and not be withdrawn acutely, as this has been shown to lead to rebound increases in myocardial ischaemia and mortality.

This patient should also be on long-term β-blocker therapy as a secondary preventative measure post-MI. In addition, he has multiple clinical risk factors. The optimal time to start therapy remains to be clearly defined, but, by starting some days prior to surgery (ideally up to 30 days), there is ample time to titrate the dose to achieve HRs within the range of 60–70 bpm and avoid hypotension. Currently, β1 selective agents with no intrinsic sympathomimetic activity, such as bisoprolol, are considered the best drugs to use. Finally, it is worth emphasizing that β-blockers are not contraindicated in patients with claudication or chronic obstructive pulmonary disease (COPD).

Antiplatelet drugs

All patients with peripheral arterial disease should be treated with an antiplatelet drug (most commonly aspirin) to reduce their long-term risk of cardiovascular complications. Historically, antiplatelet therapy was stopped prior to elective surgery to reduce the risk of haemorrhage. However, it is now appreciated that one of the factors contributing to a perioperative MI is the prothrombotic state that develops around the time of surgery. It has been suggested that antiplatelet therapy may reduce the likelihood of perioperative myocardial ischaemia by altering this procoagulant state. Indeed, the withdrawal of aspirin therapy in the perioperative period is associated with an increased incidence of MACE, and, whilst the incidence of bleeding complications may be increased by a factor of up to 1.5 by continuing aspirin, the severity of these complications is not increased. Therefore, it has been suggested that aspirin should only be discontinued if the risks of bleeding outweigh the potential cardiac benefits.

This patient scores four RCRI points and so is in a higher risk category. He is currently complaining of claudication symptoms, which may have a significant impact on his lifestyle but are neither life nor limb-threatening. These important facts must be borne in mind when weighing up the potential benefits and risks of any treatment strategy. Many surgeons, given the non-limb-threatening ischaemia that he is experiencing, would not proceed with aortic surgery in this situation. Alternative options are conservative management that includes exercise and formal smoking cessation strategies or to proceed with a less major form of revascularization treatment such as a right femoral to left femoral artery cross-over graft.

Summary

Reconstructive aortic surgery for aorto-iliac occlusive disease is a very major surgical undertaking, with risks that exceed those associated with an elective aortic aneurysm repair. The anaesthetist should play a significant role in the preoperative assessment of patients being considered for this type of surgery. They should ensure that all co-existing diseases have been optimized and that appropriate secondary preventative medications have been started in advance of any surgical procedure. They should also play an active role in the multidisciplinary team (surgeons, radiologists, and anaesthetists) that discusses treatment options and decides on the optimal treatment plan.

Further reading

Fleisher LA, Beckman JA, Brown KA, *et al.* (2007). ACC/AHA 2007 Guidelines on perioperative cardiovascular evaluation and care for noncardiac surgery: a report of the American College of Cardiology/American Heart Association task force on practice guidelines (writing committee to revise the 2002 guidelines on perioperative cardiovascular evaluation for noncardiac surgery). *Circulation*, **116**, e418–99.

Lee TH, Marcantonio ER, Mangione CM, *et al.* (1999). Derivation and prospective validation of a simple index for prediction of cardiac risk of major noncardiac surgery. *Circulation*, **100**, 1043–9.

POISE study group, Devereaux PJ, Yang H, Yusuf S, *et al.* (2008). Effects of extended-release metoprolol succinate in patients undergoing non-cardiac surgery (POISE trial): a randomised controlled trial. *Lancet*, **371**, 1839–47.

Chapter 10

Cardiothoracic anaesthesia

Dr Alistair Gibson
Dr Colin Moore
Dr Sheena Millar

Lung isolation techniques

Background

This case aims to highlight the available lung isolation techniques for pulmonary resection, the indications for their use, and troubleshooting commonly occurring problems.

Learning outcomes

1 Outline the pre-assessment principles for a patient preparing for intrathoracic surgery

2 Discuss the different techniques for employing one-lung ventilation (OLV) anaesthesia.

CPD matrix matches

2A01; 2A03

Case history

You are scheduled to anaesthetize a 61-year-old gentleman for a right-sided pneumonectomy and have been called to see him in the pre-admission clinic. He has a diagnosis of non-small cell lung cancer, and his surgery is intended to be a curative procedure. He is a lifelong heavy smoker and suffers from hypertension, AF, and angina. He has a BMI of 22.

The pre-assessment nurse has taken some baseline observations and performed an ECG for you on your arrival. Current observations are: BP 176/110 (remains raised on three repeated measurements in clinic), pulse rate 58 bpm, RR 21 breaths/min, temperature 36.8°C. His ECG shows rate-controlled AF, with no obvious signs of current or previous ischaemia.

How would you assess this patient's fitness for surgery?

This patient should be assessed, based on the recommendations set out by the British Thoracic Society guidelines of 2001 and the more recent NICE guidelines of 2011 (lung cancer).

- Patients should be assessed, using a global risk score such as THORACOSCORE
- Age is not a barrier to surgery; it is, however, known that patients of advancing age will require greater levels of perioperative support and, as a result, have higher morbidity and mortality rates
- Assessment should be made of the cardiovascular function, and surgery delayed if the patient has had an MI within 30 days. If the patient has an active cardiac condition or three or more risk factors, they should be seen preoperatively by a cardiologist. If they have no active conditions and two or fewer risk factors, no further cardiac investigation is indicated
- Respiratory function should be measured. This should be done in the sequence outlined below for patients undergoing a pneumonectomy

  1 Spirometry: if normal spirometry and good exercise tolerance, no further investigation is required. If, however, the post-bronchodilator FEV_1 is <55% of the predicted value (<2 L), further investigation is required

  2 Perform a quantitative perfusion scan, and calculate the patient's estimated post-operative FEV_1

  3 Perform the transfer factor test TLCO, and calculate the estimated post-operative transfer factor

  4 Express both post-operative transfer factor and FEV_1 as a percentage of predicted values, and assess oxygen saturations on room air. If these variables are <40% predicted, then the patient is considered high risk, and surgery should only be offered if the patient accepts the risk of complications and persistent dyspnoea post-operatively. If the measured values are >40% predicted, then surgery should be undertaken without further assessment. Any other combination of findings should precipitate further exercise testing

  5 Exercise testing should take the form of a full CPET; however, if this is not available, then the shuttle walk test may be conducted. If the patient has a VO_2 max of >15 mL/kg/min, then surgery should proceed as planned, or alternatively if they manage >25 shuttles with <4% oxygen desaturation, they should be listed for theatre. If they do not meet either of these criteria, consideration should be given to a less extensive resection or to radical radiotherapy.

What information would you like to obtain from this patient in the pre-admission clinic?

- Current level of dyspnoea
- Exercise tolerance

- Smoking status
- Presence of cardiac risk factors
- Associated comorbid conditions
- Nutritional status: a poor nutritional status has known associations with increased post- operative complications
- Treatment to date
- Medication history
- Anaesthetic history
- Presence or absence of reflux disease.

What examination will you undertake?

- Cardiorespiratory exam looking specifically for signs of congestive cardiac failure or pulmonary hypertension which are associated with high levels of perioperative morbidity and mortality
- Airway assessment
- Assessment of dentition.

What investigations will you request?

- ECG
- Pulmonary function tests (as outlined earlier in the text)
- ABG (if the pulmonary function test results are borderline)
- Baseline haematology, coagulation, and biochemistry blood tests; ensure that cross-matched blood will be available.

The patient will already have had a plain CXR film and high-resolution CT thorax, and these should be reviewed by the anaesthetist.

Case update

Your patient has three cardiovascular risk factors in the form of rhythm other than sinus, uncontrolled hypertension, and mild angina pectoris; you therefore arrange for the patient to be seen by a cardiologist. Following review by your cardiology colleagues, who have rationalized the patient's antihypertensives and continued all the other cardiac medications, you ask for the patient to undergo pulmonary function testing. Based on the steps mentioned earlier, the patient is declared fit for pneumonectomy.

What are the principles of anaesthetic management for patients undergoing a pneumonectomy?

+ Patients will require general anaesthesia with mandatory ventilation which, in most centres, will be combined with a regional technique such as an epidural, a paravertebral block, or intercostals nerve blocks
+ The ability to isolate the lungs and perform OLV, although not an absolute requirement, is highly desirable
+ Aims are to avoid inhibition of hypoxic pulmonary vasoconstriction, reduce airway irritability, and maintain cardiovascular stability
+ Intraoperative fluid administration should be restricted as far as possible, as the handling of the lung tissue impairs pulmonary capillary function, placing the patient at high risk of post-operative pulmonary oedema
+ Consideration should be given to patient positioning in the lateral decubitus position.

What techniques are available to facilitate one-lung ventilation?

There are three devices which allow lung isolation and therefore OLV.

1 Double-lumen tubes (DLTs):

  • These are the most commonly used devices to achieve lung isolation. Their popularity stems from the fact that they allow independent control of each lung
  • These devices can be either right- or left-sided and come in several different sizes and designs
  • As the name suggests, the tube has two lumens, one of which is long enough and appropriately angulated to reach the right or left main bronchus, and the other lumen is shorter and terminates in the distal trachea. The bronchial lumen has a bronchial cuff which allows separation of the lungs. The tube also has a tracheal cuff that separates the lungs from the oropharynx and the environment
  • Anatomically, the left main bronchus is longer than the right, making it much easier to correctly position a left-sided tube
  • The DLT has two curves; the bronchial lumen curve, being orientated initially anteriorly in order to pass into the tracheal inlet and then being rotated in the direction of the bronchus you are aiming to intubate
  • After $ETCO_2$ has been detected, appropriate tube positioning is confirmed by visual inspection of chest movement and by auscultation of the chest, whilst alternately clamping one lumen and ventilating the other. A fibreoptic bronchoscope is used to further check appropriate tube positioning

2 Bronchial blockers:

- These are reserved for use in situations where DLTs are deemed unsuitable. For example, in children where DLTs may be too large, in distorted airway anatomy that prevents the passage of the DLT, in critically ill patients who already have single-lumen ETT *in situ* and in whom a tube change is deemed dangerous, or when DLT insertion has been difficult or impossible
- Bronchial blockers are single-lumen, balloon-tipped endoluminal catheters
- A single-lumen, cuffed orotracheal tube is placed first, and, through it, the bronchial blocker is advanced into the main bronchus under direct vision using a bronchoscope
- The selected bronchus is then occluded by inflating the balloon
- The central lumen allows passive lung deflation, suction, and insufflations with oxygen, if required
- The main disadvantage to the use of bronchial blockers is that, in order to ventilate both lungs, the isolation of the lungs is lost

3 Endobronchial intubation with single-lumen ETT:

- Mainly reserved for the emergency separation of the two lungs, e.g. in severe pulmonary haemorrhage
- An uncut single-lumen ETT is used and will normally intubate the right main bronchus if it is not guided using a bronchoscope.

Can you list the indications for one-lung ventilation?

Absolute indications

- Isolation of the lungs to prevent cross-contamination, particularly in cases of pulmonary haemorrhage or in the presence of infections affecting a single lung
- Bronchopleural fistula where OLV allows a controlled distribution of ventilation.

Relative indications

- Facilitation of surgical procedure.

Case update

You have opted to use a double-lumen tube in order to achieve lung separation in your patient. You have selected a 39F left-sided DLT and successfully placed it within the left main bronchus, confirmed by using $ETCO_2$ monitoring, auscultation, visual inspection, and bronchoscopy. The patient has been positioned and draped for surgery, and the surgeon asks you to initiate OLV.

How would you establish one-lung ventilation? What ventilator strategy would you employ?

1 Establishing one-lung anaesthesia using a DLT:
  - A clamp is placed on the tracheal lumen to ensure all ventilation is delivered to the dependent (left) lung
  - The tracheal lumen of the DLT is then opened to air to facilitate the deflation of the right lung

2 Ventilator strategies for OLV:
  - ALI, following pneumonectomy, occurs in 2–4% of cases, despite fluid restrictive management, and is associated with a mortality of 25–50%; it has been established that this may be due to volutrauma and barotrauma during OLV
  - Maintain FiO_2 as low as possible
  - Avoid atelectasis with frequent recruitment manoeuvres
  - Tidal volume 5–6 mL/kg; external PEEP of 4–10 cmH_2O; RR of 15–20 breaths/min
  - Pressure control ventilation (peak inspiratory pressure <35 cmH_2O)
  - Permissive hypercapnia is an accepted consequence of lung-protective strategies.

Case update

Your patient has been established on OLV for approximately 40 min, and surgery is progressing well. However, you notice that his oxygen saturations have begun to fall from 96%, with an FiO_2 of 0.4, to 88%.

How would you approach the management of hypoxia and one-lung ventilation?

- Hypoxaemia affects post-operative outcomes, with an increased incidence of cognitive dysfunction, AF, renal failure, and pulmonary hypertension
- Increase FiO_2 to 1.0
- Confirm the position of the DLT, using a fibreoptic bronchoscope, and confirm that the anaesthetic machine and equipment are functioning appropriately
- If airway pressures are high, suctioning to clear any blood or secretions from the tube and an assessment for bronchospasm should be performed

- Ensure adequate cardiac output and Hb for oxygen delivery
- Supply passive oxygen flow to the non-ventilated lung, e.g. 2–4 L/min via a C-circuit. This may be enough to reduce the V/Q mismatching and improve oxygenation
- If hypoxaemia is persistent, then applying CPAP of 5–10 cmH$_2$O to the non-ventilated lung would be the next step. However, this may impede surgical progress, and so communication of the situation with the surgeon is important
- Intermittent ventilation of both lungs may be required
- Clamping of the appropriate pulmonary artery will essentially remove the shunting of blood through the non-ventilated lung and treat the hypoxaemia.

Summary

Anaesthesia for lung resection and lung isolation are challenging techniques and should only be carried out by those individuals who are familiar with the use of lung isolation equipment and the techniques required to trouble-shoot any resultant complications. An in-depth knowledge of cardiorespiratory anatomy and physiology is an absolute requirement, and the thoracic anaesthetist should be involved in patient selection and meticulous preparation.

Further reading

British Thoracic Society and Society of Cardiothoracic Surgeons of Great Britain and Ireland Working Party (2001). Guidelines on the selection of patients with lung cancer for surgery. *Thorax*, **56**, 89–108

Eastwood J and Mahajan R (2002). One-lung anaesthesia. *British Journal of Anaesthesia CEPD Reviews*, **2**, 83–7.

Karzai W and Schwarzkopf K (2009). Hypoxaemia during one lung ventilation. *Anesthesiology*, **110**, 1402–112.

Kilpatrick B and Slinger P (2010). Lung protective strategies in anaesthesia. *British Journal of Anaesthesia*, **105**, 108–16.

National Institute for Health and Clinical Excellence (2011). *Lung cancer: the diagnosis and treatment of lung cancer. Clinical guidelines, CG121.* Available at: <http://guidance.nice.org.uk/CG121>.

Ng A and Swanevelder J (2011). Hypoxaemia associated with one-lung anaesthesia: new discoveries in ventilation and perfusion. *British Journal of Anaesthesia*, **106**, 761–3.

Weiskopf R (2002). Current techniques for perioperative lung isolation in adults. *Anaesthesiology*, **97**, 1295–301.

Case 10.2

Off-pump cardiopulmonary bypass

Background

This case aims to elicit knowledge and understanding of off-pump coronary artery bypass graft (OPCABG) surgery.

Learning outcomes

1 Outline differing degree of coronary artery disease and treatment options for each

2 Discuss advantages and disadvantages of OPCABG

3 Describe an anaesthetic plan for such a case.

CPD matrix matches

2A03; 2A07

Case history

You are asked to anaesthetize a 64-year-old lady for coronary bypass graft surgery on your elective list tomorrow. She has presented to the cardiothoracic ward the evening prior to surgery, having already been assessed at a surgical pre-admission clinic.

Following discussion with the surgical team, she has opted to have her coronary bypass grafting done 'off pump'. The surgeon has indicated that she will require three grafts to be performed.

Her past medical history includes symptomatic ischaemic heart disease, hypertension, hyperlipidaemia, and type II non-insulin-dependent diabetes mellitus. She has a raised BMI of approximately 32 and is a lifelong smoker of 20 cigarettes per day.

What are the indications for coronary artery bypass grafting?

- The aim of CABG is to improve survival and to relieve the symptoms of myocardial ischaemia; these occur when an area of the myocardium receives an inadequate blood supply due to the occlusion (partial or full) of a coronary artery by atheromatous plaque or thrombus

- Emergency CABG is recommended in patients with acute MI, in whom a primary PCI has failed or cannot be performed
- CABG is recommended for patients with >50% stenosis of the left main coronary artery to improve survival
- CABG is advisable in patients who have a >70% stenosis in three or more coronary arteries or if the proximal left anterior descending artery is stenosed plus one other coronary artery
- CABG is advised in patients who are unable to tolerate antiplatelet therapy and are thus precluded from PCI.

What do you understand by the term 'off-pump'?

- 'Off-pump' indicates that the patient will not require cardiopulmonary bypass (CPB) in order to have her CABG carried out
- This means that the patient's surgery will be performed on a beating heart.

What are the perceived potential advantages of off-pump coronary artery bypass grafting?

- The intended benefits of OPCABG relate to the avoidance of CPB and not needing to cross-clamp the ascending aorta
- Reduced systemic inflammatory response
- Reduced incidence of consumptive coagulopathy
- Reduced incidence of neurological dysfunction
- Reduced incidence of renal dysfunction
- Reduced blood loss and requirement for transfusion of red blood cells and coagulation factors.

What makes off-pump coronary artery bypass grafting technically possible?

- Cardiac stabilization devices are used to stabilize a small area of the myocardium around the area where the anastomosis between the coronary artery and the graft is being carried out
- Myocardial protection from ischaemia is achieved through the use of a surgical shunt that is placed in the coronary artery to facilitate distal perfusion, whilst the anastomosis is being carried out. The shunt is then removed prior to completion of the anastomosis

• Myocardial protection is also facilitated by anaesthetic technique by reducing the myocardial oxygen demand by preventing tachycardia and also by maintaining the coronary perfusion pressure through the maintenance of an adequate MAP.

What complications should you be aware of when anaesthetizing patients for off-pump coronary artery bypass grafting?

• The most significant complications of OPCABG relate to the movement of the heart in order to access the distal, lateral, and posterior coronary arteries. This can result in haemodynamic instability via three mechanisms:

1 Moving the heart into a vertical position causes a dramatic fall in cardiac output due to changes in right heart pressures and ventricular filling having to occur through flow against gravity, and therefore an increased reliance on atrial contraction for ventricular filling. There is also a concomitant reduction in venous return

2 Cardiac wall stabilization devices apply pressure to the ventricular wall, which results in localized areas of ventricular wall motion abnormality

3 The vertical heart distorts the tricuspid and mitral valves, which result in a significant increase in valvular regurgitation

• Patients are also at risk of intraoperative ischaemia, as there will be a period where the already threatened myocardium will have its blood supply reduced or even stopped

• Arrhythmias: these can be either atrial or ventricular, although there is a higher incidence of tachyarrhythmias than of bradyarrhythmias

• Sustained haemodynamic instability or persistent ventricular fibrillation may require the patient to be stabilized on CPB. Facilities for urgent conversion from off-pump to on-pump should be available in theatre.

What information would you like to obtain during your preoperative visit?

History

• Presence of symptoms relating to their ischaemic heart disease and the severity of these symptoms, i.e. whether they have stable or unstable angina or nocturnal symptoms

• Functional capacity or exercise tolerance

• Frequency with which they have to use sublingual GTN

♦ Concurrent comorbid conditions

♦ Previous anaesthetic history

♦ Current medication history, including potential allergies and if still taking any anticoagulant or antiplatelet therapy

♦ History of reflux symptoms

♦ Smoking history.

Examination

♦ Airway assessment, including assessment of dentition

♦ Cardiorespiratory examination, with particular emphasis on identifying signs of congestive cardiac failure or concurrent respiratory disease

♦ Baseline vital observations: NIBP, HR, temperature, RR

♦ Height, weight, BMI

♦ Ease of vascular access, given her raised BMI

♦ Ease of palpation of radial arteries (preoperative coronary angiography is often done via the right radial artery that can be difficult to palpate for a period afterwards).

Case update

This lady describes angina symptoms of chest tightness on exertion, usually precipitated when she is in a hurry to arrive somewhere on time and has to walk briskly for >200 yards. Her angina does not come on at rest, and it is relieved by using her GTN spray. She has previously had a general anaesthetic for an emergency Caesarean section and reports that, other than discomfort, she had no adverse reaction to her general anaesthetic. She normally takes aspirin but has stopped this 3 days ago. She is also taking atenolol, lisinopril, bendroflumethiazide, metformin, and rosiglitazone.

Her BP is 162/88, HR 58 bpm, temperature 36.2°C, and RR 18 breaths/min.

What investigations would you wish to have been performed?

Many investigations will have been done prior to referral for CABG, and those results should be available to you.

♦ Coronary angiography: used to identify and quantify coronary artery lesions

♦ Exercise tolerance test: also known as the treadmill test, which uses the Bruce protocol of increasing physical activity to determine if ischaemia is reproducible. Not always performed, as it is used more often as a diagnostic tool for individuals with less severe disease

- Echocardiography: will allow the assessment of LV function and identify any areas of regional wall motion abnormality. It will also allow the identification and assessment of any valvular lesions. Stress echocardiography may be of use to identify areas of inducible ischaemia.

Other investigations that you will need with up-to-date results are:

- ECG: indicates the presence of LV hypertrophy, conduction abnormalities, the presence of a sinus rhythm or an underlying arrhythmia, and ischaemic changes. An ECG should be done on admission to the cardiothoracic unit and should serve both as a diagnostic aid and as a baseline for comparison with subsequent ECGs

- Blood tests: FBC, coagulation studies, U&E, including calcium and magnesium, and blood glucose, as a minimum, and any others that are deemed necessary, based on the patient's concurrent comorbid conditions or current medications. A blood sample should be sent to blood bank to ensure that cross-matched blood will be available

- CXR: may demonstrate cardiomegaly or signs of congestive cardiac failure. Also any lung lesions or lung disease should be looked for

- Pulmonary function tests: a useful baseline, especially in smokers.

What information would you like to provide to the patient during your preoperative visit?

- Planned anaesthetic technique, including risks and benefits, in order to gain informed consent

- Which of their usual medications to take or withhold. It is important to give explicit instructions to both patient and nursing staff and to document clearly in the prescription record. In this patient, it is important to continue their β-blocker, and this should be administered on the morning of surgery. They should also have in place a perioperative plan for the control of their blood glucose; this is usually achieved through the administration of an insulin infusion

- Antiplatelet therapy is usually stopped 7 days prior to surgery; however, this practice varies, according to surgical preference. In high-risk patients, aspirin may be continued purposefully, with the knowledge that this may increase the risk of intra- and post-operative blood loss

- Information as to invasive monitoring

- Information regarding the use of TOE intraoperatively

- Post-operative ventilation and critical care, although one of the advantages of OPCABG is the possibility of extubation at the end of the procedure

- Post-operative analgesia
- Premedication
- Fasting guidelines
- Answers to any questions that the patient may have.

How would you conduct anaesthesia for this patient?

- It is common to prescribe premedication to patients for cardiac surgery, and this may take the form of: anxiolysis, e.g. benzodiazepines; anti-reflux, e.g. a proton pump inhibitor (PPI) or H2 receptor antagonist; or analgesic medication, e.g. paracetamol or opioid medications. In this instance, the premedication should be with short-acting agents, as one of the goals of 'off-pump' CABG is extubation at the end of the case

- Inform the anaesthetic team of your management plan, with emphasis on any particular risks or concerns regarding the patient's care

- Draw up and clearly label all drugs and infusions prior to the patient's arrival

- Check the anaesthetic machine and equipment are functioning appropriately and that the monitoring equipment is present and functional

- On the patient's arrival in the anaesthetic room, check the patient's identification, and comply with the WHO and local checklist protocols

- Site a large-bore peripheral cannula, and insert an arterial line under local anaesthetic

- Central venous cannulation (for CVP monitoring and the administration of vasoactive infusions) ± pulmonary artery catheter placement (for monitoring pulmonary artery pressures and measuring the cardiac output) are usually carried out after the induction of anaesthesia but can be carried out under local anaesthetic in the more unwell patient

- Any of the common induction agents would be suitable, but it is the dose and rate of administration that are important. Opioids and benzodiazepines are commonly used co-induction agents

- A neuromuscular-blocking agent is used to facilitate endotracheal intubation

- Either TIVA or a volatile-based anaesthetic for maintenance would be equally acceptable

- The core temperature should be monitored, and an aggressive approach to maintaining normothermia undertaken, including the use of warmed IV fluid, forced air warmers, and raised theatre ambient temperature

- A urinary catheter is inserted to allow accurate monitoring of the urine output

- TOE is considered by many to be routine for patients undergoing cardiac surgery (except if there is a specific contraindication, e.g. oesophageal disease)

- ABGs are performed, as indicated or as per unit protocols. Parameters that are specifically looked for are K^+ levels ($\geq$4.5 mmol/L), Hb, acid–base status, and glucose

- Heparin 150 IU/kg (half of the dose given to patients requiring CPB) is given on instruction of the surgeon in the aim of achieving an activated clotting time (ACT) of >300 s.

When compared to on-pump coronary artery bypass grafting, does off-pump coronary artery bypass grafting result in reduced incidence of morbidity and mortality?

- A recently published systematic review and meta-analysis by the Cochrane trials group has indicated:

  1 OPCABG showed an increase in all-cause mortality

  2 OPCABG showed a reduction in the incidence of AF

  3 There was no statistical difference in the incidence of MI, stroke, or renal insufficiency

- The authors concluded that CABG should be carried out on-pump, using sternotomy, CPB, and cardiac arrest, unless there are contraindications to aortic cannulation and CPB

- The majority of studies into OPCABG indicated a reduction in the number of transfusion products required.

Summary

Cardiac anaesthesia for OPCABG should only be performed by cardiac anaesthetists who are familiar with the indications for the procedure and with the complications associated with the manipulation of the beating heart and the resultant cardiovascular instability. Expertise in intraoperative TOE is helpful and can be used to both monitor the patient and make diagnoses that may assist the surgical team. OPCABG is indicated in those patients in whom there are contraindications to aortic cannulation and/ or CPB.

Further reading

Chassot PG, van der Linden P, Zaugg M, Mueller XM, and Spahn D (2004). Off-pump coronary bypass surgery: physiology and anaesthetic management. *British Journal of Anaesthesia*, **92**, 400–13.

Hett DA (2006). Anaesthesia for off-pump coronary artery surgery. *Continuing Education in Anaesthesia, Critical Care & Pain*, **6**, 60–2.

Hillis LD, Smith PK, Anderson JL, *et al.* (2011). 2011 ACCF/AHA Guideline for coronary artery bypass graft surgery: executive summary: a report of the American College of Cardiology Foundation/American Heart Association Task Force of Practice Guidelines. *Circulation*, **124**, 2610–42.

Moller CH, Penninga L, Wetterslev J, Steinbruchel DA, and Gluud C (2012). Off-pump versus on-pump coronary artery bypass grafting for ischaemic heart disease. *Cochrane Database Systematic Reviews*, **3**, CD007224.

Case 10.3

Valve replacement surgery

Background

This case aims to highlight the principles of cardiac risk assessment, aortic valve surgery, and CPB.

Learning outcomes

1 Preoperative assessment for cardiac surgery

2 Principles of CPB and myocardial protection

3 Techniques of aortic valve surgery.

CPD matrix matches

2A03; 2A04; 2A07

Case history

You are scheduled to anaesthetize a 69-year-old gentleman for an elective aortic valve replacement (AVR) for aortic stenosis. He has presented to the cardiothoracic ward for assessment on the afternoon prior to surgery, having previously attended a pre-assessment surgical clinic. You meet him and his family on the cardiothoracic ward, following his clerk-in by the foundation doctor.

What are the three main causes of aortic stenosis?

1 Calcific aortic stenosis: previously considered a degenerative disease, but now considered to be similar in pathogenesis to atherosclerosis. Risk factors for coronary artery disease are the same for calcific aortic stenosis, namely male sex, hyperlipidaemia, and age. These patients normally present in the 6th, 7th, or 8th decade of life in those with trileaflet valves

2 Congenital aortic disease:

   (a) Congenital aortic stenosis that is diagnosed in infancy and childhood is most often due to unicuspid valve, although it can occasionally remain undetected until adulthood. The incidence of unicuspid aortic valve is between 0.02 and 0.04% and is associated with other congenital abnormalities such as an abnormal coronary artery anatomy, patent ductus arteriosus, and coarctation of the aorta

(b) Bicuspid aortic valve is the most common congenital cardiac malformation, with an incidence of around 2%. It usually presents in the 4th or 5th decade of life with stenosis and, less frequently, with regurgitation

(c) Quadricuspid aortic valves occur very rarely and can present in adulthood with aortic stenosis

3 Rheumatic valve disease: rare in developed countries. When rheumatic disease causes aortic stenosis, the mitral valve is often involved as well.

What are the signs and symptoms of aortic stenosis?

◆ Asymptomatic

◆ Characteristic ejection systolic murmur radiating to the carotids

◆ Exertional shortness of breath

◆ Angina

◆ Dizziness

◆ Syncope

◆ Sudden death.

The presence of symptoms is a poor prognostic indicator and is associated with significant mortality rates.

The pathophysiological process behind symptomatic aortic stenosis relates to LV outflow obstruction, resulting in an increased LV afterload and an increase in wall stress which, in turn, results in concentric LV hypertrophy and eventually LV overload and failure. LV hypertrophy results in an impairment of the coronary blood flow and reduces the diastolic function, leading to a mismatch between the oxygen supply and demand, resulting in ischaemic symptoms. LV filling becomes more dependent on atrial contraction, with the cardiac output becoming fixed and thus dependent on the SVR.

You note that your patient is documented to have severe aortic stenosis. How do you classify the degree of severity in aortic stenosis?

◆ There is no universally agreed definition. Recommended echocardiographic measurements are outlined in Table 10.1.

Table 10.1 Echocardiographic assessment of aortic valve stenosis: reference ranges for grading aortic stenosis

	Mild	Moderate	Severe
Aortic jet velocity (m/s)	<2.6–2.9	3.0–4.0	>4.0
Mean gradient (mmHg)	<20	20–40	>40
Aortic valve area (cm²)	>1.5	1.0–1.5	<1.0
Indexed aortic valve area (cm²/m²)	>0.85	0.6–0.85	<0.6
Velocity ratio*	>0.5	0.25–0.5	<0.25

* Velocity ratio = LVOT Vmax/AV Vmax.

Reprinted from *Journal of the American Society of Echocardiography*, 22, 1, Baumgartner H et al., 'Echocardiographic assessment of valve stenosis: EAE/ASE recommendations for clinical practice', pp. 1–23, Copyright 2009, with permission from Elsevier.

What information would you look to elicit in the preoperative visit?

History

- Presence of symptoms relating to aortic stenosis, as outlined earlier
- Functional capacity or exercise tolerance.
- Concurrent comorbid conditions
- Previous anaesthetic history
- Current medication history, including potential allergies and if still taking any anticoagulant or antiplatelet therapy
- History of reflux symptoms and dysphagia (relevant for the use of TOE)
- Smoking history.

Examination

- Airway assessment, including the assessment of dentition
- Cardiorespiratory examination, with particular emphasis on identifying signs of congestive cardiac failure
- Slow rising and low volume pulse
- Ejection systolic murmur which may radiate to the carotids, apex, or 2nd right intercostal space
- Baseline vital observations: NIBP, HR, temperature, RR
- Height, weight, BMI.

Case update

Your patient describes exertional dyspnoea, angina, and one occasion of syncope. He is a lifelong smoker and has reduced his level of activity to 'pottering around the house' due to breathlessness. He is a non-insulin-dependent type II diabetic and is normally hypertensive. His current medications include furosemide, lisinopril, simvastatin, metformin, and aspirin. His BMI is 32, and his baseline observations are HR 76 bpm, BP 154/96, temperature 36.4°C, and RR 18 breaths/min.

What investigations would you wish to have been performed?

The majority of investigations should already have been done in the preoperative work-up of the patient, prior to the decision to proceed with AVR surgery, and should include those outlined here:

- Echocardiography: has been established as a vital tool in the diagnosis and assessment of the severity of aortic stenosis and is thus mandatory prior to AVR surgery. A focused study of the aortic valve, including Doppler echocardiography to assess the flow characteristics, is considered to be the standard technique. Points of particular interest should include the valve area, mean and peak pressure gradients across the valve and left ventricular measurements, and an assessment of LV function.

- ECG: indicates the presence of LV hypertrophy, conduction abnormalities, the presence of a sinus rhythm or an underlying arrhythmia, and ischaemic changes. An ECG should be done on admission to the cardiothoracic unit and should serve as both a diagnostic aid and as a baseline for comparison with subsequent ECGs

- Blood tests: FBC, U&E, including calcium and magnesium, coagulation studies, and blood glucose, as a minimum, and any others that are deemed necessary, based on the patient's concurrent comorbid condition or current medications

- CXR: may demonstrate cardiomegaly or signs of congestive cardiac failure

- Coronary angiography: coronary artery disease must be looked for. A CT coronary angiography (less invasive) may be considered in younger patients who are at lower risk for coronary artery disease

- Pulmonary function tests: useful in identifying those with restrictive or obstructive lung deficits, in addition to their cardiac conditions.

This patient has severe aortic stenosis, as determined by his echocardiogram. He has LV hypertrophy present on his ECG and a moderate renal impairment, with cardiomegaly apparent on his CXR.

Other investigations that are common, but not routine, include:

- Dobutamine stress echocardiography may assist in determining the degree of severity of the valvular defect in patients with poor LV function
- Exercise testing is contraindicated in symptomatic patients but is useful in the risk stratification of asymptomatic patients with severe lesions.

How would you quantify this patient's operative risk for aortic valve replacement surgery?

The validated European System for Cardiac Operative Risk Evaluation (Euro-SCORE) provides medical staff with a projected operative mortality for patients undergoing cardiac surgery and assesses patients under the headings of patient-related factors, cardiac-related factors, and operation-related factors.

This patient's operative mortality, based on EuroSCORE, is <5%.

What information will you give to the patient during your preoperative visit?

- Planned anaesthetic technique, including risks and benefits, in order to gain informed consent
- Which of their usual medications to take or withhold. It is important to give explicit instructions to both patient and nursing staff and to document clearly in the prescription record
- Information as to invasive monitoring
- Information regarding the use of TOE intraoperatively
- Post-operative ventilation and critical care
- Post-operative analgesia
- Premedication
- Fasting guidelines
- Answers to any questions that the patient may have
- Information about the likelihood of a blood transfusion.

How would you prepare for the conduct of anaesthesia for aortic valve replacement surgery?

- It is common to prescribe premedication to patients for cardiac surgery, and this may take the form of: anxiolysis, e.g. benzodiazepines; anti-reflux, e.g. PPI or H2 receptor antagonist; or analgesic medication, e.g. paracetamol or opioid medications
- Inform the anaesthetic team of your management plan, with emphasis on any particular risks or concerns regarding the patient's care

- Draw up and clearly label all drugs and infusions prior to the patient's arrival
- Check the anaesthetic machine and equipment are functioning appropriately and that the monitoring equipment is present and functional
- On the patient's arrival in the anaesthetic room, check the patient's identification, and comply with the WHO and local checklist protocols
- Site a large-bore peripheral cannula, and insert an arterial line under local anaesthetic
- Central venous cannulation (for CVP monitoring and the administration of vasoactive infusions) ± pulmonary artery catheter placement (for monitoring pulmonary artery pressures and measuring the cardiac output) are usually carried out after the induction of anaesthesia but can be carried under local anaesthetic in the more unwell patient
- Any of the common induction agents would be suitable, but it is the dose and rate administered that are important. Opioids and benzodiazepines are commonly used co-induction agents
- A neuromuscular-blocking agent is used to facilitate endotracheal intubation
- Either TIVA or a volatile-based anaesthetic for maintenance would be equally acceptable
- The core temperature should be monitored
- A urinary catheter is inserted to allow accurate monitoring of the urine output
- TOE is considered by many to be routine for patients undergoing valvular surgery (except if there is a specific contraindication, e.g. oesophageal disease)
- Remote defibrillation pads are attached if the patient has had previous cardiac surgery
- ABGs are performed, as indicated or as per unit protocols. Parameters that are specifically looked for are K^+ levels, Hb, acid–base status, and glucose
- Heparin (300 IU/kg) is given on instruction of the surgeon, in the aim of achieving an ACT of >450 s.

What are the haemodynamic goals in anaesthetizing someone with aortic stenosis?

- Ensure that myocardial oxygen demand does not exceed supply: this is achieved by recognizing that the coronary blood flow takes place during diastole and relies on an adequate SVR. Therefore, it is preferable to maintain a sinus rhythm at a rate of 60–80 bpm

- Minimize vasodilatation associated with anaesthesia, either through the use of an opioid-based technique or the use of α-agonists
- Arrhythmias should be treated aggressively.

This patient is undergoing aortic valve replacement surgery through a midline sternotomy incision and will require a period of time on cardiopulmonary bypass. What are the main reasons for using cardiopulmonary bypass for cardiac surgery?

- Motionless heart
- Bloodless field
- Excellent surgical access.

What does a cardiopulmonary bypass circuit consist of?

- An extracorporeal circuit which aims to replicate the functions of the patient's heart and lungs
- A venous tubing which usually drains under gravity into a reservoir
- A systemic blood pump which can be a roller or centrifugal pump. The aim of the pump is to ensure blood flow against the resistance of the CPB circuit. It should create no stasis or turbulent flow and be able to adjust for different sizes of the CPB tubing
- A heat exchanger
- An oxygenator: typically provided by membrane oxygenators. Gas exchange is less efficient than in the human lung, as the surface area is approximately one-tenth and the diffusion distance is greater than in the normal lung
- An arterial filter
- An arterial cannula for the return of blood to the patient.

An example of a CPB circuit is shown in Figure 10.1.

What steps will you have to take in order to prepare your anaesthetized patient for cardiopulmonary bypass?

- Ensure the bypass circuit is primed, usually with a crystalloid solution. RCC may be added if the patient has pre-existing anaemia. Heparin is usually added to the circuit
- Ensure adequate anticoagulation with heparin to achieve an ACT of >450 s
- Obtain baseline ABGs to assess the acid–base balance
- Ensure the vaporizer is mounted on the CPB circuit or TIVA is established

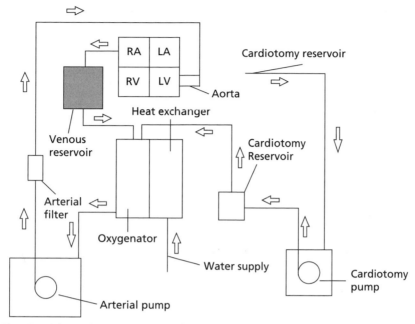

Fig. 10.1 Schematic representation of a standard CPB circuit.

- Ensure that the patient is not hypertensive in order to prepare for aortic cannulation—usually a systolic pressure of 100 mmHg is acceptable

- Be prepared for potential cardiovascular instability.

What are the forms of myocardial protection available for use, in conjunction with cardiopulmonary bypass, and why are they required?

- Myocardial protection is required as the aortic cross-clamp is applied on the ascending aorta, effectively ceasing coronary circulation. It is for this reason that myocardial protection is used to prevent hypoxic insult and cell death

- Cardioplegia applied to the coronary circulation results in the cessation of electrical, and thus mechanical, activity of the heart, resulting in greatly reduced oxygen and metabolic demands. This can be applied both ante-gradely, via the aortic root or directly into the coronary ostia, or retrogradely via the coronary sinus. Cardioplegic solutions are often infused at timed intervals to maintain electromechanical arrest and to maintain optimal operative conditions

- Cardioplegic solutions are most often given as cold infusions and are either crystalloid or blood solutions. Blood solutions are thought to provide the advantage that they deliver oxygen, buffer H$^+$ ions, and scavenge free radicals

- Other techniques, often used in conjunction with cardioplegia solutions, are the use of systemic moderate hypothermia (approximately 32°C) and reducing aortic cross-clamp times.

Why do we use systemic hypothermia for patients undergoing cardiopulmonary bypass?

- Decreases myocardial oxygen consumption
- Improves resistance to ischaemic insult
- Allows for low-flow CPB, without organ damage secondary to reduced perfusion pressures.

What are the potential problems associated with cardiopulmonary bypass?

- CPB induces a systemic inflammatory response: this is due to the prolonged exposure of the patient's blood to foreign materials and to the frictional forces applied to blood cells during their passage through the bypass circuit. Attempts have been made to coat the surface of bypass circuits with biocompatible coatings, in an effort to reduce the incidence and severity of SIRS through a reduction in the release of pro-inflammatory mediators such as cytokines and the complement system
- Modern CPB machines incorporate suction pumps that are used to reintroduce blood spilled into the surgical field to the bypass machine, and thus the patient's circulation. However, despite their usefulness in reducing waste and loss in CPB, they also allow the retransfusion of fat and leucocytes
- Haemodilution, and thus iatrogenic anaemia, due to the volume of crystalloid required to prime the CPB pump, although some haemodilution may be advantageous to improve flow characteristics in the hypothermic patient
- Pump-induced haemolysis: lower incidence of this with centrifugal pumps than with roller pumps
- Poor control of acid–base balance and oxygenation: modern bypass machines now have in-line monitoring of ABGs, in order to reduce the risk of gross acid–base disturbance
- Air embolism
- Post-operative confusion, brain injury, or stroke: commonly described as 'pumphead' which is thought to be due to macro- or microemboli of atheromatous plaques from the aorta.

Your patient has had an uncomplicated procedure. Where should he be cared for post-operatively?

◆ Specialist cardiothoracic ICU.

What should the aims of post-operative care in this patient be?

◆ Re-warming

◆ Cardiovascular stability

◆ Close monitoring and swift recognition of post-operative complications

◆ Analgesia

◆ Safe environment for emergence from anaesthesia and extubation.

What are the common post-operative complications associated with this type of aortic valve replacement surgery?

◆ Bleeding

◆ Tamponade

◆ Arrhythmias

◆ Heart block that may require cardiac pacing: it is common for surgeons to leave epicardial pacing wires *in situ* post-operatively

◆ Air embolus: most commonly in the right coronary artery. This can lead to arrhythmias or to right heart failure.

Summary

Anaesthesia for valvular surgery requires expertise in the areas of pre-assessment of cardiac risk and the pathophysiology of valvular disease, familiarity with CPB, and the ability to perform a comprehensive TOE study intraoperatively. Anaesthetic techniques should focus on ensuring myocardial oxygen demand does not exceed supply by avoiding tachycardia and vasodilatation.

Further reading

Alston RP (2005). Pumphead or not! Does avoiding cardiopulmonary bypass for coronary artery bypass surgery result in less brain damage? *British Journal of Anaesthesia*, **94**, 699–701.

Bonow RO, Carabello BA, Chatterjee K, *et al*. (2008). 2008 Focused update practice incorporated into the ACC/AHA 2006 guidelines for the management of patients with valvular heart disease. A report of the American College of Cardiology/American Heart Association Task Force on Practice Guidelines. *Circulation*, **118**, 523–661.

Breisch EA, White FC, and Bloor CM (1984). Myocardial characteristics of pressure overload hypertrophy: a structural and functional study. *Laboratory Investigations*, **51**, 333–42.

Carabello BA and Paulus WJ (2009). Aortic stenosis. *Lancet*, **373**, 956–66.

Chacko M and Weinberg L (2012). Aortic valve stenosis: perioperative anaesthetic implications of surgical replacement and minimally invasive interventions. *Continuing Education in Anaesthesia, Critical Care & Pain*, **12**, 295–301.

Joint Task Force on the Management of Valvular Heart Disease of the European Society of Cardiology, European Association for Cardio-Thoracic Surgery (EACTS), Vahanian A, Alfieri O, Andreotti F, *et al*. (2012). Guidelines on the management of valvular heart disease (version 2012). *European Heart Journal*, **33**, 2451–96.

Machin D and Allsager C (2006). Principles of cardiopulmonary bypass. *Continuing Education in Anaesthesia, Critical Care & Pain*, **6**, 176–81.

Otto CM, Kuusisto J, Reichenbach DD, Gown AM, and O'Brien KD (1994). Characterization of the early lesion of 'degenerative' valvular aortic stenosis: histological and immunohistochemical studies. *Circulation*, **90**, 844–53.

Roach GW, Kanchuger M, Mangano CM, *et al*. (1996). Adverse cerebral outcomes after coronary bypass surgery. *New England Journal of Medicine*, **335**, 1857–63.

Vahanian A, Baumgartner H, Bax J, *et al*.; Task Force on the Management of Valvular Heart Disease of the European Society of Cardiology; ESC Committee for Practice Guidelines. Guidelines on the management of valvular heart disease. *European Heart Journal*, **28**, 230–68.

Transcatheter cardiac valve surgery

Background

This case aims to highlight the indications for, and the anaesthetic implications of, a transcatheter aortic valve implantation (TAVI).

Learning outcomes

1 Discuss the anaesthetic implications of different operative approaches for aortic valve disease

2 Outline an appropriate anaesthetic technique for a transcatheter valve procedure.

CPD matrix matches

2A07

Case history

A 72-year-old female patient has been scheduled for TAVI for aortic stenosis, which has been classified as severe on echocardiography. You have been asked to anaesthetize her for this procedure.

What are the indications for performing an aortic valve replacement using the transcatheter aortic valve insertion technique?

◆ The operative morbidity in patients undergoing AVR through sternotomy and CPB, who have concomitant LV dysfunction, renal disease, respiratory disease, and previous sternotomy, increases from 4% in the population without these comorbidities to approximately 22%

◆ Based on the increased risk, NICE produced guidelines on those patients who should be considered for a TAVI procedure:

1 A EuroSCORE of >20 (i.e. the percentage of predicted operative mortality for cardiac surgery)

2 Severe respiratory disease

3 Refused surgery by two cardiac surgeons

4 Previous sternotomy and patent coronary bypass grafts ('hostile chest')

- The European Society of Cardiology recommendations are outlined as follows:

    1 TAVI should only be undertaken following assessment by both cardiologists and cardiac surgeons

    2 TAVI should only be performed in hospitals with cardiac surgery services on site

    3 TAVI is indicated in symptomatic patients who have been refused surgery and who are expected to achieve an improvement in quality of life and have a life expectancy of >1 year.

What are the contraindications to transcatheter aortic valve implantation?

- An estimated life expectancy of <1 year
- Comorbidities likely to limit the quality of life, regardless of TAVI success
- Disease of other valves which require surgical repair
- An inadequate aortic valve annulus size (i.e. very small or very large)
- LV thrombus
- Active endocarditis

Relative contraindications include:

- Bicuspid valve
- Untreated coronary artery disease
- Cardiovascular instability
- LV ejection fraction of <20%.

There are three different approaches to TAVI that can be considered by the TAVI team:

- Transfemoral (TF)
- Transaortic (TAo)
- Transapical (TAp).

TF TAVI is the most straightforward and commonly used approach, involving bilateral groin punctures. Those suitable for TAVI, but with small femoral vessels or with atheromatous disease of the femoral vessels or the abdominal or thoracic aorta, may be considered for TAo TAVI. This is done via a small anterior upper right thoracotomy or an upper sternal wound. However, if the ascending aorta is inaccessible via either of these wounds or the ascending aorta is heavily calcified or atheromatous, then TAp TAVI, via a small left thoracotomy over the apex of the heart, may be possible.

Your patient has met the above criteria for aortic valve replacement using a transcatheter aortic valve implantation technique. What are the potential advantages to her of having her procedure in this manner?

- A full sternotomy is not required: this has implications for reduced post-operative pain and recovery time. There is a lower incidence of post-operative wound infection
- No need for CPB and the associated complications
- Reduced stay in critical care and reduced hospital stay: these patients would have previously been in the subgroup of patients who had prolonged periods of post-operative mechanical ventilation and critical care management.

Your patient has severe respiratory disease in the form of chronic obstructive pulmonary disease. She has symptomatic aortic stenosis, chronic kidney disease stage 3, and a EuroSCORE of 23. How would you approach this patient's perioperative care?

Preoperative assessment

- A thorough history and examination, ensuring that the medical therapy is optimized for all comorbid conditions
- A focused anaesthetic history and examination
- A 12-lead ECG
- Haematological and biochemistry blood tests
- A blood sample sent to blood bank for cross-matching
- A detailed transthoracic echocardiogram
- CXR
- Gated CT angiogram of the aortic valve, thoracic and abdominal aorta, and iliofemoral vessels
- Coronary angiography ± angioplasty may be indicated
- Aspirin is prescribed preoperatively
- No sedative premedication is generally required, but, on an individual basis, a light, short-acting sedative may be indicated.

How would you prepare to anaesthetize your patient for her transcatheter aortic valve implantation?

- Ensure familiarity with the facilities provided for TAVI procedures, as these are often carried out in distant or isolated sites where additional help is not readily available. The facility (usually a cardiac catheter laboratory or hybrid theatre) should therefore have a piped gas supply, scavenging capability, anaesthetic machines, difficult airway equipment, access to anaesthetic and emergency drugs, and full patient and anaesthetic monitoring equipment

- The facility should also contain some means of supporting the circulation mechanically, e.g. with an intra-aortic balloon pump (IABP), an ECMO circuit, or a CPB circuit, with a perfusionist dedicated to the facility

- Anaesthetic and emergency drugs should be prepared and be ready for use prior to the patient's arrival in the anaesthetic room

- The monitoring equipment, anaesthetic machine, and emergency equipment should be checked to ensure adequate function and identify any potential problems

- When working in an isolated environment with a team of cardiothoracic surgeons, cardiologists, pacing technicians, and catheter laboratory staff, it is especially important to have a comprehensive team briefing. Everyone has to be aware of, and agree with, the escalation plan and the level that treatment will be taken to for each individual patient, in the event of complications arising.

Can you outline the intraoperative management of this patient?

- Most procedures are carried out under general anaesthesia, but, in a small subset of patients, it may be possible to perform TF TAVI under local anaesthesia and sedation

- Monitoring should be established, and a large-bore peripheral cannula sited

- An arterial line should be placed prior to induction

- Following induction and tracheal intubation, central venous cannulation is performed

- A urinary catheter is inserted

- Remote defibrillator pads must be attached

- Temperature monitoring and active maintenance of normothermia with patient- and fluid-warming devices

- 150 U/kg of heparin is given (aiming for an ACT of >300 s) after the initial vessel punctures are made
- TOE (ideally three-dimensional) is used, in conjunction with radiological screening, to permit constant visualization of the aortic valve throughout the procedure, thus assisting in the correct placement of the replacement valve.

Outline the post-operative plan

- The patient will be extubated at the end of the procedure, unless there has been a complication
- Admission to critical care post-operatively is advised for a period of close monitoring
- Analgesia can be provided with the use of a long-acting local anaesthetic to the operating site (local infiltration and intercostal nerve blocks, as indicated) and simple analgesics, e.g. paracetamol. Long-acting opiates may be required for the TAo and TAp patients
- Antiplatelet therapy is required.

No procedure is without risk, and it is imperative that you are aware of the potential risks associated with a transcatheter aortic valve implantation in order to identify and manage them swiftly. Can you identify the major risks of the transcatheter aortic valve implantation procedures?

- The technique involves the passage of a wire across the aortic valve, and then a balloon valvuloplasty is performed to dilate the valve. At this point, rapid ventricular pacing is initiated to reduce the LV ejection and cardiac motion; this can result in prolonged cardiovascular instability, possibly requiring inotropic support and/or mechanical support
- TAVI placement can result in an obstruction of the coronary blood flow, causing ischaemia of the myocardium. A rapid diagnosis on coronary angiography and stent deployment can be lifesaving
- Haemorrhage: blood and blood products should be easily available from blood bank. Cardiothoracic surgeons can deal with haemorrhage from chest wounds, whilst vascular surgeons may be required to assist if there has been damage to the femoral vessels
- Pericardial tamponade: the echocardiographer will diagnose this quickly on TOE, and relief, either by percutaneous drainage or by an open procedure, may be required

- Stroke due to embolization of atheromatous plaques from the aorta
- Arrhythmias and, in particular, complete heart block: the temporary ventricular pacing wire used for the procedure can be left *in situ*, if required.

Summary

Patients selected for TAVI procedures are high-risk surgical candidates with multiple comorbidities. They require a comprehensive preoperative assessment and optimization carried out by a multidisciplinary team, consisting of cardiac anaesthetists, cardiac surgeons, and cardiologists. Anaesthesia is conducted in unfamiliar surroundings in remote locations, requiring forward planning to ensure equipment and appropriate staff are immediately available. The technique requires coordinated teamworking of the cardiac anaesthetists, cardiac surgeons, cardiologists, and catheter laboratory staff. Full knowledge of the potential complications and appropriate management are essential for patient safety in this setting.

Further reading

European System for Cardiac Operative Risk Evaluation. Available at: <http://www.euro-score.org>.

Klein AA, Webb ST, Tsui S, Sudarshan C, Shapiro L, and Densem C (2009). Transcatheter aortic valve insertion: anaesthetic implications of emerging new technology. *British Journal of Anaesthesia*, **103**, 792–9.

National Institute for Health and Clinical Excellence (2012). *Transcatheter aortic valve implantation for aortic stenosis. NICE interventional procedure guidance 421.* Available at: <http://www.nice.org.uk/nicemedia/live/11914/58611/58611.pdf>.

Smith CR, Leon MB, Mack MJ, *et al.* (2011). Transcatheter versus surgical aortic valve replacement in high-risk patients. *New England Journal of Medicine*, **364**, 2187–98.

Chapter 11

Hepatobiliary and transplant anaesthesia

Dr Neil H Young
Dr Rory Mayes

Case 11.1

Anaesthesia for major liver resection

Background

The liver is a highly vascular organ with a blood flow of 1500 mL/min, the portal vein contributing 75% and the hepatic artery 25% of the total flow. The liver can be divided into eight functional segments, based on their blood supply and biliary drainage, and this forms the basis of the various types of liver resection that may be possible. Large volumes of the liver may be resected, without the subsequent development of liver failure, due to the liver's capacity to regenerate, a process that starts as early as 24 hours post-resection.

Prior to resection taking place, a preoperative assessment must establish that a sufficient liver remnant will be left post-resection. This is done radiologically. For patients with a normal liver, a remnant of approximately 20% is required; for those with significant steatosis or hepatic dysfunction, a much larger remnant is required. Patients requiring a resection that would leave an inadequate liver remnant may undergo selective portal vein embolization 6 weeks prior to resection, to facilitate hypertrophy of the proposed remnant.

Learning outcomes

1 Outline the preoperative assessment of a patient for liver resection

2 Discuss the anaesthetic and surgical techniques to minimize complications such as blood loss

3 Appreciation of the possible post-operative complications.

CPD matrix matches

2A03; 2A07

Case history

A 68-year-old man is listed for an extended right hepatectomy for metastatic disease. Eighteen months previously, he had an anterior resection for carcinoma of the colon. Follow-up imaging at 12 months revealed metastatic deposits in liver segments 4 and 8. He has recently completed a course of neoadjuvant chemotherapy. He is a lifelong smoker, with mild COPD, and takes regular inhaled beclomethasone and tiotropium. He has a moderate alcohol intake.

What important factors must be considered during the preoperative assessment?

- The general cardiorespiratory reserve for major laparotomy, including the effects of chemotherapy
- The hepatic function
- The extent of resection.

Which investigations are recommended?

- FBC, U&E, LFTs, coagulation screen, cross-match, ECG, CXR
- Pre-chemotherapy computed tomography (CT) or MRI to assess the extent of liver resection required and the size of the liver remnant
- Positron emission tomography (PET) scan to exclude extrahepatic disease.

What are the potential major intraoperative problems?

- Major haemorrhage requiring massive transfusion
- Cardiovascular instability secondary to vascular isolation during resection
- Air embolism.

Which anaesthetic technique should be used?

- General anaesthesia, with either a thoracic epidural or PCA for post-operative analgesia
- Large-bore venous access
- A rapid infusion device should be available
- Arterial and central venous pressure monitoring
- A urinary catheter
- Normothermia
- Intraoperative ABG and ROTEM® analysis may be useful
- Prophylactic antibiotics.

How is blood loss minimized?

- Inflow vascular occlusion, including Pringle manoeuvre
- Maintaining a low central venous filling pressure
- Avoidance of acidosis, hypothermia, and hypocalcaemia.

Case update

The patient's surgery has proceeded uneventfully, and he has been subsequently extubated and transferred to the HDU. The intraoperative blood loss was 800 mL. On admission to the HDU, routine blood analysis demonstrates Hb 98 g/L, Plt 145 × 10^9/L, Na$^+$ 135 mmol/L, K$^+$ 4.0 mmol/L, urea 7.8 mmol/L, Cr 112 micromoles/L, PT 14 s, and lactate 2.8 mmol/L. He has an epidural *in situ*, and initial observations are HR 65 bpm, BP 100/50 mmHg, CVP 5 mmHg, and urine output 30–40 mL/hour.

Over next few hours, the patient becomes hypotensive with a low CVP. A total of 1000 mL of Gelofusine® is administered, and an ABG sampling at this time demonstrates Hb 94 g/L, H$^+$ 56 nmol/L, PaO$_2$ 14 kPa on 4L/min of oxygen, PaCO$_2$ 5.8 kPa, and lactate 3.9 mmol/L.

The patient fails to respond to the fluid bolus, and, over the next hour, he has a further 2000 mL of Gelofusine® and a noradrenaline requirement of 0.2 mcg/kg/min. His HR is 110 bpm, BP 85/50 mmHg, and CVP 3 mmHg. Blood tests show Hb 84 g/L, Plt 101 × 10^9/L, PT 19 s, lactate 7.8 mmol/L, and BM 2.8 mmol/L.

What are the next appropriate management steps?

◆ Continue cardiovascular resuscitation

◆ Dextrose bolus

◆ The patient requires immediate return to theatre, as there are concerns regarding the vascular supply to the liver remnant. Ensure blood for transfusion will be available in theatre

◆ ROTEM® may help direct point-of-care management of evolving coagulopathy.

Case update

On reopening, a congested liver remnant was found, with an obstructed outflow noted. Surgical correction of this results in a dramatic reduction in fluid and noradrenaline requirement. The patient returns to ICU, intubated and ventilated, with a plan to remain so overnight. Readmission bloods are Hb 78 g/L, WCC 15 × 10^9/L, Plt 98 × 10^9/L, PT 18 s, lactate 5.6 mmol/L, and BM 6.8 mmol/L.

He remains cardiovascularly stable overnight, requiring maintenance fluid only and no blood or blood product administration. Lactate continues to fall, and the acidosis resolves, allowing the noradrenaline to be weaned in parallel. The following morning, his routine bloods show Hb 81 g/L, Plt 108 × 10^9/L, PT 15 s, lactate 2.9 mmol/L, BM 5.9 mmol/L, and ALT 980.

What should be done next?

- Extubate
- Continue the epidural for further 24 hours, then remove if the platelet count and PT are within the normal range
- Monitor liver function: ALT may rise further but should decrease over the next few days, unless further problems
- Look out for any evidence of sepsis: a further liver 'hit' could be devastating
- DVT prophylaxis and peptic ulcer prophylaxis
- Establish enteral feeding.

Case discussion

Liver resection was previously associated with significant mortality, primarily due to major blood loss. Change in anaesthetic and surgical techniques has now reduced mortality to approximately 3%. Indications for hepatic resection include:

1 Metastatic colorectal carcinoma

2 Primary hepatocellular carcinoma (HCC)

3 Cholangiocarcinoma

4 Neuroendocrine tumours

5 Live donor liver transplantation.

Perioperative anaesthetic considerations

All patients will be intubated and ventilated. Intra-arterial BP and CVP monitoring is essential in all major resections, as is wide-bore venous access. Both an epidural or opioid PCA may be used for post-operative analgesia, and each has its advantages and disadvantages.

Surgical techniques to reduce blood loss include vascular isolation techniques such as the Pringle manoeuvre which involves occlusion of the hepatic artery and portal vein. This inflow occlusion means that an intraoperative blood loss is primarily from the hepatic veins. Therefore, fluid restriction and maintenance of a low CVP are required to reduce blood loss. The cardiovascular effects of inflow occlusion include a significant increase in the SVR and a reduction in the cardiac index.

The use of laser coagulation and ultrasound aspiration during resection has also been instrumental in the reduction of intraoperative blood loss.

The development of a coagulopathy is more likely in patients who are hypothermic, hypocalcaemic, or have pre-existing cirrhosis or steatosis, or have had chemotherapy. Blood sugars should be monitored, especially if there is a prolonged period of vascular occlusion.

Post-operative complications

All patients are monitored in a critical care area following a major liver resection. Mortality rates have significantly reduced and are now in the region of 2–3%. Significant morbidity remains a concern, particularly in patients who have a small liver remnant or have pre-existing liver disease.

Early post-operative haemorrhage may require immediate return to theatre, following the correction of coagulopathy. Bile leaks are relatively common but should respond to antibiotics if they are of small volume. Larger volumes of bile leaks will require endoscopic retrograde cholangiopancreatography (ERCP) and biliary stenting. Sepsis from any cause will delay the liver regeneration; therefore, a high index of suspicion is required, and early diagnosis and treatment are essential.

Small-for-size syndrome may develop in patients who have extended resections or a poorly functioning remnant. It usually presents with evidence of sepsis and the derangement of LFTs. Management is conservative, with organ support, appropriate antibiotic therapy, and the control of sepsis. Mortality is high.

Summary

The main indications for liver resection are colorectal metastases or HCC. Therefore, significant cardiorespiratory comorbidities may co-exist.

Good communication between the surgeon and the anaesthetist is essential throughout the perioperative period. Intraoperative invasive monitoring and wide-bore venous access are essential, as haemodynamic instability and significant blood loss may occur.

Post-operative management initially requires a period of critical care, and complications, such as bleeding and sepsis, must be identified and managed urgently.

Further reading

Jones C, Kelliher L, Thomas R, and Quiney N (2011). Perioperative management of liver resection surgery. *Journal of Perioperative Practice*, **21**, 198–202.

McNally SJ, Revie E, Massie LJ, *et al.* (2012). Factors in perioperative care that determine blood loss in liver surgery. *HPB (Oxford)*, **14**, 236–41.

Sutcliffe R, Antoniades CG, Deshpande R, Tucker O, and Heaton N (2009). *Liver and pancreatobiliary surgery: with liver transplantation (Oxford Specialist Handbooks in Surgery)*. Oxford University Press, Oxford.

Tympa A, Theodoraki K, Tsaroucha A, Arkadopoulos N, Vassiliou I, and Smymiotis V (2012). Anaesthetic considerations in hepatectomies under hepatic vascular control. *HPB Surgery*, 2012, 720754.

Case 11.2

Acute liver failure

Background

Acute liver failure (ALF) can be defined as the development of coagulopathy and encephalopathy in a patient with previous normal liver function, over a period of <24 weeks. There are over 40 definitions of ALF in the published literature, but virtually all include the development of coagulopathy and encephalopathy. The most common cause of ALF in Europe and North America is paracetamol overdose. Other causes include drug-induced liver injury, autoimmune hepatitis, viral hepatitis, Budd–Chiari syndrome, Wilson's disease, and pregnancy-induced ALF. In 15% of cases, the diagnosis can be unknown or indeterminate.

Learning outcomes

1 Identify the initial management steps in a patient with fulminant hepatic failure

2 Discuss the challenges in the anaesthetic and critical care management for patients with ALF receiving liver transplantation.

CPD matrix matches

2C04

Case history

A 33-year-old woman (Mrs L) is an inpatient on an acute medical ward, 72 hours following an overdose with 20 g of paracetamol. She did not present until 48 hours after the paracetamol ingestion. You have been asked as the intensive care registrar to assist with sedation, as she is becoming agitated.

What would your initial assessment points be?

- ◆ ABCD assessment
- ◆ FBC
- ◆ Coagulation profile

- LFTs
- Laboratory and bedside glucose
- Paracetamol level
- Lactate
- Will need a full liver work-up, including hepatitis serology and human immunodeficiency virus (HIV) test.

Case update

An ABCD assessment reveals that she is protecting her airway and has a RR of 24, peripheral oxygen saturations of 98% on air, HR of 130 bpm, BP of 95/40 mmHg, and GCS of 13/15 (E4 M5 V4).

Basic laboratory investigations include:

- Hb 100 g/L, WCC 11.2×10^9/L, Plt 45×10^9/L, PT 70 s (INR 5.8), APTT 36 s (APTT ratio 1.2), fibrinogen 0.9 g/L
- Na$^+$ 137 mmol/L, K$^+$ 3.4 mmol/L, urea 12.5 mmol/L, Cr 180 micromoles/L
- ALT 28 000 U/L, ALP 150 U/L, Bil 80 micromoles/L, albumin 32 g/L
- Glucose 3.1 mmol/L.

Where should she be managed?

- She should be managed in an ICU
- She should be considered for transfer to a centre with a liver transplantation programme.

At what stage should intubation be considered?

- Tracheal intubation should be undertaken before transfer
- If already in a transplantation centre, a further period of observation could be considered.

What precautions are necessary around the time of intubation and transfer?

- Cerebral oedema is a common cause of death in ALF, and measures to prevent rises in ICP and preserve CPP should be undertaken
- A modified RSI technique, including a short-acting opioid, should be used
- Patients should be nursed in a neutral 30° head-up position
- Tracheal tubes should be taped, rather than tied

- Ventilation should aim for a low normal $PaCO_2$ (4.5 kPa) and avoid hypoxaemia
- Hypotension should be avoided; ALF patients are vasodilated, and vasopressor support with noradrenaline is very commonly required.

The patient is intubated, mechanically ventilated, and transferred to the intensive care unit of a centre with a liver transplantation programme. Which criteria can be used to determine whether or not liver transplantation will be necessary?

- The King's College criteria (KCC) may be used
- KCC are good at predicting patients with a poor outcome, but less good at predicting those with a good outcome
- A full psychiatric assessment would also be necessary prior to listing for liver transplantation.

What should the basic goals of intensive care be in patients with acute liver failure?

- Maintain normoxia
- Target low-normal $PaCO_2$ (4.5 kPa)
- Maintain MAP >65 mmHg (may need to target higher MAP if intracranial hypertension)
- Very likely to need renal replacement therapy: this should be continuous veno-venous haemofiltration (CVVH), not intermittent haemodialysis, for the sake of cardiovascular stability and to prevent large swings in the ICP
- Meticulous attention to aseptic precautions and prophylactic antibiotics: sepsis with multiple organ failure is the most common cause of death in patients with ALF
- Tolerance of coagulopathy: unless there is frank bleeding or invasive procedures planned, coagulopathy should generally be tolerated, to allow monitoring of liver function. If coagulopathy is profound, advice should be sought from the transplantation centre.

Your patient reaches the King's College criteria and is listed for a super urgent liver transplantation. Should she have an intracranial pressure monitoring device placed? What are the risks and benefits of this?

- The placement of an ICP monitoring device in ALF remains controversial

- Cerebral oedema is a common cause of death in ALF, and an ICP monitor may allow treatment strategies to control this
- There are risks of precipitating a catastrophic intracranial bleeding during device placement, and correction of coagulopathy prior to this is necessary.

Mrs L has an intracranial pressure monitoring device placed. The opening pressure is 30 mmHg. Which treatments can be used to control her intracranial pressure?

- Mannitol
- Hypertonic saline
- Therapeutic hypothermia
- Barbiturate coma
- Indomethacin: this has been used in specialist centres as a rescue therapy for refractory raised ICP, though there is limited evidence for this, and it should only be used by clinicians with considerable expertise in managing ALF.

Mrs L receives an offer of a liver within 24 hours of being listed for transplantation. What are the stages of this operation, and what challenges do these present to the anaesthetist?

- Major procedure in a critically unwell patient
- ICP may be elevated and needs to be controlled intraoperatively
- Laparotomy, dissection, and hepatectomy in a coagulopathic patient lead to major blood loss, and massive transfusion is not uncommon
- An adequate large-bore central IV access is mandatory
- Intraoperative TEG can be utilized to optimize the coagulation status
- Patients often have a large vasopressor requirement from the outset, and cardiac output monitoring, such as a pulmonary artery catheter, is usually used
- During the anhepatic phase, hypothermia and hypoglycaemia can be severe
- When reperfusion of the liver occurs, there can be a massive reperfusion syndrome, manifest as electrolyte abnormalities, arrhythmias, and cardio-vascular collapse
- K^+ rises significantly during reperfusion, and, if CVVH has been needed preoperatively, this often needs to be continued intraoperatively. CVVH is more effective in this patient group, as intermittent filtration therapies may be associated with a surge in the ICP.

Mrs L goes on to receive an orthotopic liver transplant. She returns to the intensive care unit after an 8-hour operation. What are the important post-operative considerations?

- Ensuring graft function by monitoring PT, lactate clearance, and glucose
- Commencement of immunosuppression therapy
- A Doppler ultrasound is usually done within the first 24 hours to assess the adequacy of the hepatic artery flow
- When the graft appears to be functioning, the patient is normothermic, with a normal acid–base status, consideration can be given to weaning sedation, ventilation, and assessment for extubation.

Case discussion

Any patient with ALF should be discussed with a transplantation centre. In the case of paracetamol overdose, it is vital to ensure that N-acetylcysteine has been administered at the earliest opportunity. Patients with encephalopathy should always be intubated prior to transfer, with precautions taken to prevent rises in the ICP during intubation and transfer. Encephalopathy can deteriorate very quickly, with patients who only appear mildly confused rapidly deteriorating to a comatose state. It is also vital to place an arterial line and central line prior to transfer—shock can develop rapidly and be profound in patients with ALF, necessitating fluid resuscitation and BP support with noradrenaline.

On arrival in a transplantation centre, an assessment will be made as to whether or not the patient is suitable to be listed for orthotopic liver transplantation. The criteria for listing for super urgent liver transplantation in the UK are based on the KCC: arterial pH <7.3 or concurrent grade III/IV encephalopathy, Cr >300 micromoles/L, and PT >100 s. Arterial lactate can now also be used, with a lactate of >3 mmol/L post-fluid resuscitation allowing listing, although there is some debate as to whether the lactate modification adds to the KCC. The decision to list a patient for super urgent liver transplantation requires close interdisciplinary liaison between intensivists, hepatologists, transplant surgeons, psychiatrists, and anaesthetists.

Summary

The survival from ALF has increased dramatically in the transplantation era, from <10% before the 1980s to around 67% now. Predicting which patients can survive without a graft remains a challenge. There are extracorporeal liver support systems available, and future trials may guide the usefulness of this therapy in patients with ALF.

Further reading

Craig DGN, Ford AC, Hayes PC, and Simpson KJ (2010). Systematic review: prognostic tests of paracetamol-induced acute liver failure. *Alimentary Pharmacology and Therapeutics*, **31**, 1064–76.

Lee WM (2012). Recent developments in acute liver failure. *Best Practice & Research Clinical Gastroenterology*, **26**, 3–16.

NHS Blood and Transplant (2014). *Liver transplantation: selection criteria and recipient registration*. Available at: <http://www.odt.nhs.uk/pdf/liver_selection_policy.pdf>.

O'Grady JG, Alexander GJ, Hayllar KM, and Williams R (1989). Early indicators of prognosis in fulminant hepatic failure. *Gastroenterology*, **97**, 439–45.

Wlodzimirow KA, Eslami S, Abu-Hanna A, Nieuwoudt M, and Chamuleau RAFM (2012). Systematic review: acute liver failure—one disease, more than 40 definitions. *Alimentary Pharmacology and Therapeutics*, **35**, 1245–56.

Anaesthesia following renal transplantation

Background

Renal transplantation is becoming ever more common, with over 2800 renal transplants performed in 2011/12. Graft and patient survival following this operation continues to improve, therefore it is not uncommon for these patients to present for elective or emergency surgery in non-transplant centres. They are a patient population who may have significant comorbidities, either as a cause or result of their long-standing renal failure that necessitated renal transplantation. Issues to consider, specific to the transplant recipient preoperatively, include:

1 Graft function

2 Evidence of rejection

3 Immunosuppression regimen and side effects

4 Evidence of end-organ damage, either as a result of the disease process or due to immunosuppression.

Learning outcomes

1 Acknowledge the potential complications in transplant recipients presenting for an unrelated surgery

2 Ensure the graft function is assessed preoperatively

3 Employ an appropriate plan for the delivery of immunosuppressive therapies through the perioperative period.

CPD matrix matches

2A03

Case history

A 56-year-old man, who had a renal transplant 3 years ago for renal failure secondary to glomerulonephritis, presents for elective right hemicolectomy for colonic carcinoma. He has a history of hypertension secondary to end-stage renal failure and takes atenolol and lisinopril. His other medications include simvastatin, aspirin, and an immunosupppression regimen of prednisolone, mycophenolate mofetil (MMF), and tacrolimus.

What are the main considerations in the preoperative assessment of a patient with a previous renal transplant?

- Evaluation of transplanted organ function
- Exclude rejection
- Exclude infection
- Evaluation of end-organ damage, secondary to either complications of renal failure or the side effects of immunosuppression
- Other side effects of immunosuppression.

How does chronic rejection present?

- Deteriorating organ function
- Non-specific symptoms, fatigue, general malaise.

What issues relating to the renal function are important to obtain from the history?

- Renal function since transplant
- Episodes of rejection
- Need for dialysis
- Presence of a working fistula.

What investigations would you perform?

- FBC, U&E, LFTs, phosphate, magnesium, glucose, coagulation screen, urinalysis, ECG.
  Basic laboratory investigations results include:
- Hb 110g/L, WCC 4.1, Plt 135
- Na$^+$ 137, K$^+$ 4.5, urea 7.4, Cr 154
- Urinalysis normal
- ECG sinus rhythm, LV hypertrophy.

What should be done regarding this patient's immunosuppression perioperatively?

- Continue the normal immunosuppression regimen
- Change from oral to IV route, if required
- Drug levels will need to be monitored if significant blood loss or fluid shifts are observed.

What anaesthetic technique should be used, and is invasive monitoring essential?

The anaesthetic technique used should ensure an adequate perfusion of the transplanted kidney. Immunosuppressive drugs may modify the effects of many drugs used in anaesthesia, including muscle relaxants; therefore, monitoring of neuromuscular blockade is essential.

Invasive monitoring is not essential and is only necessary if the type of surgery or the patient's clinical status demands it. Immunosuppressed patients are more prone to infection; therefore, attention to strict asepsis during line insertion is essential, and all lines should be removed as soon as possible.

How should analgesia be provided?

- Multimodal technique
- Avoid NSAIDs
- Epidural is not contraindicated, but again attention to an aseptic technique, normal coagulation, and platelet function
- Morphine or fentanyl PCA.

What issues must be addressed post-operatively?

- Ensure adequate filling and perfusion of graft
- Ensure immunosuppression is maintained; monitor levels, and have a high index of suspicion of toxicity, especially if the renal function deteriorates
- Remove all invasive monitoring as soon as possible
- DVT prophylaxis and early mobilization, as a hypercoagulable state may exist.

Case discussion

Successes with public awareness campaigns and advances in transplantation techniques will result in increasing numbers of transplant recipients presenting for unrelated elective and emergency surgery in the future. A key consideration is the assessment of graft function during preoperative consultation. Renal graft function is assessed by adequacy of urine output and improving or stable biochemistry. Graft rejection may present as deteriorating biochemistry or as minimal non-specific symptoms such as lethargy or fatigue.

All patients will be immunosuppressed; the regimen will vary slightly from centre to centre, but it is imperative that this is continued in the perioperative period. Change of route of administration may be required, as may measurements of therapeutic levels, especially in surgery where there are significant fluid shifts or blood loss. Ciclosporin should be given 4–7 hours preoperatively.

The side effects of immunosuppression therapies are listed in Table 11.1, but, in addition, these patients are more susceptible to infections, including opportunistic infections, and have an increased incidence of malignancy, including post-transplant lymphoproliferative disorder.

Elective surgery should be deferred if an infection or a rejection is diagnosed preoperatively.

Intraoperative issues

General or regional anaesthesia may be used, as indicated. If a regional technique is used, attention must be given to strict asepsis, platelet and coagulation function, and the effect of hypotension on graft perfusion. IV access can be challenging. Patient positioning is important, as these patients may have hyperparathyroidism and osteoporosis.

Table 11.1 Side effects of immunosuppressive therapies

Immunosuppressant agent	Side effect
Steroid	Hypertension, hyperlipidaemia, diabetes, neurotoxicity
Azathioprine	Bone marrow suppression, hepatotoxicity, pancreatitis
Ciclosporin	Nephrotoxicity, neurotoxicity, hypertension, hyperlipidaemia, diabetes, hypomagnesaemia, hyperkalaemia, gingival hyperplasia
MMF	Bone marrow suppression, GI disturbance
Tacrolimus	Nephrotoxicity, neurotoxicity, hypertension, hyperlipidaemia, diabetes, hypomagnesaemia, hyperkalaemia
Sirolimus	Bone marrow suppression, hyperlipidaemia

Adapted from Killenberg PG et al., *Medical care of the liver transplant patient*, Third edition, p. 509, Copyright 2006, with permission from Wiley.

These patients are at slightly increased risk of aspiration; therefore, intubation should be considered. Orotracheal intubation is preferred, rather than the nasotracheal route, due to the increased risk of infection from the nasal flora.

Routine antibiotic prophylaxis is all that is necessary, and supplemental steroid is not usually required.

Monitoring of neuromuscular blockade is essential, as immunosuppression has a variable effect on the metabolism of muscle relaxants. Suxamethonium is safe, unless hyperkalaemic.

Invasive monitoring should only be used if dictated by the type of surgery or the patient's clinical status. It should be removed as soon as possible, due to the increased risk of infection.

Ensure an adequate fluid status and renal perfusion pressure throughout the perioperative period, and avoid all potentially nephrotoxic drugs, e.g. NSAIDs. If a blood transfusion is required, leucocyte-depleted blood is preferred.

Summary

Patients who have had a renal transplant will usually have multiple comorbidities, related either to the disease process that necessitated the transplant, or the long-term effects of haemodialysis, or the side effects of immunosuppression. It is imperative that the graft function is assessed preoperatively. Transplant recipients are usually well known to the transplant centre where the transplant was performed and have regular follow-up. Information regarding patient and graft progress can easily be accessed by contacting the transplant unit, as can advise on all matters of perioperative management.

Further reading

Bellamy MC and Scott A (2012). Therapeutic issues in transplant patients. *Anaesthesia and Intensive Care Medicine*, **13**, 259–62.

Mason LJ (2004). *Paediatric transplant patients and their medical conditions/therapies: implications for perioperative management*. Available at: <http://www.pedsanesthesia. org/meetings/2004winter/pdfs/mason_Transplant.pdf>.

NHS Blood and Transplant. *Organ donation*. Available at: <http://www.organdonation.nhs.uk>.

Kostopanagiotou G, Sidiropoulou T, Pyrsopoulos N, *et al*. Anesthetic and perioperative management of intestinal and multivisceral allograft recipient in nontransplant surgery. *Transplant International* 2008, **21**, 415–27.

Case 11.4

Management of the brainstem-dead organ donor

Background

Active organ donor management can increase the number of organs suitable for transplantation and allow planned and unhurried removal of organs. It is vital that active organ donor management is continued throughout the perioperative period. Good organ donor management should benefit all organs, and conflict should be avoided between strategies that aim to optimize thoracic or intra-abdominal organs.

Learning outcomes

1 Describe the perioperative critical care and anaesthetic management of the brainstem-dead heart-beating organ donor

2 Acknowledge the process and potential anaesthetic difficulties during organ retrieval surgery.

CPD matrix matches

2C06

Case history

A 37-year-old man (Mr T), who sustained a subarachnoid haemorrhage 48 hours ago, has been confirmed brainstem-dead. You are the anaesthetic registrar on call and have been asked to provide anaesthetic support for a multiorgan retrieval procedure.

What are the physiological changes associated with brainstem death?

+ A preceding period of rising ICP

+ Compensatory arterial hypertension to attempt to restore CPP, the Cushing response, resulting in the stimulation of arterial baroreceptors and a vagally mediated bradycardia

- A 'catecholamine storm' immediately following brainstem death, with tachycardia and vasoconstriction
- Loss of vascular tone and hypotension following catecholamine storm
- Apnoea will occur if ventilation is not controlled.

How should you assess this patient prior to anaesthesia for a multiorgan retrieval procedure?

- You should adopt a similar approach as you would for any other ventilated ICU patient requiring major body cavity surgery
- A thorough bedside ABC assessment, including assessment of the tracheal tube position, ventilator parameters, cardiovascular status, and inotrope requirement
- Collateral history from case-notes and ICU staff
- Review of recent blood results, including ABGs, FBC, coagulation profile, U&E, Cr, and LFTs
- Review of CXR
- Review of any cardiac investigations, e.g. echocardiography
- Review of paperwork relating to brainstem death tests and the authorization for organ donation.

Case update

Your patient has a predicted body weight of 70 kg. He is currently on volume-controlled ventilation of 700 mL at 12 breaths/min, with a PEEP of 5 cmH$_2$O and an FiO$_2$ of 0.5. His ABG shows PaO$_2$ of 15 kPa, PaCO$_2$ of 4.0 kPa, HCO$_3^-$ of 20 mmol/L, and BE of −6.

What can be done to optimize his pulmonary function?

- Lung-protective ventilation should be used, and his tidal volume should be reduced to 6–8 mL/kg; lung-protective ventilation as part of a package of care, has been shown to increase the number of transplantable lungs
- The lowest FiO$_2$ to achieve normoxia should be used. Lowering the FiO$_2$ may prevent bronchiolitis obliterans syndrome in the recipient
- Fluid balance management can be complex, and, whilst the circulating volume must be adequate, pulmonary oedema should be avoided.

Case update

Mr T has an arterial BP of 80/40 mmHg, a CVP of 5 mmHg, a lactate of 2 mmol/L, and warm peripheries. He is not currently receiving any inotropes.

How can he be optimized from a cardiovascular point of view?

◆ He is likely to need BP support in the form of a catecholamine infusion such as noradrenaline

◆ It can be very difficult to get a balance between an adequate intravascular volume and avoiding excessive extravascular lung water

◆ Cardiac output monitoring may be useful to guide fluid boluses; pulmonary artery catheters, oesophageal Doppler monitoring, and techniques based around arterial waveform analysis have all been used

◆ There is no good evidence to guide the type of fluid used for a fluid bolus; however, starch solutions have been associated with an increased incidence of renal dysfunction in some groups of critically ill patients.

Case update

You review Mr T's ICU chart. He has been passing 500 mL/hour of urine for the last 3 hours. His Na^+ has increased to 155 mmol/L.

What condition has likely developed? What are the other endocrine changes that occur following brainstem death?

◆ Mr T has developed central diabetes insipidus

◆ Posterior pituitary function is commonly lost

◆ Anterior pituitary function can be preserved or only partially lost

◆ Insulin secretion is decreased, and hyperglycaemia is common

◆ Hypothalamic temperature regulation is lost.

What drugs can be given as part of 'hormonal resuscitation'?

◆ Methylprednisolone is commonly given to brainstem-dead organ donors, to moderate the inflammatory response that occurs with brainstem death

◆ Glucose levels are often high; an infusion of a short-acting insulin should be given to target normoglycaemia

◆ Central diabetes insipidus may be treated with desmopressin or vasopressin. If the patient has a significant inotrope requirement, then adding vasopressin makes physiological sense

◆ Some organ retrieval teams also administer thyroid hormones, although this is not supported by a recent systematic review.

You transfer Mr T through to theatre. What are the key considerations before the retrieval procedure commences?

- Positioning: usually arms by side
- Large-bore IV access
- Arterial and central lines are mandatory
- Consider cardiac output monitoring
- A surgical pause should occur: you and the retrieval team may well not have worked together before. Issues to be discussed should include the timing of antibiotics, methylprednisolone, and heparin. The documentation relating to brainstem death and the authorization for organ donation should also be reviewed at this time.

What anaesthetic technique should be used?

- Reflex movements can occur, and muscle relaxation is necessary
- If hypertension and tachycardia occur, they can be well treated by the use of a volatile anaesthetic agent. There may also be a beneficial preconditioning effect in the transplanted organs.

What are the surgical stages of a multiorgan retrieval procedure?

- Laparotomy and an initial inspection of abdominal organs
- Median sternotomy: the organ donor should be disconnected from the ventilator during this, then reconnected with a recruitment manoeuvre
- Abdominal dissection continues with the aid of a sternal retractor
- The cardiothoracic team will inspect the heart
- If lung retrieval is planned, then a bronchoscopy will be performed, and differential blood gases from the right and left pulmonary veins will be taken
- The final stage is organ perfusion and retrieval. If the thoracic organs are not being retrieved, then the aorta will be cross-clamped, and perfusion of the abdominal organs commenced below the cross-clamp. Ventilation can be discontinued at this stage
- If the thoracic organs are being retrieved, then the heart will be arrested by the use of a cardioplegia solution. If lung retrieval is planned, pulmoplegia will follow this.

Case discussion

A systems approach is useful in active organ donor management. Lung-protective ventilation should be used. If lung retrieval is planned, then the lowest possible FiO_2 to achieve a PaO_2 of >10 kPa should be used. Fluid management can be challenging, with a difficult balance between an adequate intravascular volume and the avoidance of excess extravascular lung water. The use of a flow-directed fluid management strategy may be of benefit. The development of central diabetes insipidus is common, and this should be treated with vasopressin to prevent dehydration and electrolyte disturbances. Hypothermia and hyperglycaemia should be avoided. The timing of antibiotics, methylprednisolone, and heparin will be guided by the retrieval team.

Summary

Perioperative goals should be centred around maintaining good critical care with lung-protective ventilation and careful fluid balance. Intraoperatively, clear communication between the retrieval team and the anaesthetist is vital. Muscle relaxation is necessary, and volatile anaesthetic agents may be useful in treating hypertension, as well as having a potential beneficial preconditioning effect that is yet to be fully elucidated. The timing of antibiotics, methylprednisolone, and heparin will be guided by the retrieval team.

Further reading

Brunkhorst FM, Engel C, Bloos F, *et al.* (2008). Intensive insulin therapy and pentastarch resuscitation in severe sepsis. *New England Journal of Medicine*, **358**, 125–39.

Macdonald PS, Aneman A, Bhonagiri D, *et al.* (2012). A systematic review and meta-analysis of clinical trials of thyroid hormone administration to brain dead potential organ donors. *Critical Care Medicine*, **40**, 1635–44.

McKeown DW. *Guidelines for donor care during multiorgan retrieval procedures. Local guideline*, Version 10, 2014. Obtained from personal communication with author.

McKeown DW, Bonser RS, and Kellum JA (2012). Management of the heartbeating brain-dead organ donor. *British Journal of Anaesthesia*, **108** (suppl 1), 96–107.

Perner A, Haase N, Guttormsen AB, *et al.* (2012). Hydroxyethyl starch 130/0.42 versus Ringer's acetate in severe sepsis. *New England Journal of Medicine*, **367**, 124–34.

Chapter 12

Urology

Dr Clair Baldie
Dr Simon Heaney

Case 12.1

Laparoscopic radical prostatectomy

Background

There is an increasing surgical preference to performing radical prostatectomy via a non-invasive laparoscopic route, as this reduces the risk of significant blood loss from pelvic bleeding, compared to an open procedure. However, laparoscopic surgery presents its own challenges for the anaesthetist, and patients presenting for this procedure often have comorbidities which exacerbate perioperative difficulties.

Learning outcomes

1 Perform an assessment of comorbidities in a patient presenting for major urological surgery

2 Discuss the haemodynamic effects of pneumoperitoneum in this patient group

3 Outline the perioperative management for a patient with diabetes.

CPD matrix matches

2A03; 2A07

Case history

You are assessing a 65-year-old, 85 kg man with localized prostate cancer, attending for a laparoscopic radical prostatectomy. His past medical history includes type II diabetes, hypertension, and an unremarkable appendicectomy.

A preoperative ECG demonstrates a sinus rhythm, with a ventricular rate of 60, and a left bundle branch block which is unchanged from an ECG 5 years previously. Bloods results include Hb 145, WCC 5.3, Plt 156, Na^+ 138, K^+ 3.8, urea 6.2, and Cr 84. His drug therapy includes lisinopril 20 mg od, bendroflumethiazide 2.5 mg od, aspirin 75 mg od, simvastatin 40 mg od, metformin 1 g bd, and Levemir® 30 U od in the morning.

How would you adapt your preoperative assessment to this patient?

Cardiovascular disease is common in diabetic patients, and clinical symptoms should be actively sought and investigated appropriately. All diabetics should be treated as having a high risk of perioperative myocardial ischaemia. Microvascular complications of interest are nephropathy and neuropathy. Impaired renal function affects the excretion of a wide variety of drugs, and any pre-existing neurological symptoms should be carefully documented, lest they be blamed on the anaesthetic! Resting tachycardias, orthostatic hypotension, constipation/diarrhoea, gustatory sweating, and impotence suggest the presence of autonomic neuropathy, which has a particular association with gastroparesis, regurgitation, and aspiration.

A recent HbA1c should be obtained to ascertain the adequacy of diabetes management in the last 2–3 months. Levels >69 mmol/mol (8.5%) indicate poor glycaemic control and have been associated with a wide range of adverse events. If time and local protocols allow, poorly controlled diabetics should be considered for preoperative optimization of their diabetes. Knowledge of a recent blood glucose is mandatory.

Your patient denies any respiratory or cardiovascular symptoms; he is independent for all activities of daily living and walks his dog daily. His latest HbA1c is 75 mmol/mol (9%), and his capillary blood gas is 13.3 mmol/L. How would you manage his diabetes on the morning of surgery?

This man is a poorly controlled diabetic, undergoing cancer surgery; cancelling the operation to optimize his diabetes is not in his best interest at this stage. Every effort should be made to maintain a good glycaemic control (blood glucose between 4 and 12 mmol/L). On the morning of surgery, metformin should be discontinued, Levemir® given with a 33% dose reduction, and, due to the fact the operation will be lengthy, a variable rate IV insulin infusion (VRIII) started.

How would you conduct an anaesthetic for your patient?

Pneumoperitoneum is required, as well as a substantial period of reverse Trendelenberg (at least 35°). The camera operator stands at the head, making access to the airway difficult. Intubation and IPPV are mandatory; however, your patient is fasted and does not report any symptoms suggesting reflux, so an RSI is not required. Two large-bore cannulae and an arterial line would be prudent. With the arms tucked under the drapes, accessing the patient intraoperatively is problematic. Estimating blood loss is notoriously difficult, as the suction contains a mixture of wash, urine, and blood.

The availability of near-patient Hb testing using HemoCue® or blood gas machine with a fitted co-oximeter would be ideal, with blood being readily drawn from the arterial line.

Maintaining cardiovascular stability is optimal in any anaesthetic, but, due to this patient's poorly controlled diabetes, this may be more difficult (autonomic dysfunction) and of particular importance (increased risk of myocardial ischaemia).

Remifentanil has attractive properties that promote cardiovascular stability and is easily titrated. Reduction in the HR is a common side effect which, when combined with peritoneal stretch and vagal stimulation, can result in dangerous bradycardias; vigilance and the appropriate use of an anticholinergic agent, such as glycopyrrolate, are required. Loading with a long-acting opioid must, of course, be completed well before the end of the operation to prevent remifentanil-induced hyperalgesia.

Case update

Induction of anaesthesia occurs with 2 mg of midazolam, a remifentanil infusion (0.1–0.2 micrograms/kg/min), 100 mg of proprofol, and 50 mg of atracurium. A size 8 portex ETT is sited. IPPV is commenced, and anaesthesia maintained with desflurane and remifentanil. A single slow bolus of gentamicin 2 mg/kg is given to prevent bacteraemia during instrumentation of the urinary tract. A total of 1 g of IV paracetamol and 10 mg morphine are administered to provide post-operative analgesia. A total of 4 mg of ondansetron is used to prevent PONV. On insufflation of the abdomen, your patient's BP increases from 105/56 to 136/72 and then drops 15 min later to 80/46. A fluid bolus and 6 + 6 mg of ephedrine restore the BP to 102/62.

Explain the pathophysiology of the fluctuations in blood pressure and another intervention that could restore cardiovascular stability

Pneumoperitoneum increases the intra-abdominal pressure and is known to have a profound effect on the cardiovascular system. Initially, cardiac output increases, due to autotransfusion of pooled blood from the splanchnic circulation which boosts venous return. The SVR rises, due to direct effects of the insufflation pressure on the vasculature and the release of catecholamines as the peritoneum is stretched. Substantial increases in the myocardial workload occur which may not be tolerated in patients with cardiovascular disease.

Ongoing increases in intra-abdominal pressure can result in the compression of the inferior vena cava, a reduction in venous return, and drop in cardiac output. This is particularly true in hypovolaemic patients or those with impaired cardiac function. The patient is fasted and, due to his high preoperative blood glucose, experienced an osmotic diuresis; he is likely to be hypovolaemic. A simple intervention to treat the cardiovascular instability is to lower the intra-abdominal pressure by releasing some, or all, of the insufflation gas. This can provide time to facilitate an adequate fluid filling.

Case discussion

Laparoscopic surgery is a well-established technique in urology, used within a wide variety of procedures, including nephrectomy, nephroureterectomy, pyeloplasty, cystectomy, varicocelectomy, and radical prostatectomy. Advantages over open surgery include improved cosmetic appearance, better visualization of the operative field, reduced analgesic requirements, improved post-operative respiratory function, and reduced recovery time. However, the raised intra-abdominal pressure, patient positioning, and carbon dioxide absorption that occur during laparoscopic surgery create particular stressors for the patient and challenges for the anaesthetist. Disruption of cardiovascular homeostasis has already been discussed. Other effects include:

- Respiratory: cephalad shift of the diaphragm, due to pneumoperitonium and Trendelenberg positioning, reduces FRC, increases the closing capacity, increases V/Q mismatch, and lowers compliance, the net effect being atelectasis, hypoxaemia, and hypercarbia. IPPV and careful titration of PEEP can help to offset these effects, but caution is advised, as large amounts of PEEP lower the cardiac output

- Renal/liver: insufflation of gas reduces renal and liver function by simple pressure effects on afferent vessels and reducing the cardiac output. An intra-abdominal pressure of 20 mmHg reduces the glomerular filtration by 25%. Patients with pre-existing renal and hepatic disease should be carefully considered before embarking on a laparoscopic procedure

- Neurological: animal models suggest that a rise in the intra-abdominal pressure plus a head-down position can lead to a 150% rise in the ICP. A rise in the ICP is believed to contribute to cerebral oedema and the temporary neurological dysfunction that is occasionally observed in patients emerging from procedures requiring prolonged Trendelenberg positioning. Pneumoperitoneum is undesirable in patients with a pre-existing raised ICP (space-occupying lesions and hydrocephalus) or those with ventriculo-peritoneal shunts

◆ Vasculature: a rare, but devastating, complication of steep Trendelenburg positioning is 'well leg compartment syndrome'. A combination of impaired venous drainage, due to pneumoperitoneum compressing the femoral veins, and impaired arterial perfusion, due to raised lower limbs, can lead to rhabdomyolysis.

Much of the morbidity and mortality associated with laparoscopic procedures can be reduced significantly by simple measures such as returning the patient to a level position for 5–10 min every 2–3 hours and limiting insufflation pressures within the abdomen. The anaesthetist should be vigilant and robust in their approach to ensure that this occurs.

Ten to 15% of surgical patients are diabetic, making diabetes one of the most common conditions faced by the anaesthetist. Recent NHS diabetes guidelines from April 2011 emphasize glycaemic control as the fundamental aim of the perioperative management of the diabetic patient. The dangers of hypoglycaemia are well known, but historically hyperglycaemia has been seen as less important, or even physiologically advantageous, 'providing added energy to damaged tissue'. Evidence supporting the dangers of hyperglycaemia perioperatively is derived from three sources:

1 Laboratory-based studies clearly demonstrate hyperglycaemia impairs innate immunity, by impairing complement and neutrophil function. Hyperglycaemia has procoagulant effects, promotes vasoconstriction, and increases blood viscosity, all of which serve to impair blood flow

2 Leuven's seminal 2001 RCT, comparing tight glycaemic control (4.4–6.1 mmol/L) to a control arm (10–11.9 mmol/L) within a critical care environment, demonstrated clear reductions in mortality and morbidity in the treatment arm. Although the larger NICE-Sugar 2009 RCT failed to repeat these results (in fact, revealing a higher mortality in the tight glycaemic group), these conflicting findings have been blamed on an increased rate of hypoglycaemia. The current consensus suggests that, if hypoglycaemia can be avoided, the avoidance of hyperglycaemia has significant benefits for patients

3 Retrospective studies in all types of surgical patients have demonstrated clear associations between hyperglycaemia and a plethora of adverse outcomes, including wound infection, DVT/PE, increased length of hospital stay, MI, UTI, and death.

Current guidelines suggest 4–12 mmol/L as an acceptable blood glucose range for all diabetic patients that balances the risks of hypo- and hyperglycaemia. Maintaining this throughout a surgical patient's hospital stay is challenging, but several simple interventions can be made:

1 Consideration of preoperative optimization of poorly controlled diabetics (HbA1c >69 mmol/mol (8.5%)) by referral to a diabetic specialist

2 Continuation of long-acting insulins and some oral hypoglycaemics on the morning of surgery and throughout the fasting period (a full list is found in the guidelines)

3 Regular blood glucose monitoring: hourly on the day of surgery, and prompt action to treat hypo- or hyperglycaemia

4 Use of subcutaneous corrective doses of short-acting insulin to correct hyperglycaemia, by either taking advice from the patient, or assuming 1 U will drop the blood sugar by 3 mmol/L in a type I diabetic, or giving 0.1 U/kg in a type II diabetic

5 Appropriate initiation and withdrawal of VRIII.

Summary

A thorough preoperative assessment and meticulous attention to detail of comorbidities will allow optimal preparation of the older patient for urological surgery. Anticipation of physiological changes associated with surgical stresses, e.g. pneumoperitoneum, should minimize the perioperative deleterious effects on the cardiovascular and respiratory systems and optimize post-operative outcomes.

Further reading

Conacher ID, Soomro NA, and Rix D (2004). Anaesthesia for laparoscopic urological surgery. *British Journal of Anaesthesia*, **93**, 859–64.

Hayden P and Cowman S (2011). Anaesthesia for laparoscopic surgery. *Continuing Education in Anaesthesia, Critical Care & Pain*, **11**, 177–80.

Midgley S and Tolley DA (2006). Anaesthesia for laparoscopic surgery in urology. *EAU-EBU Update Series*, **4**, 241–5.

NHS Diabetes (2011). *Management of adults with diabetes undergoing surgery and elective procedures: improving standards*. Available at: <http://www.rcoa.ac.uk/system/files/PUB-MGMT-DIABETES.pdf>.

Turina M, Fry DE, and Polk HC Jr (2005). Acute hyperglycemia and the innate immune system: clinical, cellular, and molecular aspects. *Critical Care Medicine*, **33**, 1624–33.

Total cystectomy with ileal conduit formation

Background

Ileal conduit (IC) is the standard urinary diversion procedure for patients undergoing cystectomy. It has been replaced more recently by bladder substitution procedures in suitable cases. However, IC is still the preferred procedure for patients with comorbidities and those less able to self-catheterize after neo-bladder formation.

A short segment of the small bowel is dissected, into which the ureters are anastomosed and a stoma is formed. This allows urine to traverse the abdominal wall and empty into a bag fixed to the skin.

Learning outcomes

1 Outline a perioperative plan for a patient having a radical cystectomy

2 Discuss potential complications, including major haemorrhage

3 Plan appropriate post-operative analgesia and fluid balance monitoring.

CPD matrix matches

2A03, 2A07

Case history

A 69-year-old man, recently diagnosed with invasive bladder cancer, is on your operating list for an open radical cystectomy and IC formation.

Past medical history includes a left MCA infarct 4 years previously, with a mild residual right-sided weakness. He is able to mobilize well with a stick, walking up to half a mile twice per week. He is hypertensive, with no history of ischaemic heart disease, but is a previous heavy smoker with COPD. His medications include tamsulosin, aspirin, Seretide®, salbutamol, lisinopril, and amlodipine. At pre-admission clinic, he is advised to omit his lisinopril on the day of surgery.

Which preoperative investigations are required?

+ FBC: Hb 145 g/L, WCC 5.2 × 10^9/L, Plt 254 × 10^9/L

+ U&E: urea 4.2 mmol/L, Cr 87 micromoles/L, Na^+ 146 mmol/L, K^+ 4.5 mmol/L

+ Normal LFTs

+ Coagulation studies: APTT ratio 1.1, PT ratio 1.0

+ Group and save: group A rhesus-positive, no antibodies detected

+ ECG shows a sinus rhythm, rate of 74 bpm, with occasional ventricular ectopics

+ Pulmonary function tests carried out at pre-admission clinic show FEV_1 of 2.95 L and FVC of 4.2 L, with a ratio of 70%.

What are the issues to discuss with the patient preoperatively?

+ Anaesthetic technique: ideally combined general anaesthetic and regional technique.

Post-operative analgesia

This gentleman would benefit from the insertion of an epidural. He has a degree of impaired respiratory function, and therefore there is an indication to recommend this procedure.

The potential risks and benefits of a perioperative epidural are discussed with the patient, in order for him to make an informed decision as to accepting this analgesic technique.

Invasive vascular access and monitoring

He has good venous access, and two large-bore cannulae should be inserted. An arterial line and CVC are indicated, as significant blood loss is expected, and they will be helpful for monitoring the BP and delivering vasopressor support in the peri- and post-operative period, if required.

Cardiac output monitoring

Oesophageal Doppler monitoring will be useful to guide fluid replacement in theatre. The perioperative administration of fluids and/or vasoactive drugs, targeted to increase the global blood flow defined by explicit measured goals, reduces mortality following surgery. The use of oesophageal Doppler perioperatively is recommended in the NICE guidelines.

Possible blood transfusion

The possibility of a blood transfusion should be discussed with the patient and documented that he agrees to receive blood products, if necessary.

Post-operative high dependency care environment

Inform the patient and his relatives that he will be nursed in the surgical HDU post-operatively.

What other alternative analgesic techniques could be discussed?

Alternative techniques are bilateral TAP blocks, morphine or fentanyl PCA, and subcutaneous ketamine infusion. Wound catheters, with regular post-operative top-ups of 0.25% bupivacaine, could also be considered.

What is the sequence of events in the anaesthetic room?

- Routine monitoring set-up for the patient (ECG, NIBP, oxygen saturation probe)
- Insert a large-bore IV cannula, and run IV fluids
- Insert a low thoracic epidural awake, with an aseptic technique: the patient either sitting or lying on his side. A test dose of local anaesthetic should be administered
- Once the epidural has been inserted, anaesthesia is induced. After the patient has been intubated and ventilated, put in the arterial and central lines.

What drugs do you want to use in your epidural?

It is best not to use the epidural during the procedure if major blood loss is expected, as it may compound hypovolaemic hypotension. An infusion of remifentanil can be used for analgesia, and then the epidural is loaded once haemostasis is achieved.

A combined opiate/local anaesthetic technique is used. A bolus of 3 mg of diamorphine is injected, followed by an infusion of 0.1% of bupivacaine with 2 micrograms/mL of fentanyl.

In the initial stages of loading the epidural, be vigilant for hypotension, continuing with IV fluids and vasopressor support, if required.

How will the patient be positioned? What else is to be done before the operation starts?

- The patient will be in a lithotomy position, with padded supports for the legs
- A urinary catheter is inserted, and a volumeter attached
- The patient should be wearing antithrombosis stockings, and calf mechanical compression applied to be used perioperatvely

- Insert an oesophageal temperature probe, and apply a warming blanket to the patient
- Remember to check all pressure areas, and check the IV/arterial lines are unkinked, before the patient's arms are wrapped by his sides and the surgical drapes are applied
- IV fluids should be delivered through a warming device
- Prophylactic antibiotics should be given before the first incision, as per local microbiology guidelines.

The surgical procedure involves an initial dissection and excision of the bladder and lymph nodes. There may be considerable blood loss during this stage. The theatre team should monitor suction and swabs for lost volumes. There will be a collection of urine in the pelvis, and the use of saline wash will confuse the amount of blood loss.

The use of bedside oesophageal Doppler monitoring of the cardiac output and regular ABG analysis are recommended to guide the perioperative fluid administration and use.

Once the bladder and prostate are removed, the pelvis will be packed with swabs, and the IC part of the procedure will begin.

A 12–15 cm segment of the ileum is dissected with its blood supply: one end opens as a stoma onto the abdominal wall, and the other end is attached to the ureters. The two ends of the small bowel from which it is dissected are anastomosed.

Case update

During theatre, despite adequate fluids and a Hb of 111 g/L, he required more regular vasopressor boluses, and therefore a noradrenaline infusion (80 micrograms/mL) was started at 3 mL/hour. This maintained his MAP at 70–80 mmHg.

The procedure finished after 7 hours, and the blood loss was estimated at 1700 mL.

The noradrenaline infusion was stopped soon after entering the recovery area, as his BP began to increase.

An FBC, U&E, coagulation, and an ABG were sent to the laboratory. The patient had a further 2 mg of diamorphine and a bag of solution top-up to the epidural, leaving him comfortable and stable cardiovascularly. There was urine output from the new stoma.

In the post-operative period, the patient was cared for in the surgical HDU where enhanced recovery protocols are used for the early introduction of an oral diet and mobilization. An effectively working epidural is very helpful in this process. VTE prophylaxis was administered 6 hours post-operatively, as per local guidelines.

The patient managed well post-operatively, as the epidural was effective and was kept in use for 3 days. For step-down analgesia, a fentanyl patch was applied, and the epidural stopped 12 hours later. Breakthrough pain was treated with short-acting oral oxycodone, as required.

He stayed in the HDU for 4 days and was then transferred to the urology ward. He continued to make a good recovery and was discharged home on the 10th post-operative day.

What post-operative complications may be expected?

Post-operative complications related to IC surgery have been reported in up to 56% of cases and relate mainly to anastomotic leaks, paralytic ileus, and fistula formation.

Later post-operative metabolic derangements are less common with IC, compared to previous ureterosigmoidostomy procedures. Hyperchloraemic acidosis, due to the absorption of Cl^- in exchange for HCO_3^- across the bowel mucosa, is less likely, as there is continual external drainage. This leads to shorter time of urine being in the bowel segment, limiting the time for anion exchange.

Summary

In general, the group of patients undergoing this procedure have a high incidence of existing comorbidity and therefore are higher-risk surgical candidates. In terms of reducing risk, standardized perioperative plans of care, in terms of enhanced recovery (ERAS) protocols, have led to improvement in post-operative morbidity. Patients undergoing IC should be included in the ERAS pathway.

Further reading

Ballantyne JC, Carr DB, deFerranti S, *et al.* (1998). The comparative effects of postoperative analgesic therapies on pulmonary outcome: cumulative meta-analyses of randomised controlled trials. *Anesthesia & Analgesia*, **86**, 598–612.

Farnham SB and Cookson MS (2004). Surgical complications of urinary diversion. *World Journal of Urology*, **22**, 157–67.

Grocott MP, Dushianthan A, Hamilton MA, Mythen MG, Harrison D, Rowan K; Optimisation Systematic Review Steering Group (2012). Perioperative increase in global blood flow to explicit defined goals and outcomes following surgery. *Cochrane Database of Systematic Reviews*, **11**, CD004082.

National Institute for Health and Clinical Excellence (2011). *CardioQ- ODM (oesophageal Doppler monitor) (MTG3)*. Available at: <http://guidance.nice.org.uk/MTG3>.

Royal College of Anaesthetists (2009). *National audit of major complications of central neuraxial block in the United Kingdom. Report and findings, January 2009*. Available at: <https://www.rcoa.ac.uk/system/files/CSQ-NAP3-Full_1.pdf>.

Percutaneous nephrolithotomy

Background

About 2% of the population have a urinary tract stone at any one time. Many people are asymptomatic, but pain is the commonest symptom. Preoperative investigations must identify the position, size, and number of stones that may be present in the renal parenchyma and/or the collecting system. Extracorporeal shock wave lithotripsy began in the 1980s and introduced a minimally invasive method of treating stones. However, this method has been found to have limitations in obese patients and those with an abnormal renal anatomy where it is difficult to put the stone in the focal zone of the wave generator. In these cases, surgical intervention is required.

Learning outcomes

1 Perform a preoperative assessment for percutaneous renal tract surgery

2 Understand patient positioning during these procedures

3 Anticipate and manage specific post-operative complications related to percutaneous nephrolithotomy (PNL).

CPD matrix matches

2A03; 2A07

Case history

A 37-year-old man presented to his GP with intermittent severe left flank pain and haematuria. Investigations by the urology team found him to have a 3.0 cm calculus in the left kidney. He was seen in pre-admission clinic for work-up for an elective PNL.

He is fit and well, with no previous medical history, is not on any medications, and has no allergies.

What are the important investigations for this man at pre-admission clinic?

- FBC
- U&E
- Urinalysis.

Case update

His results show Hb 141 g/L, WCC 8.5 × 10^9/L, Plt 289 × 10^9, urea 4.5 mmol/L, Cr 76 micromoles/L, Na^+ 140 mmol/L, and K^+ 4.3 mmol/L. Despite his haematuria, his ultrasound is normal. His renal function is also normal. Urinalysis shows blood ++, nitrite ++, and leucocytes ++.

What must the staff in the pre-admission clinic do after seeing the urinalysis result?

Send off a urine sample for culture and sensitivity (C&S), as it indicates this gentleman has a urine infection. The microbiology must be followed up pre-operatively and appropriate antibiotics started, before the patient comes in for the procedure. The urine will be re-tested on the day of admission.

Case update

The gentleman was advised to visit his GP 2 days later and be prescribed a suitable antibiotic from the C&S sample taken at the pre-admission clinic. However, due to work commitments, he had only managed to visit his GP 2 days before coming in for surgery. The GP had started him on a course of ciprofloxacin. On admission, his urinalysis was similar to the previous result.

The surgeon and the anaesthetist discussed the case and thought it best that the procedure be cancelled. He would be rescheduled after he had completed the course of antibiotics.

The patient was annoyed and argued against this decision—he felt fine and had made considerable plans to cover his business whilst in hospital and recovering from his procedure.

Further discussion ensued, and a review of his observations made—the patient was systemically well; he had a normal WCC and was apyrexial.

The decision was made to continue with the procedure.

What are the main issues for the anaesthetist for this type of procedure?

- Renal function (drug metabolism considerations)
- Positioning

- Sepsis
- Bleeding
- The possibility of a prolonged procedure: stones have differing chemical make-up and require variable lengths of time for their destruction by ultra-sonics or laser
- A change/delay of procedure: occasionally, at cystoscopy, it may be noted that there is an overt infection present, and the PNL procedure will not be perfomed. Instead, a nephrostomy will be performed and a post-operative course of appropriate antibiotic prescribed
- Crowded theatre: the procedure involves a urologist, a radiologist, and a radiographer. Equipment includes an X-ray C-arm with screens and a fibre-optic scope stack.

What is your plan for managing the airway for this procedure?

The patient should be intubated, preferably using a reinforced tube. The procedure involves two positions. First, the patient will go into a lithotomy position for the urologist to perform cystoscopy and insert a ureteric balloon catheter to be used for the retrograde study.

The patient will then be put into a prone position. The radiologist will perform access through the flank to the kidney, under radiological guidance. Initially, a needle is inserted, followed by dilators, then followed by a telescope sleeve inserted into the calyx of the kidney. It is through this access sleeve that the urologist is able to pass a scope and the ultrasound device or laser that will break up the stone.

What drugs will you draw up for the case?

- Consider midazolam 1–3 mg
- Propofol 2–4 mg/kg
- Remifentanil to be run as an infusion
- Atracurium 0.5 mg/mL
- Ondansetron 4 mg
- Morphine 10 mg
- Ephedrine and metaraminol.

What is the standard antibiotic prophylaxis for urological procedures?

Each anaesthestist should check with the local antimicrobial policy, but generally gentamicin 2 mg/kg is used if the renal function is normal. If there is significant renal impairment, then the alternative is ciprofloxacin 400 mg which should be given prior to the start of cystoscopy.

What are the issues in positioning for this case?

For the prone position, take care with regard to pressure areas, i.e. ankles, knees, male genitalia, breasts, and face. Use a pillow under the upper chest area, pelvis, and ankles. Ensure there is no pressure on the eyes and there is adequate padding where contact occurs. There are many types of face protectors available. The arms should be placed on boards in front of the head. Ensure the shoulders are positioned, so there is no stretch on the neck or brachial plexus.

Are there any other perioperative interventions and monitoring to consider?

◆ An active patient warming device, such as a Bair Hugger®, is imperative: this procedure may be prolonged, and there is often a lot of irrigation fluid that may soak through to the sheets

◆ Temperature probe

◆ The patient should be wearing thromboembolism deterrent (TED) stockings, and a mechanical calf compression device should be applied.

What would you prescribe for post-operative medication?

◆ Analgesia:
  • Morphine PCA, with a loading dose prescribed
  • Regular paracetamol
  • For young patients with normal renal function: consider regular NSAID
◆ Antiemetics: ondansetron and cyclizine
◆ VTE prophylaxis 6 hours post-operatively
◆ Buscopan® 10 mg, as required, for urinary tract spasm.

Case update

The urologist has almost finished the process of stone breakdown. So far, the procedure has been uneventful. However, the patient begins to require more regular doses of pressor and inotropic support with metaraminol and ephedrine. The BP remains no more than 70/40, despite these drugs and turning off the remifentanil infusion.

What is the most likely cause of hypotension for this patient, and what should the anaesthetist do next?

The most likely cause is septic shock:

- Give colloid boluses, and start a vasopressor infusion
- Give antibiotics, as per local hospital guideline for severe urinary sepsis.

Case update

Within 15 min, the procedure is complete, but the patient is now on an infusion of metaraminol (0.5 mg/mL) running at 45 mL/hour. The anaesthetist has managed to put in a radial arterial line. His vital signs are: HR 85 bpm, BP 90/45 mmHg, SpO_2 98% on FiO_2 0.5. An ABG has been sent for analysis, demonstrating: H^+ 54 nmol/L, pCO_2 5.1 kPa, pO_2 13.5 kPa, HCO_3^- 24.5 mmol/L, BE –8.2, and lactate 3.1 mmol/L.

What should be the next course of action?

Refer to the critical care consultant, and arrange admission to the ICU. This patient has severe urosepsis and should be admitted for continued ventilation, vasopressor support, and monitoring. Insert a CVC, and change the vasopressor support to a noradrenaline infusion.

Case update

The patient was stabilized in theatre and then transferred to the ICU. He was kept intubated and ventilated for 2 days, and he required vasopressor support for 3 days. His renal function deteriorated and reached a plateau of urea 15 and Cr 198, but he did not require haemofiltration. He was discharged from hospital 5 days after leaving the ICU.

Summary

PNL was established in the 1970s and is considered to be the best technique for removing large and multiple stones in the inferior calyx. A 2007 review of >1000 cases showed the incidence of post-operative fever is 21–32% and that of septicaemia of 0.3–4.7%. A careful selection of patients is recommended to reduce complications. PNL is contraindicated in patients with a UTI or pyonephrosis.

Further reading

Michel MS, Trojan L, and Rassweiler JJ (2007). Complications in percutaneous nephrolithotomy. *European Urology*, **51**, 899–906.

Transurethral resection of the prostate

Background

Transurethral resection of prostatic tumours require specific consideration for potential electrolyte disturbance throughout the perioperative period. Patients may present for surgery with an obstructive nephropathy, with elevated urea and creatinine, and are at risk of dilutional hyponatraemia, resulting in water intoxication syndrome, both during and following the procedure, due to the absorption of hypotonic 1.5% glycine irrigation fluid.

Learning outcomes

1 Recognize the post-operative transurethral resection of the prostate (TURP) syndrome

2 Differentiate other causes of post-operative neurological impairment

3 Outline the correct management plan for post-operative hyponatraemia.

CPD matrix matches

2A06; 2A07

Case history

A 70 kg, 79-year-old man with benign prostatic hypertrophy has presented for an elective TURP. He was known to have glaucoma, recurrent UTIs, AF, and a mild degree of cognitive impairment. However, he lived alone in the community, with support from his daughter. He had an excellent exercise tolerance and frequently went for long walks. He managed all his activities of daily living. His medications included aspirin, digoxin, tamsulosin, oxybutynin, doxazosin, and timolol.

A preoperative ECG demonstrated AF, with a ventricular rate of 72. Pre-operative investigations were as follows:

◆ Hb 134 g/L, WCC 6.5, Plt 232

◆ Na^+ 132 mmol/L, K^+ 4.5 mmol/L, urea 5.5 mmol/L, Cr 62 micromoles/L.

Induction of anaesthesia occurred with 50 micrograms of fentanyl and 100 mg of propofol. A size 4 LMA was placed correctly. A self-ventilating anaesthetic was maintained with sevoflurane, with 1 g of IV paracetamol, a further 50 micrograms of fentanyl, and 5 mg of morphine as intraoperative analgesia. A single slow bolus of gentamicin 2 mg/kg was given to prevent bacteraemia during instrumentation of the urinary tract.

The urology registrar struggled to resect the hyperplastic tissue and required help from his consultant. Ninety minutes later, the operation finished, and the patient entered the recovery room. A further 30 min later, the recovery nurse informs you that she cannot waken your patient.

What is your differential diagnosis for the delayed recovery of consciousness?

1 Pharmacological:

- Opioids: produce sedation and respiratory depression, the intensity of which can be difficult to predict in the elderly
- Volatile anaesthetic agent: emergence from anaesthesia depends on the pulmonary elimination, MAC awake being typically 30% of MAC. Opioid-induced hypoventilation lengthens the time taken to exhale the anaesthetic agent

2 Metabolic:

- Hypoglycaemia: post-operatively most often results from poorly controlled diabetes, starvation, and alcohol consumption
- Hyperglycaemia: blood hyperosmolality and hyperviscosity predispose to cerebral oedema and thrombosis
- Hyponatraemia: <120 mmol/L causes confusion; in this context, the most likely cause would be TURP syndrome
- Hypothermia: confusion at <35°C unconsciousness at <30°C

3 Respiratory failure: resulting in hypoxia, hypercapnia, or both

4 Neurological:

- Intraoperative cerebral insult, secondary to an inadequate cerebral perfusion, due to a low MAP, thrombosis, or intracranial haemorrhage
- Central anticholinergic syndrome, antihistamines, antidepressants, and anti-parkinsonian drugs are common culprits.

What would be your initial management?

- ABC: secure the airway, 100% oxygen, manual ventilation
- D: assess GCS, capillary blood glucose

♦ E: measure the temperature, and warm if <35.5°C; clinical examination with particular attention to the respiratory and nervous systems (focal or lateralizing neurology)

♦ Investigations:
  • ABG: correct hypoxia, hypercapnia, or acidosis
  • A point-of-care assessment of Hb values if a co-oximeter measurement is not included in the ABG, e.g. HemoCue® (blood loss is inevitable during TURP and difficult to estimate intraoperatively, due to the large amounts of irrigation fluid used)
  • Blood tests: FBC, U&E, osmolality, and glucose.

Case update

After a further 15 min, your patient started to regain consciousness but was confused, complaining that he could not see properly. Over the next few minutes, he became increasingly agitated, before slipping into a self-limiting 2-min grand mal seizure. Meanwhile, the blood gas results are available, demonstrating a Na^+ of 114 mmol/L (later confirmed on formal bloods).

What is your diagnosis?

Severe TURP syndrome.

What is your management?

Secure the airway, and support ventilation, as required, typically with tracheal intubation and PPV. Inotropes or vasopressors should be administered via a central line, as required, to maintain normotension for the patient, with invasive pressure monitoring via arterial access.

Further seizures can be controlled with IV diazepam, in 2 mg increments, up to 10 mg, or repeated once after 15 min. Consider a bolus of 2 g IV magnesium sulfate if seizures are uncontrolled.

You may consider administering a small dose of hypertonic saline (3% NaCl), typically in the dose of 1–1.5 mL/kg, infused over 1 hour.

The patient should be subsequently admitted to intensive care for ongoing therapy.

Case discussion

Most often associated with TURP, a similar phenomenon has been described with other procedures requiring irrigation fluids such as endometrial ablation and ureteroscopy.

The most common irrigation fluid used in the UK is 1.5% glycine which has an osmolality of 220 mOsmol/kg, hypotonic relative to plasma (280–300 mOsmol/kg). Rapid intravascular infusion of this hypotonic fluid can trigger a variety of pathological processes.

1 Intravascular volume shifts:

Absorption rates of irrigation fluid can approach 200 mL/min, leading to a rapid intravascular volume expansion, with consequent hypertension, reflex bradycardia, LV failure, and pulmonary oedema. This may be followed by profound hypotension, as dilutional hyponatraemia and hypertension lead to a net water flux, along osmotic and hydrostatic pressure gradients, out of the intravascular space. Fluid shifts should be anticipated in the patient with TURP syndrome, necessitating invasive monitoring and careful fluid management in a critical care setting post-operatively.

2 Hyponatraemia and plasma osmolality:

Rapid infusion of sodium-free fluid produces hyponatraemia, via an initial dilutional effect, followed by natriuresis. Although undoubtedly hyponatraemia contributes to the pathology of TURP syndrome, current thinking suggests that plasma hypo-osmolality may be the more important factor. The clinical consequences of hyponatraemia are due to water moving from a relatively hypo-osmolar ECF into the hyperosmolar cell interior, cerebral oedema being the most serious complication. The Nernst equation predicts that a decrease in the extracellular Na^+ concentration, from 140 to 100 mmol/L, has only a modest effect on membrane excitability, increasing the resting membrane potentials by a modest 9 mV. Therefore, the likely explanation for TURP symptoms, such as headache, altered level of consciousness, nausea and vomiting, seizures, coma, and death, is not the low levels of Na^+ per se, but the plasma hypo-osmolality resulting in cerebral oedema. Measuring and correction of plasma osmolality should be a key aspect in the management of TURP syndrome.

In practice, Na^+ levels below 120 mmol/L are likely to be associated with low plasma osmolality and severe TURP syndrome, requiring treatment. Infusion of hypertonic saline, commonly 3%, is the conventional treatment used. Regimes vary, but the following has been suggested:

- Calculate total body water (TBW) as 0.6 × body weight (kg), e.g. 70 kg man = 42 L
- 2 × TBW / 1000 as the number of mL of 3% NaCl which will raise serum [Na^+] by 1 mmol/L
- For example, 2 × 42 / 1000 = 84 mL of 3% NaCl
- Usually given over 1 hour.

The rate of correction has traditionally been advocated to be no more than 1 mmol/L/hour, to avoid the most feared complication of central pontine myelinolysis (CPM). Most authors suggest stopping hypertonic saline on the resolution of symptoms and not waiting for Na^+ levels to be fully corrected.

3 Hyperglycinaemia:

Glycine is a known inhibitory neurotransmitter, present in the midbrain, spinal cord, and retina. These depressant effects on the CNS make hyperglycinaemia the most likely culprit for the visual aberrations described during TURP syndrome. Symptoms can range from blurred vision to complete blindness and will usually resolve within 24 hours as the glycine is metabolized. No specific treatment is required, except for reassurance.

Glycine also potentiates the action of NMDA receptors which can result in paradoxical excitatory symptoms such as seizures. Consideration of magnesium therapy for glycine-induced encephalopathy is a rational approach. In addition to its well-known membrane-stabilizing properties, magnesium exerts a negative action on NMDA receptors, and plasma levels are likely to be low, due to the dilutional effects of the irrigation fluid.

Anaesthetic considerations

Spinal anaesthesia is regarded as the technique of choice for TURP (2.5–3.0 mL of plain 0.5% bupivacaine), despite a lack of objective evidence demonstrating clear benefit over general anaesthesia. Perceived advantages are good post-operative analgesia, reduced surgical stress response, and, most importantly, the early identification of TURP syndrome. Sedation can be provided with midazolam or propofol, though these drugs could mask the early signs of TURP syndrome. Additionally, the profound sympathetic blockade from a spinal anaesthetic can worsen the cardiovascular consequences of profound fluid shifts.

If a general anaesthetic technique is selected, a single-shot caudal epidural injection with 20–25 mL of 0.375% plain bupivacaine could be considered for post-operative analgesia. A valid criticism of this case would be the failure to consider a regional technique.

Summary

There are several benefits to the use of regional anaesthesia in urological surgery in the elderly patient group. The generic advantages of a central–neuraxial block, including reduction in post-operative respiratory complications, reduced venous thrombosis risk (particularly important in patients with prolonged lithotomy positioning), and reduced blood loss, are boosted by the benefit of the ability to continually monitor central neurological function in patients undergoing TURP, under regional anaesthesia alone.

Further reading

Duffty J and Hilditch G (2009). Anaesthesia for urological surgery. *Anaesthesia and Intensive Care Medicine*, **10**, 307–12.

Gravenstein D (1997). Transurethral resection of the prostate (TURP) syndrome: a review of the pathophysiology and management. *Anesthesia & Analgesia*, **84**, 438–46.

O'Donnell A and Foo I (2009). Anaesthesia for transurethral resection of the prostate. *Continuing Education in Anaesthesia, Critical Care & Pain*, **9**, 92–6.

Reeves MD and Myles PS (1999). Does anaesthetic technique affect the outcome after transurethral resection of the prostate? *BJU International*, **84**, 982–6.

Sinclair R and Falerio R (2006). Delayed recovery of consciousness after anaesthesia. *Continuing Education in Anaesthesia, Critical Care & Pain*, **6**, 114–18.

Vaidya C, Ho W, and Freda BJ (2010). Management of hyponatremia: providing treatment and avoiding harm. *Cleveland Clinic Journal of Medicine*, **77**, 715–26.

Chapter 13

The difficult airway

Dr Caroline Brookman
Dr Vanessa Humphrey

Introduction: the difficult airway

Difficulty with airway management can be encountered in all anaesthetic sub-specialties. A difficult airway may be due to difficulty in mask ventilation, supraglottic device ventilation, tracheal intubation, or all three. Difficult face mask ventilation has a reported incidence of 0.01–5%. Failed intubation has an incidence of 1:2230 in the general population, but this does not take into account the number of attempts, technique or device used, or the degree of skill and experience of the operator.

The cases in this chapter serve as examples of management, based on the clinical experiences of the authors. There is a lack of evidence for specific techniques in those who are truly difficult, and each set of circumstances is unique. However, recent national audits (NAP4), published guidelines, and prominent cases in the media have demonstrated the need for careful airway assessment, planning and communication of airway management, and improved training in airway management techniques.

The development of new airway devices, e.g. indirect and videolaryngoscopes, may provide alternatives in some cases, but there is limited evidence for their use in difficult airways, and designs are still evolving.

In all cases, certain rules apply, despite the variety of approaches:

1 **Oxygenation** is the priority. Failure to provide it will cause hypoxic brain injury, followed by death

2 Develop an airway strategy to avoid progression to a 'can't intubate, can't ventilate' (CICV) situation

3 Repeated attempts at airway manipulation cause trauma, oedema, and morbidity. Make your first attempt your best attempt, e.g. optimize direct laryngoscopy through optimal positioning, alignment, and use of adjuncts such as the Oxford Head Elevating Laryngoscopy Pillow™ in obese patients

4 Be aware of the influences of human factors such as task fixation. Since a difficult airway is a rare occurrence, it can lead to denial or reinforcement of a high-risk approach

5 Aim to improve training and personal experience with the wide variety of equipment and techniques in use. Become highly competent in the core airway skills

6 Careful preoperative assessment, planning, and communication are para-mount, including backup plans and a plan for extubation. Follow-up and documentation of difficult airways should be thorough

7 National guidelines from the Difficult Airway Society are readily available—know and use them.

Further reading

Cook TM, Woodall N, and Frerk C; on behalf of the Fourth National Audit Project (2011). Major complications of airway management in the UK: results of the Fourth National Audit Project of the Royal College of Anaesthetists and the Difficult Airway Society. Part 1: anaesthesia. *British Journal of Anaesthesia*, **106**, 617–31.

Cook TM, Woodall N, Harper J, and Benger J; on behalf of the Fourth National Audit Project (2011). Major complications of airway management in the UK: results of the Fourth National Audit Project of the Royal College of Anaesthetists and the Difficult Airway Society. Part 2: intensive care and emergency departments. *British Journal of Anaesthesia*, **106**, 632–42.

Difficult Airway Society Extubation Guidelines Group: Popat M, Mitchell V, Dravid R, Patel A, Swampilla C, and Higgs A (2012). Difficult Airway Society Guidelines for the management of tracheal extubation. *Anaesthesia*, **67**, 318–40.

Henderson J, Popat M, Latto I, and Pearce A (2004). Difficult Airway Society guidelines for management of the unanticipated difficult intub*ation. Anaesthesia*, **59**, 675–94. Also available at: <http://www.das.uk.com/guidelineshome.html>.

Popat M (2009). *Difficult airway management*. Oxford University Press, Oxford.

Sudheer P and Stacey M (2002). Anaesthesia for awake intubation. *British Journal of Anaesthesia CEPD Reviews*, **2**, 139–43.

Cervical spine injury

Background

Between 2 and 5% of blunt trauma patients have a cervical spine injury, and this should be assumed, until proven otherwise. Immobilization, with an appropriately sized hard collar, sandbags, and tape, should be checked in the primary survey. With this full combination, spinal movement is decreased to about 5% of normal. Ten per cent of those with a cervical spine injury have another vertebral fracture, so the patient should be 'log-rolled' on a spinal board to maintain vertebral column alignment.

Learning outcomes

1 Acknowledge the incidence of cervical spine injury in the polytrauma patient
2 Discuss the risks and benefits of conventional vs video-assisted intubation techniques in a patient with a neck injury.

CPD matrix matches

1C01; 2A01

Case history

A 19-year-old male driver presents to the ED, following a head-on collision with another vehicle at 60 mph. He is alert and talking, but he has a scalp laceration and obvious bruising over his chest. Initial observations include HR 72, BP 90/60, RR 24 breaths/min, SpO_2 98% on high-flow oxygen, and a GCS of 14/15 due to confusion. He is in a hard collar with spinal board and sandbag immobilization.

What should be the initial management strategy in the emergency department?

Initial management of the trauma victim with a potential spinal cord injury uses ATLS principles. This includes assessment and sequential treatment of:

- Airway with cervical spine control
- Breathing

◆ Circulation and control of haemorrhage

◆ Disability

◆ Exposure.

Airway patency should be assessed, high-flow oxygen applied, and a jaw thrust used to open the airway, if necessary. If the airway or breathing is compromised, the decision to intubate should be made early to maximize oxygen delivery and limit secondary hypoxic damage to the injured spinal cord.

In the hypotensive trauma patient, haemorrhage should be excluded. This may be difficult, as concurrent injuries may be masked by spinal cord injury. The goals of spinal cord resuscitation should be cervical spine stabilization, prevention of secondary injury, fracture reduction, and spinal cord protection. This may involve early ventilation, maintaining spinal perfusion, temperature control, and glycaemic control. Cervical spine injury can have both mechanical and vascular components to it, leading to hypoperfusion. The vertebral arteries, due to their course, are often compromised in cervical trauma.

What are the airway considerations in cervical spine trauma?

The urgency of airway intervention is the most important factor in planning airway management for patients with potential cervical spine injuries. Other considerations include the risk of worsening spinal cord injury during laryngoscopy, the airway anatomy, the degree of patient cooperation, and the anaesthetist's expertise. Airway instrumentation may need to be as an emergent procedure for airway obstruction, respiratory failure, or management of severe head injury. At a later stage, airway management for surgical treatment of the fractured spine or other injuries may be necessary. The main aim during airway management in patients with potential cervical spine injuries is to cause the least amount of spinal movement possible.

Concurrent head injury, with reduced consciousness and pharyngeal tone, is the commonest trauma-related cause of airway obstruction. The airway may also be soiled with blood or regurgitated matter. Blunt or penetrating injuries that can obstruct the airway include maxillary, mandibular, and laryngotracheal fractures and large anterior neck haematomas. Vigilant reassessment with immediate restoration and protection of airway patency are essential.

A difficult intubation should be anticipated, due to:

◆ Suboptimal positioning, due to immobilization of the cervical spine

◆ Requirement for an RSI with cricoid pressure

◆ Potential for prevertebral swelling, due to haematoma and soft tissue oedema

◆ Poor visibility at laryngoscopy, due to debris or distorted anatomy in maxillofacial trauma.

Case update

The patient's GCS rapidly dropped to 8. He is still breathing spontaneously, with an SpO_2 of 96%, but now requires an oropharyngeal airway to maintain his airway. The working diagnosis is that of an expanding intracranial haematoma. The patient now needs to be intubated and ventilated to protect his airway and ensure adequate oxygenation and control of carbon dioxide.

What are the options for airway management?

Rapid sequence induction and direct laryngoscopy

For patients requiring immediate airway control, where there are no other anticipated difficulties, RSI with cricoid pressure and manual in-line stabilization (MILS) may be the best option, due to speed and familiarity. All airway manoeuvres will produce some degree of cervical spine movement, and mask ventilation (with chin lift and jaw thrust) is known to produce more movement than direct laryngoscopy.

Precise cervical spine MILS should be maintained throughout by an allocated second individual. This opposes the rotation of the occipito-atlanto-axial complex that is generated by direct laryngoscopy. Movement is primarily at C1–3 during elevation of the laryngoscope blade. The front of the hard collar should be removed; otherwise, it will impede mouth opening, jaw thrust, laryngeal manipulation, and supraglottic/surgical airway insertion, if required. It will also increase the proportion of Cormack and Lehane grade 3 or 4 laryngeal views. It does not contribute significantly to neck stabilization during laryngoscopy. MILS allows for a better view and less cervical spine movement than a hard collar. Bimanual cricoid pressure is advised, if there is a fracture in the C4–6 region, but does require another anaesthetic assistant. Cricoid pressure itself has little effect on the upper cervical spine. Standard RSI precautions are necessary and a backup plan identified.

Intubation is difficult in nearly 10% of RSIs undertaken in the ED. Problems may be avoided by assessing for potential difficulties pre-induction. Pre-oxygenation may be difficult, due to poor mask seal, patient confusion, maxillofacial trauma, and airway obstruction. Mechanical trismus may hinder the supraglottic airway (SGA) or laryngoscope insertion. MILS and cricoid pressure increase the incidence of Cormack and Lehane grade 3 laryngeal views to 20%. No particular laryngoscope blade has shown a superior benefit, except the McCoy levering laryngoscope, which will improve the view at laryngoscopy in the neutral position by up to 50% in simulated cervical spine injuries. Application of the lever avoids maximal elevation of the blade, and so less force is required for laryngoscopy. This also has the additional benefit of producing less of a haemodynamic response during laryngoscopy. The use of backward, upward, and rightward pressure (BURP) may also improve the laryngoscopic view. A gum elastic bougie can then aid intubation, following minimal glottic exposure. The use of a straight blade may exert less vertebral movement than a curved blade in experienced hands. The role for the newer indirect (including 'video') laryngoscopes is less clearly defined. They may provide better glottic visualization, but do not necessarily reduce movement of the cervical spine, and may have a longer intubation time. Further evidence is required regarding these devices.

Awake fibreoptic intubation

AFOI with adequate local anaesthesia has the advantage of avoiding movement of the unstable cervical spine. It may also be performed with cervical spine immobilization and allows neurological assessment, following intubation. It may also be the best option where difficulty is anticipated for anatomical reasons. However, this method requires skill and specialist equipment, and it is impractical in the urgent situation. Blood, saliva, and vomitus can make fibreoptic visualization impossible. Patient coughing can be disastrous for cervical spine stability and the ICP. Therefore, airway anaesthesia should be careful and thorough. Judicious opioids can be used, in addition to suppressing coughing, e.g. a remifentanil infusion. The technique is usually reserved for the controlled situation of a planned surgical fixation.

Asleep fibreoptic intubation

An alternative technique in the planned situation is that of an asleep fibreoptic intubation. Again, this can be achieved with a cervical spine immobilization in place. A Berman™ intubating airway may act as a useful conduit. Alternatively, an SGA/Aintree™ technique may be considered. The latter can also be useful in the failed or unanticipated difficult intubation. The forces applied during SGA insertion can cause a posterior displacement of the cervical spine, but the movement is less than that seen in direct laryngoscopy.

Surgical airway

In the emergency situation, waking a patient up after the return of spontaneous breathing is rarely appropriate, especially if an RSI is undertaken for an inadequate airway patency, ventilation, or oxygenation. A surgical airway may therefore be necessary in a 'can't intubate' situation. In some situations, e.g. laryngotracheal disruption with an impending airway obstruction, an emergency tracheostomy is the initial treatment of choice and should be done by an experienced operator from the outset. Surgical airway manoeuvres can produce a posterior displacement of the cervical spine, but this should not prevent the use of this lifesaving procedure. Creating a surgical airway is harder with a restricted neck extension, laryngotracheal disruption, subcutaneous emphysema, or an anatomical distortion by a penetrating injury or haematoma. Needle cricothyroidotomy may be difficult in this situation. Therefore, a surgical technique is indicated, with a horizontal stab incision through the skin and cricothyroid membrane, followed by a blunt enlargement of the wound to pass a cuffed tube.

Case update

The hard collar was replaced with MILS, and the patient underwent an RSI with thiopentone, fentanyl to obtund the haemodynamic response, and suxamethonium. (Suxamethonium is safe to use within the first 24, and possibly up to 72, hours after an acute spinal injury.) He had an uneventful intubation over a bougie, using a McCoy laryngoscope. He then went on to have an emergency craniotomy and evacuation of an extradural haematoma.

Summary

The optimal strategy for airway management in cervical spine injury remains controversial. There is no evidence of superiority for one technique over another, with respect to neurological outcome. The technique chosen will primarily depend on the urgency of the situation. A familiar technique done well and in a timely manner is the most appropriate.

Further reading

Cranshaw J and Nolan J (2006). Airway management after major trauma. *Continuing Education in Anaesthesia, Critical Care & Pain*, **6**, 124–7.

Crosby E (2006). Airway management in adults after cervical spine trauma. *Anesthesiology*, **104**, 1293–318.

Leemans M and Calder I (2011). The unstable cervical spine. In: Johnston I, Harrop-Griffiths W, and Gemmell L, eds. *AAGBI core topics in anaesthesia*, pp. 88–104. Wiley-Blackwell, Oxford.

Theron A and Ford P (2012). Acute cervical spine injuries in adults: initial management. *Update in Anaesthesia*, **28**, 112–18.

Trauma.org. Available at: <http://www.trauma.org>.

Veale P and Lamb J (2002). Anaesthesia and acute spinal cord injury. *British Journal of Anaesthesia CEPD Reviews*, **2**, 139–43.

Case 13.2

Acromegaly

Background

Acromegaly is a syndrome caused by oversecretion of growth hormone after long bone epiphyseal fusion. The pathology is usually an anterior pituitary tumour, but it can also arise from other hormonally active tumours. Acromegaly affects males and females equally. It has an incidence of 3–4 per million per year, and a prevalence of 50–70 cases per million population. It has an insidious onset and usually presents in middle age with the classical physical appearance of bony overgrowth of the hands, feet, and facial bones, and soft tissue enlargement of the upper airway.

Learning outcomes

1 Discuss the airway difficulties and comorbidities that present in a patient with acromegaly

2 Outline a plan for the induction of anaesthesia in an acromegalic patient for elective surgery.

CPD matrix matches

1C01; 2A01

Case history

A 45-year-old male with acromegaly presents for transphenoidal removal of a pituitary tumour. Airway assessment reveals normal dentition, a large tongue, Mallampati class 3, an interincisor gap of 3 cm, mandibular protrusion class A, thyromental distance of 7 cm, and good atlanto-occipital movements.

What are the characteristic features of acromegaly?

Musculoskeletal

- ◆ Coarsening of features
- ◆ Large hands and feet

- Prominent supraorbital ridges
- Wide nose
- Nerve compression syndromes
- Kyphoscoliosis
- Skin thickening, increased sweating/sebum production
- Arthropathy
- Myopathy.

Airway

- Macroglossia
- Prognathism with malocclusion
- Hypertrophy of pharyngeal and laryngeal soft tissue—epiglottis, aryepiglottic folds
- Fixation and thickening of the vocal cords
- Recurrent laryngeal nerve palsy
- Decreased width of the cricoid arch
- Glottic/subglottic stenosis.

What are the other associated conditions?

Cardiovascular

- Hypertension—40%
- LV hypertrophy
- Ischaemic heart disease
- Congestive cardiac failure
- Cardiomegaly
- Conduction defects and arrhythmias.

Other

- Diabetes—25%
- Obstructive sleep apnoea—70%
- Pulmonary function tests—extrathoracic obstruction
- Visceromegaly
- Mass effects from tumour—visual field defect (optic chiasm compression), headache.

What are the potential difficulties with airway management?

The nature of airway difficulty can be unpredictable and difficult to accurately identify. First, there may be a problem in maintaining a patent airway with a face mask, due to the large tongue and general upper airway soft tissue hypertrophy, when muscle tone is lost under general anaesthesia. This is particularly relevant in those with a history of obstructive sleep apnoea. In addition, the application of a face mask may be awkward, due to a large head and jaw. Second, direct laryngoscopy and tracheal intubation may also be difficult. SGAs may not be helpful, due to soft tissue hypertrophy.

The following statistics have been previously reported:

- 39% of acromegalics had some degree of airway difficulty (Seidman)
- 26% (Schmitt) to 33% (Hakala) had a Cormack and Lehane grade 3 or 4 view at laryngoscopy
- 10% were a difficult intubation (Schmitt, Nemergut/Zuo)
- Asleep fibreoptic intubation may fail (Hakala).

Routine airway assessment may also give an inaccurate prediction. Twenty per cent of acromegalics with a Mallampati class 1 or 2 may be difficult to intubate.

What are the options for airway management?

Patients with acromegaly require a very careful and thorough airway assessment. If there is any concern regarding the ability to maintain a patent airway, then a technique whereby the airway is secured awake is the safest option. In practice, this means an AFOI.

An airway strategy should be formulated with a plan A, and a backup plan should that fail. This must be communicated to the anaesthetic assistant. All equipment should be checked with regard to its availability, cleanliness, and functionality.

A reinforced (armoured) ETT is best to avoid the risk of kinking. (A pre-formed south-facing ETT may not be long enough in an acromegalic.) The ETT should be taped to the opposite side from the nostril used for surgical access. A throat pack should be inserted, and its use documented, as per local protocol. Documentation of the Cormack and Lehane grade under direct laryngoscopy post-AFOI is useful for any future intubations.

Case update

This patient underwent an uneventful AFOI, using a spray-as-you-go technique, with remifentanil 0.1 micrograms/kg/min sedation.

What is the plan for extubation?

Much is written and talked about with regard to difficult intubation. Often, less attention is paid to extubation. This is potentially a very risky time. This patient will have nasal packs in and a throat pack which should be removed and documented as done. The oropharynx should be carefully suctioned under direct vision, including the posterior nasopharynx. There will probably be blood present which has the risk of causing laryngeal obstruction post-extubation—commonly referred to as a 'coroner's clot'.

Any residual neuromuscular block must be reversed, and discontinue general anaesthesia. Adequate long-acting analgesia should have been given. A smooth emergence is the aim to minimize the chance of increased venous pressure from coughing, causing further bleeding. Continuing the remifentanil infusion is very helpful in achieving this. (Remifentanil is commonly used intraoperatively to obtund the hypertensive response to periods of intense surgical stimulation. Its context-insensitive half-life ensures a rapid offset, regardless of the rate and duration of infusion.) The patient should obey commands and have regular spontaneous respiration before the ETT is removed. The patient should be extubated in the sitting position to optimize airway and respiratory function. There will be obligate mouth breathing, due to the nasal packs.

After every extubation, there should be a clear plan for reintubation, should that be necessary, with appropriate equipment and staff available.

Post-operative airway care

Supplemental oxygen, ideally via a capnography mask, is given in the immediate post-operative period. A more prolonged period of observation will be required for those with a history of obstructive sleep apnoea.

Summary

Due to the potential problems of airway maintenance and intubation, AFOI has increasingly become the technique of choice. As such, there is little recent evidence regarding the optimal method of securing the airway under general anaesthesia, and nothing published regarding the use of videolaryngoscopes in these patients. A Plan A and an escape plan for extubation should be formulated as a routine in patients with advanced airway management at induction.

Further reading

Hakala P, Randell T, and Valli H (1998). Laryngoscopy and fibreoptic intubation in acromegalic patients. *British Journal of Anaesthesia*, **80**, 345–7.

Menon R, Murphy PG, and Lindley AM (2011). Anaesthesia and pituitary disease. *Continuing Education in Anaesthesia, Critical Care & Pain*, **11**, 133–7.

Nemergut EC, Dumont AS, Barry UT, and Laws ER (2005). Perioperative management of patients undergoing transsphenoidal pituitary surgery. *Anesthesia & Analgesia*, **101**, 1170–81.

Nemergut EC and Zuo Z (2006). Airway management in patients with pituitary disease. A review of 746 patients. *Journal of Neurosurgery and Anesthesiology*, **18**, 73–7.

Reddy R, Hope S, and Wass J (2010). Acromegaly. *BMJ*, **341**, 400–1.

Schmitt H, Buchfelder M, Radespiel-Tröger M, and Fahlbusch R (2000). Difficult intubation in acromegalic patients: incidence and predictability. *Anesthesiology*, **93**, 110–14.

Seidman PA, Kofke WA, Policare R, and Young M (2000). Anaesthetic complications of acromegaly. *British Journal of Anaesthesia*, **84**, 179–82.

Smith M and Hirsch NP (2000). Pituitary disease and anaesthesia. *British Journal of Anaesthesia*, **85**, 3–14.

Thyroid tumour

Background

Communication with the patient and surgical team is of paramount importance in the emergency situation where the patient has a threatened airway. The anaesthetist should also be experienced in the technique of AFOI before attempting a difficult airway in an unusual position. This case demonstrates how one must then adapt to a particular situation.

Learning outcomes

1 Make an initial assessment of the acutely compromised airway.
2 Formulate a plan for emergency management of the difficult airway.

CPD matrix matches

2A01

Case history

A 71-year-old female presented with increasing shortness of breath over 3 weeks. She now has severe dyspnoea and a choking sensation which is relieved by lying prone. Her only past medical history is that of hypothyroidism. On examination, she is lying prone, propped up on her elbows. She is maintaining her own airway, is able to talk in short sentences, and has an inspiratory stridor. She has an obvious large neck mass, originating on the left and causing a tracheal deviation to the right. She is referred for an urgent tracheostomy.

What is your initial management?

The airway is in a critical condition. Supplemental oxygen should be given. IV dexamethasone and nebulized adrenaline (1 mg in 5 mL of saline) will help to reduce any associated mucosal oedema and buy some time for the preparation of equipment, drugs, and staff.

Case update

Initial nasendoscopy by an ENT surgeon showed a normal larynx and normal vocal cords. Therefore, the entire obstructive lesion was below the cords. Further investigation was necessary to determine the extent of the lesion, prior to definitive treatment. The patient underwent emergency radiological investigations, comprising ultrasound and CT scans (performed whilst the patient remained prone). These demonstrated a large solid mass arising from the thyroid, deviating and compressing the trachea to approximately 5 mm, but with no retrosternal component. The carotid artery was also displaced. Upper airway assessment was unremarkable, with good mouth opening, full dentition, and a Mallampati class 2. The surgical plan is for a tracheostomy and biopsy of the lesion. For this, the patient will need to be turned supine.

What are the problems?

The airway is in a critical condition and at risk of sudden total obstruction. The patient is now becoming exhausted, both by the work of breathing and that of keeping herself propped up on her elbows. The trachea is severely deviated, possibly kinked, and is significantly compressed. Whether this compression is fixed or not is unknown.

The tumour is potentially causing venous congestion, further hazarding the airway and increasing the bleeding risk on both airway manipulation and surgery. The patient can only maintain her airway in the knee–elbow prone position. This partially relieves the compression on the trachea, due to the weight of the tumour. Any airway manipulation will need to be done in this position.

What are the options to secure the airway?

1 Is it possible to do a tracheostomy under local anaesthesia?

No. It is not technically possible to perform this in the prone position. It is also likely to be an extremely difficult procedure, due to the large tumour in the way, the potential bleeding, and the extent of the tracheal deviation and compression.

2 Is it possible to intubate under general anaesthesia?

No. It is not possible to do this prone, as the patient's position will collapse. Supine, there is an unsurmountable risk of a CICV and 'can't achieve front of neck access' situation.

Therefore, the plan is to intubate her awake, whilst she remains self-supporting.

What are the problems of an awake fibreoptic intubation in this case?

A topical 'spray-as-you-go' technique is required, as superior laryngeal nerve blocks and a cricothyroid puncture are obviously not possible. There is a risk of causing bleeding and laryngospasm, or the patient might panic, causing a sudden loss of airway.

Sedation is contraindicated, as the patient's airway is dependent on her being fully awake and self-supporting. The unusual position creates additional complications. Although experienced in fibreoptic intubation, this operator had never performed the procedure in that position before.

How are you going to perform the procedure?

It is very important to build up a rapport with the patient and gain her confidence. An explanation of the plan and the fact that it is the only safe option available is essential. All members of the theatre team must remain calm. Your plan must be communicated and discussed with the rest of the team.

Routine monitoring, IV access, and supplemental oxygen are applied. An antisialogogue, such as glycopyrrolate, is necessary, given as early as possible. All equipment should be prepared and checked.

The patient will be positioned prone on the operating table, supporting herself on her elbows, as far up the table as possible, allowing easy access to her head for the operator to sit on the floor beneath her.

Topical anaesthesia, using 4% lidocaine, can be carefully applied to the upper airway, using whatever method the operator is experienced in. This can be supplemented by further instillations via the working channel of the fibrescope.

What size and type of endotracheal tube should be selected?

A small-diameter, atraumatic ETT is preferred such as a size 6.0. This will minimize the gap between the fibrescope and the ETT, with less chance of encountering resistance passing through the cords and traumatizing the compressed trachea. If available, a bullet-tipped reinforced ETT, e.g. Fastrach™, will also have the advantage of resisting compression by the tumour on turning the patient supine.

The only adult ETT available with a smaller diameter would be a microlaryngoscopy tube, sizes 5 and 5.5. Their compatibility would need to be checked with the particular make/size of the fibreoptic scope used.

What is your plan B?

In this case, there is really not any other option, and an emergency cricothyroidotomy will not be possible. However, an experienced consultant ENT surgeon was present and scrubbed, with surgical instruments immediately to hand.

Case update

The procedure was well tolerated and straightforward. Below the cords, the trachea was 'slit-like', but the fibreoptic scope passed through, and a 6.0 Portex™ Ivory ETT was gently railroaded with ease.

Once the airway was secured, the patient was anaesthetized and turned supine. She underwent an uneventful surgical tracheostomy, using a size 8.0 adjustable flange tracheostomy tube, positioned laterally due to the tumour.

Subsequent pathology results of the biopsy were returned as a high-grade lymphoma. The patient received chemotherapy but unfortunately died within a month.

Summary

If conscious, patients with acute airway compromise will automatically adopt the easiest position in which to breathe. In this case, the patient's position (equivalent to that of the quadrupedal animal) creates an airway alignment with an atlanto-occipital extension, opening the airway up, along with gravity displacing the soft tissues. Securing the airway with the patient awake and self-supporting is the only safe option.

Further reading

Neal MR, Groves J, and Gell IR (1996). Awake fibreoptic intubation in the semi-prone position following facial trauma. *Anaesthesia*, **51**, 1053–4.

Morquio's syndrome

Background

Morquio's syndrome is one of the mucopolysaccharidoses (MPS), which is a group of inherited multisystem storage disorders. Specific enzyme deficiencies cause an incomplete degradation of complex glycosaminoglycans and the storage of acid mucopolysaccharides. Clinical manifestations reflect the accumulation of specific MPS derivatives in various organs. It is subdivided into types:

- Type I: Hurler, Scheie, and Hurler–Scheie syndromes
- Type II: Hunter's syndrome
- Type III: Sanfilippo syndromes A, B, C, and D
- Type IV: Morquio's syndrome, types A and B
- Type VI: Maroteaux–Lamy syndrome
- Type VII: Sly syndrome.

Learning outcomes

1 Acknowledge the difficulties in an adult with a congenital syndrome affecting the airway

2 Discuss the difficulties in managing paediatric-sized patients in the adult setting.

CPD matrix matches

1C01; 2A01

Case history

A 40-year-old female presents with left pelvi-ureteric junction obstruction with marked hydronephrosis. She has a nephrostomy *in situ* and requires a ureteroscopy and endopyelotomy. She has Morquio's syndrome. She has had multiple orthopaedic procedures as a child. Her most recent anaesthetic was 10 years ago, and her notes are not available. She has no other past medical history. She is active and has no overt cardiorespiratory symptoms.

What are the key features of Morquio's syndrome?

All of the MPS are primarily characterized by the following clinical features:

- Physical deformities
- Skeletal abnormalities
- Cardiac defects
- Ocular defects
- Neurological/mental disabilities
- Reticuloendothelial abnormalities.

Morquio's syndrome has an incidence of <1 in 250 000. It is autosomal recessive, therefore affecting males and females equally. There is an accumulation of keratan sulphate. The diagnosis is made by the characteristic clinical features, keratan sulphaturia, and specific enzymatic assays. The main features are skeletal abnormalities.

What are the general skeletal abnormalities?

- Short stature
- Pectus carinatum (pigeon chest)
- Lower rib flaring
- Genu valgus
- Valgus deformity of the elbow
- Ulnar deviation of the wrist
- Metacarpal deformities
- Ligamentous laxity and hypermobile joints (but not hips, knees, elbows)
- Flat feet
- Waddling gait.

What are the spinal abnormalities?

- Short trunk and neck
- Platyspondyly universalis (flattened vertebrae)
- Wide intervertebral disc spaces
- Progressive spinal deformity: lumbar lordosis, dorsal kyphosis, and barrel-shaped chest
- Odontoid hypoplasia and subluxation of C1 on C2, leading to spinal cord compression.

What are the other features?

- ◆ Restrictive lung defect secondary to thoracic spine problems
- ◆ Aortic and mitral regurgitation
- ◆ Corneal clouding
- ◆ Conductive hearing loss
- ◆ Hepatosplenomegaly
- ◆ Mid-face hypoplasia and a depressed nasal bridge, resulting in a broad, flat face
- ◆ Enamel dysplasia
- ◆ Death from spinal cord problems or cor pulmonale in 3rd to 4th decade.

Case update

On examination, this patient has the typical stature of Morquio's syndrome. She is 100 cm tall and weighs 25 kg. Her heart sounds are normal, and her chest is clear. Her airway examination reveals moderate mouth opening (Mallampati class 2), moderate jaw protrusion, and a full set of teeth. She has a very short neck, with no cervical extension and minimal flexion.

Her investigations show the following:

- ◆ Normal blood biochemistry and haematology
- ◆ ECG: sinus tachycardia; rate of 120
- ◆ Pulmonary function tests: FEV_1 0.5 L, FVC 0.75 L, ratio 66.7%
- ◆ Echocardiogram: normal valves, good LV function.

Her C-spine X-rays show the following:

- ◆ Very limited movement
- ◆ Abnormal, reduced height vertebrae
- ◆ The anterior arch of the atlas and C2 fused inferiorly
- ◆ Central subluxation, appears stable
- ◆ Bony protruberance into the hypopharynx by the anterior arch of the atlas.

What are the general problems in anaesthetizing this patient?

This lady is a paediatric-sized patient; her height is equivalent to that of a 4-year-old and her weight to that of an 8-year-old child.

- ◆ Positioning for surgery will require the Lloyd–Davies set-up
- ◆ Paediatric-sized equipment

- Temperature control
- Fluid balance
- Difficult, prolonged surgery
- Drug dosing.

What are the specific airway problems?

She is going to be difficult to both maintain an airway and to intubate. Conventional direct laryngoscopy will not be possible, due to:

- Facial abnormalities
- Excess pharyngeal mucosa
- Atlas protruberance into the hypopharynx
- Lack of C-spine mobility
- Atlanto-axial subluxation.

What are the options available to secure the airway?

Since this lady is an adult with normal intelligence, her management will be different to that seen in paediatric practice. The safest way is to secure the airway awake. However, there are some specific issues to be considered in this case.

Equipment

Regarding the size of the ETT, a 4-year-old child would normally take a 5.5, and an 8-year-old a 6.5 internal diameter ETT. Although this lady has a relatively large head, in comparison to her body, a small ETT is preferable for fibreoptic intubation to minimize the difficulty in railroading the tube. Appropriately sized rescue equipment also needs to be sourced and be immediately available for the duration of the perioperative period.

Local anaesthesia of the airway

A spray-as-you-go technique is the safest approach, using whatever method of topicalization with which the operator is most familiar. The maximum dose needs to be carefully calculated, since she is only 25 kg: 9 mg/kg = 225 mg = 5.5 mL of 4%, or 11 mL of 2%, lidocaine.

Sedation

This should be cautious. The aim is to achieve a cooperative and relaxed patient and maintain verbal contact. Drugs should be titrated very carefully, as doses (particularly of anxiolytics) cannot be directly extrapolated from paediatric dose calculations. The agent used will depend on individual preference and experience, e.g. midazolam or TCI propofol or remifentanil.

The patient will also require a preoperative anticholinergic (such as glycopyrrolate 150 micrograms) and supplemental oxygen. The cervical spine should be protected by keeping the neck in a neutral position.

Case update

This patient had an AFOI under sedation which was technically very difficult. After topicalization of the airway, the oral route was attempted. However, there was very little air space, due to a large epiglottis, excess pharyngeal mucosa, and the protrusion of an osteophyte into the hypopharynx. The vocal cords were visualized, but the fibrescope was unable to pass through, due to the very acute angle. The level of sedation had to be reduced, as the patient's airway tended to obstruct very easily. The nasal route was then attempted after further topicalization. (A total of 200 mg of lidocaine was administered.) This approach was much easier, due to the less acute angle of the airway. A size 6.0 ETT was railroaded with ease.

How are you going to extubate this patient?

Muscle relaxation should be reversed, and any residual drugs in the IV line must be adequately flushed through. This lady had a brief apnoea after her cannula was flushed, probably due to residual remifentanil. Dexamethasone 4 mg was given intraoperatively to reduce any airway swelling, in view of the prolonged airway instrumentation in the presence of a pre-existing narrow airway. The cuff was deflated to check for a leak around the tube prior to extubation. The patient was extubated awake in the sitting position. Due to the local anaesthesia, the nasal ETT is usually well tolerated.

What is the appropriate post-operative care plan for this lady?

The patient should have supplemental oxygen and regular observations. Ideally, she should be nursed in a high dependency area. Non-opioid analgesia should be maximized, with judicious parenteral opioid, if necessary. Transcutaneous carbon dioxide monitoring may be useful. The doses of all drugs and fluids will need to be carefully calculated.

What was your plan B if a fibreoptic intubation was not achievable?

Abandon the procedure. This is non-lifesaving surgery. Any further attempts will cause trauma and oedema to an already narrow airway. This patient would need very careful planning for a future date and may need the assistance of experts from a specialized unit.

In retrospect, the nasal route should have been the initial plan. It is easier to anaesthetize with a smaller dose of local anaesthetic, and it provides a straighter approach to the larynx. The osteophyte had also been noted on the C-spine X-ray, but its relevance not appreciated until during the procedure.

Summary

This case highlights some of the problems in dealing with a congenital syndrome within an adult hospital setting. It also reminds us that, on occasion, we may need to abandon the procedure and do no further harm.

Further reading

Williams KA, Barker GL, Harwood RJ, and Woodall NM (2005). Combined nebulization and spray-as-you-go topical local anaesthesia of the airway. *British Journal of Anaesthesia*, **95**, 549–53.

Chapter 14

Transport and retrieval medicine

Dr Jon McCormack

Case 14.1

Pre-hospital management of a multiply injured trauma victim

Background

The recent recognition of pre-hospital emergency medicine as a certified sub-specialty by the Royal College of Anaesthetists and the Royal College of Emergency Medicine will increase exposure to, and opportunities for, anaesthetists working in a field traditionally dominated by emergency medicine physicians. The key aspects of this discussion relate to the vital lifesaving procedures that anaesthetists may be expected to perform, functioning as single-handed practitioners, with limited resources in a high pressure and an unfamiliar environment.

Learning outcomes

1 Effective and safe operation in the pre-hospital environment
2 Initial assessment and resuscitation of the polytrauma patient
3 On-scene interventions
4 Transfer to definitive care.

CPD matrix matches

2A02; 2A11

Case history

During an intensive care medicine attachment you are on a rota shared with the ED to provide a pre-hospital medical team, in response to a request from paramedics on scene for a physician's attendance. One evening you are tasked for an emergency medical response to a high-speed road traffic collision, in which a car has left a motorway at high speed after aquaplaning and rolled over several times in a field. No specific details have been provided, other than there are multiple severely injured casualties.

What are the key principles relating to responding safely and effectively to a pre-hospital request like this?

Team composition

Requests for a pre-hospital medical response team should have defined staff identified on a specific trauma team rota. Teams should not be hastily brought together on receipt of such a tasking, as team dynamics are likely to be suboptimal. The team should be a minimum of two members, typically a doctor and an ED nurse, though enhanced role paramedics and critical care practitioners are increasingly filling this role. All team members must be appropriately trained in emergency anaesthesia and advanced emergency interventions, extrication, communication, and scene safety. Neither of these team members should ideally be involved in driving to the scene of an accident, as ongoing communication and navigation will impede safe driving.

Equipment

Pre-hospital medical equipment should be comprehensively detailed and checked regularly. This should include equipment for intubation and ventilation, vascular access, splints, dressings, thoracocentesis and minor surgical procedures, and drugs to facilitate these procedures. However, pre-hospital medical equipment should be restricted to that which may actually be used on scene; for example, advanced airway devices, invasive pressure lines, multiple infusion pumps, and complex ventilators are unnecessary in the pre-hospital environment. The appropriate equipment and drugs should be available to hand immediately and packaged securely in a bag which is dedicated for the pre-hospital team's use only.

Communication

On arrival at the scene of the accident, the medical team should identify themselves immediately to the senior fire officer who has overall command of the scene safety. Do not assume that all vehicles have been made safe from movement or fire hazard. After ascertaining it is safe to approach the casualties, identify yourself and colleagues to the ambulance incident officer; obtain a summary of casualties involved and a brief nature of the injuries. Consider a coordinated review of multiple casualties, and perform a rapid trauma triage before committing the team's resources to any specific patient.

Personal protective equipment

This should be donned before arrival on scene. As a minimum, it should include a hard hat, with identification of the wearer as a member of the medical team, clear eye protection, a high-visibility waterproof jacket, protective footwear, and protective gloves. Be particularly vigilant for the use of cutting equipment, which

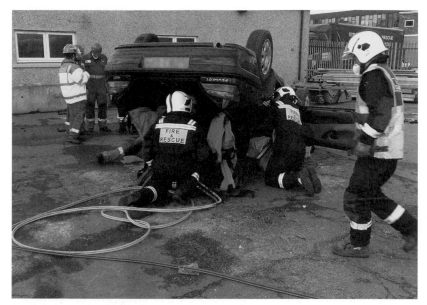

Fig. 14.1 Example of appropriate personal protective equipment to be donned during a patient extrication from an overturned vehicle. Note the spray of glass shards displaced during the cutting process. (Reproduced with kind permission from the Emergency Medical Retrieval Service.)

may cause shards of metal and glass to be violently dispersed and may cause significant injury to inappropriately placed limbs or digits (see Figure 14.1).

Case update

On arrival at the scene, you are updated by the lead paramedic that there are three casualties and one fatality. The most seriously injured patient is a 15-year-old male who was ejected from the hatchback as the car rolled over. He was only recently found over 30 m from the vehicle, face down in a muddy field. He has clearly sustained head and facial injuries, has blood and mud in his airway and laboured respirations, is peripherally shut down, and is minimally responsive to painful stimulus. He has had no interventions as yet from the paramedics.

What life-threatening injuries should your primary survey aim to identify at this stage?

Airway

Prior to any manoeuvres, the patient requires spinal immobilization. This patient, found lying face down, should have a cervical hard collar applied and subsequently be log-rolled onto a scoop stretcher. Definitive immobilization with head blocks and tapes, and chest, pelvic, and leg fixation straps will be required prior to movement but are likely to impede the primary assessment so should be deferred in favour of MILS initially. The airway should be inspected for broken teeth, foreign bodies, blood or secretions, and controlled suction performed under direct vision, if appropriate. Avoid deep blind suctioning at this stage, due to concerns of pushing debris deeper into the airway. High-flow oxygen should be administered through a trauma mask with a reservoir bag. It is now accepted practice to insert nasopharyngeal airways as an airway adjunct in the multiply injured patient.

Breathing

Rapid assessment of life-threatening chest injuries includes determination of the presence of flail chest, tension pneumothorax, haemothorax, or tamponade. All will be difficult to assess in the pre-hospital environment, due to poor lighting and ambient noise from vehicles and machinery. There should be a very low threshold for performing thoracostomies in severely injured casualties with possible chest injuries if they will be ventilated for transfer to definitive care.

Circulation

Assessment of the cardiovascular status may be limited to peripheral or central pulse checks, until monitoring can be established and ECG and BP measurements are performed. Peripheral capillary refill is likely to be significantly prolonged in trauma victims, due to hypovolaemia and the rapid onset of hypothermia.

Disability

Where possible, an accurate three-component GCS should be documented early in the assessment process to form a baseline from which to assess the response to therapeutic interventions. Frequently, an AVPU system is communicated by paramedics, briefly detailing whether the casualty is **a**lert, responsive to **v**oice or **p**ain, or **u**nconscious. A motor response to pain only is suggested to equate to a GCS of 8. The pupils should be examined at this stage. A brief scan of the limbs may reveal obvious gross deformities which should be considered and managed later, as part of the secondary survey.

Case update

Your rapid primary survey elicits that the patient has a compromised airway, due to blood and secretions; he has laboured breathing, with an obvious flail chest on the left side and a reduced air entry. The carotid pulse is present, but peripheral pulses are impalpable, and the capillary refill is >5 s. He is minimally responsive to pain, with some abnormal hand flexion, and has a slightly dilated pupil on the left side. He has gross lower limb deformities.

Outline the immediate management priorities for this patient

This patient will require emergency anaesthesia for intubation and ventilation for his chest and head injuries, decompression of a probable haemopneumothorax, vascular access with volume support, fracture immobilization, and packaging for transport.

Intubation

A drug-assisted intubation is the priority to maintain oxygenation, prevent hypercarbia, and protect the airway in the face of depressed consciousness.

Location

Where possible, the patient should have any interventions performed on the ambulance trolley, rather than on the ground, to minimize difficulties. This should be in an area away from the immediate scene of the accident, ideally with privacy from the general public, with dedicated assistance from the ambulance and fire services. Where possible, any engines or generators should be turned off to minimize disruption on critical verbal communication during the induction of anaesthetic. The area should be as well lit as possible.

Equipment

A preparation area should be identified, and all necessary intubation equipment and drugs laid out in an orderly fashion (see Figure 14.2). The location of emergency adjuncts or surgical airway equipment should be identified to team members. Oxygen reserves and battery-operated suction units must be immediately to hand. All monitoring, including capnography, should be established and confirmed as operational, prior to the commencement of the induction of anaesthesia. The choice of anaesthetic drugs for induction may be varied, dependent on the clinical situation, but agents which minimize cardiovascular instability, e.g. ketamine, are often favoured by pre-hospital physicians.

Team resource management

Defined roles should be allocated for airway management, anaesthetist assistance, drug administration, cricoid pressure, and manual in-line neck stabilization. Typically, the medical team will consist of two staff; hence it will be necessary to request the support of ambulance, police, or fire service colleagues for some of these roles. The entire team should be briefed on the planned sequence of the induction, and roles defined in the event of an escape plan

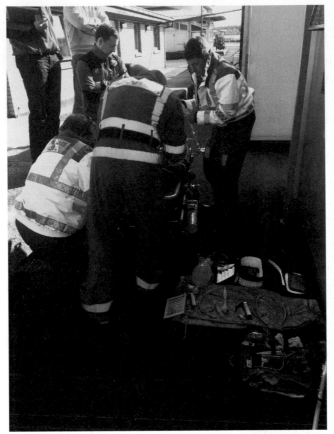

Fig. 14.2 Example of an appropriate 'airway kit dump' for a pre-hospital RSI.

needing to be activated. Many pre-hospital emergency services use a checklist to ensure equipment availability and team role definition, such as that shown in Figure 14.3.

Chest decompression

With the finding of a flail chest and the commencement of IPPV, thoracic decompression is indicated in the patient. Needle decompression is generally ineffective beyond immediately releasing a tension pneumothorax in a peri-arrest situation. The favoured approach in the pre-hospital settings is formal thoracostomy, without an intercostal chest drain insertion. The open wound can be immediately re-explored with a gloved finger if there is concern of re-accumulation of blood or air. The timing of this procedure should be carefully considered. Pre-intubation thoracostomy will likely lead to a sucking chest wound in a patient with respiratory distress. However, deferring the procedure

	EMRS Emergency Anaesthesia Checklist
✓	**PLAN**
	Rapid sequence induction (RSI) indicated?
	Airway assessment - ABCD and LEMON
	Modifications to standard RSI considered?
✓	**PREPARE PATIENT**
	Optimise patient position including 360° access where possible
	Establish monitoring (BP, Sp02, ECG) and ensure visible to team leader
	IV access x 2 and fluids running freely
	Connect nasal cannula to pt & wall O_2-5L (apnoeic O_2study)–NOT Pre-Hosp pt
	Optimum pre-oxygenation – 3–5mins of high flow O_2
✓	**PREPARE EQUIPMENT**
	Suction - accessible on right side of patient
	Endotracheal tube x 2 (Size 8.0 male, 7.0 female + smaller size)
	Endotracheal tube cuffs checked and lightly lubricated
	20ml syringe
	2 working laryngoscopes (standard or video) – Macintosh size 3 & 4 blades
	Tube tie or Thomas tube holder
	Catheter mount
	Filter
	Capnograph attached to filter and monitor
	Stethoscope
	Bougie & stylet
	Magills forceps, LMA and surgical airway in sight
✓	**PREPARE TEAM–ALLOCATE ROLES**
	Airway/intubation
	Cricoid pressure
	Intubator's assistant (pass equipment)
	Drug administration
	Manual inline stabilisation (if indicated)
	Drug Administrator to turn on nasal cannula O_2 to 15 L immediately after paralysing agent given
✓	**TEAM BRIEFING INCLUDING FAILED INTUBATION PLAN**
	Plan A e.g. Intubation
	Plan B e.g. LMA insertion
	Plan C e.g. Bag Mask Ventilation
	Plan D e.g. Surgical Airway
✓	**DRUGS**
	Estimate patient's weight in kg
	Suxamethonium 1.5 mg/kg or Rocuronium 0.6 – 1.0 mg/kg
	Etomidate 0.3 mg/kg⁻ or Ketamine 2 mg/kg
	Atropine / Ephedrine / Epinephrine prefilled syringes available
	Modifications to standard drugs / dosage considered
✓	**CONFIRMATION OF AIRWAY**
	Check ETC02 trace on monitor
	Listen for air entry – Team Leader verifies airway secure
✓	**PREPARE FOR TRANSFER**
	Maintain anaesthesia, analgesia and paralysis for journey
	Insert Guedel airway as bite block if not using Thomas tube holder

Fig. 14.3 An example of a pre-induction checklist. (Reproduced with kind permission from the Emergency Medical Retrieval Service.)

until after intubation runs this risk of air accumulation and intrathoracic pressure effects. The often favoured approach is for one team member to perform intubation; then as soon as correct tracheal tube placement is confirmed, a second team member performs a thoracostomy. Where serious chest injury is suspected and a unilateral thoracostomy has been performed, due consideration should be given to decompressing the contralateral side as a default, as clinical examination in the pre-hospital or transport environment is likely to prove difficult to confirm or exclude the presence of a contralateral pneumothorax.

Vascular access

In a multiply injured shocked patient, vascular access will be a challenging task. Difficulties include hypovolaemia reducing venous filling, hypothermia causing peripheral vasoconstriction, and long bong fractures disrupting venous flow. At least two good venous access points should be established prior to the emergency induction of anaesthesia. Where multiple limb injuries are evident, avoid siting cannulae distal to the fractures, as extravasation of drugs and fluids into the fracture haematoma is predictable. A proximal intraosseus needle insertion may be of value, with the humeral head being an optimal site for this. Small boluses of crystalloid should be infused to achieve perfusion that generates at least a palpable radial pulse, but caution should be exercised to avoid overinfusion that may result in relative hypervolaemia and clot disruption. Availability to blood and blood products is at present limited in most pre-hospital medical services, but, where available, early transfusion is likely to improve outcome.

Fracture immobilization

Blood loss from lower limb long bone fractures will contribute significantly to hypovolaemia, and the legs should be splinted prior to transport. There are a variety of commercially available devices, in the style of box splints or modified Thomas splints, carried in the pre-hospital settings which can be rapidly applied. Similarly, where the mechanism of injury has been significant, it is valuable to consider applying a pelvic splint prior to moving the patient.

Packaging

Adequate packaging of the patient, prior to transfer to definitive care, aims to serve two functions: to reduce potential fractures, so limiting further blood loss, pain, or neurological injury; and to maximize the safety and security of ventilatory equipment and IV fluid and drug lines. This patient requires general immobilization on a scoop stretcher or vacuum mattress, with straps across the chest, pelvis, knees, and feet, and additional cervical spine stabilization with head blocks and tapes. Patients should not be transported over any distance on extrication boards, sometimes referred to as 'spinal boards'. The splinted legs and pelvis should be incorporated in this spinal immobilization package. Access to two IV lines should be preserved during packaging, such that these are readily accessible during transport, without the need to undo any retaining straps. In the pre-hospital setting, it is common that manual ventilation with a bag and mask is used over transport ventilators, but whichever is used, continuous end-tidal capnography, attention to tube fixation and the protection of the gas supply tubing is paramount to minimize the risk of accidental extubation.

Case update

Your patient has undergone an RSI with ketamine and rocuronium. On laryngoscopy, the airway was found to be contaminated with blood and foreign debris, but he has been intubated and had subsequent bilateral thoracostomies. He has markedly reduced pulmonary compliance, but, with manual ventilation, it is possible to achieve an SpO_2 >90%. Full monitoring is established which demonstrates tachycardia and hypotension, though the physiological parameters are relatively stable and you have administered appropriate doses of sedation, analgesia and muscle relaxant. He has been fully immobilized for both leg fractures and spine and is now packaged for transport to your satisfaction. A road ambulance and rotary wing air ambulance are on scene, and you are 5 miles from the nearest district general hospital and 15 miles from the nearest major trauma centre.

How should this patient's transfer to definitive care be undertaken?

There are many factors influencing the decision making on transport platforms, and, in many cases, the air ambulance may not always be the most rapid transport modality (see Figure 14.4).

Speed

Air ambulances will travel considerably faster than road ambulances, but there are often time delays built into air transfer that limit the benefits of faster relative ground speed. There will be carrying time and loading time into the aircraft; typical start-up and shutdown procedures take several minutes at each end of the flight. Many major trauma centres have on-site helipads which do not require secondary (road) transfer to the ED, but this is not uniform and may not be serviceable due to maintenance, staffing, or weather issues. A journey of 15 miles may take 20–25 min by road out with congested areas/times. A flight of this similar distance may only take 6–8 min, but there is likely to be at least 10 min added by loading/unloading and start-up/shutdown procedures, so the time difference over a road transfer for these sorts of distances becomes marginal.

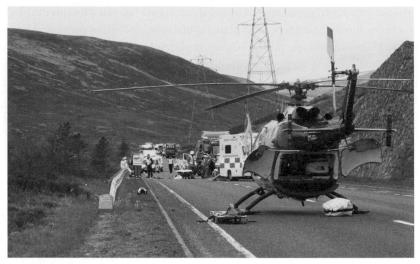

Fig. 14.4 Air ambulances will often be present at the scene of major road traffic collisions. (Reproduced with kind permission from Scotland's Charity Air Ambulance.)

Patient management

Access to the patient and additional equipment is usually restricted in air ambulances, and the potential to perform interventions beyond manual ventilation and administering drugs is limited. If it is anticipated that major interventions may be required on transport, consider land transport. This also allows the opportunity to stop the vehicle and for staff to come out of their safety restraints to perform procedures from an optimal position, which is not possible in a helicopter.

Safety

Any team member flying in an air ambulance must have the appropriate certification for safety standards, including operating around the aircraft with rotors running, communication, evacuation drills, and operation of medical equipment within the aircraft. If these have not been completed, then these staff should not fly, and road transport should be used. The pilot may refuse to transport any team member without the necessary safety training.

Handover

A verbal summary of the injuries and interventions should be prepared, whilst en route to the receiving trauma unit. This should be clear and succinct, ideally in an SBAR type format (**s**ituation, **b**ackground, **a**ssessment, **r**ecommendation) or ideally ATMIST for trauma patients (**a**ge, **t**ime of incident, **m**echanism of injury, **i**njuries, **s**igns (vitals), **t**reatment so far). This handover should be delivered to the receiving team leader, with all team members' attention, prior to any transition of ventilation or monitoring. A copy of the pre-hospital medical notes, interventions, and drug administration should be presented to the receiving team.

Summary

Performing emergency anaesthesia and critical care interventions in the pre-hospital environment is a challenging and high-risk process which should only be undertaken by practitioners with suitable training and experience in scene safety, communication, team resource management, ambulance assets, and a solid understanding of triage principles and how logistics may influence transport or destination decisions. These services must be regulated by strict governance systems and internal training processes. However, with the rapid delivery of critical care interventions prior to hospital arrival, the potential for improved outcomes for critically injured trauma victims may be recognized.

Further reading

Ellis D and Hooper M (2010). *Cases in pre-hospital and retrieval medicine*. Churchill Livingstone, Chatswood.

Institute for Healthcare Improvement. *SBAR technique for communication: a situational briefing model*. Available at: <http://www.ihi.org/knowledge/Pages/Tools/SBARTechni queforCommunicationASituationalBriefingModel.aspx>.

Intensive Care Society (2011). Guidelines for the transport of the critically ill adult, 3rd edn. Available at: <http://www.ics.ac.uk/ics-homepage/guidelines-standards/>.

The collapsed neonate

Background

Whilst the definitive management of a critically ill neonate involves complex therapeutic interventions delivered by teams led by neonatologists, the geography of modern living dictates that a collapsed neonate may present to any acute care facility across the country which may have very limited medical, nursing, and anaesthetic resources. Seemingly well neonates may have been discharged home, within hours to days of birth, to remote, rural or island communities, and medical teams in those areas may have to deliver fundamental neonatal intensive care for a considerable period of time before a transport team can retrieve the patient. This discussion serves to outline the key diagnoses presenting in the collapsed neonate and what interventions could be offered by the anaesthetic team whilst awaiting retrieval.

Learning outcomes

1 Recognize the common presenting features in a collapsed neonate and identify the likely causes
2 Commence an appropriate therapy
3 Stabilize the child whilst awaiting the retrieval team arrival.

CPD matrix matches

2D01; 2D07

Case history: presenting features and common diagnoses

You are fast-paged to your small district general hospital's ED, immediately following the arrival of a term 10-day-old, previously well female neonate brought in by the paramedics in a collapsed state. On arrival, you find the patient to be intermittently gasping, with apnoeic pauses, peripherally cyanosed, and drowsy.

What are the likely differential diagnoses that may explain this collection of symptoms?

The key factors to consider when formulating a differential diagnosis include:

◆ Age: by definition of being under 28 days old, this patient is a neonate; however, certain pathologies are more likely within certain time frames of the neonatal period. Within the first few hours or days of birth, severe congenital anatomical anomalies are likely to manifest, e.g. tracheo-oesophageal fistulae or diaphragmatic herniae, presenting with respiratory distress or impaired feeding. At around days 7–14 of age, the initial physiological closure of the ductus arteriosus is subsequently followed up by the anatomical duct closure. This is a key development, resulting in the manifestation of duct-dependent cardiac lesions. Sepsis and metabolic disorders may manifest at any time throughout this neonatal period but tend to initially present with non-specific symptoms, including poor feeding, drowsiness, and apnoeas

◆ Apnoea: this is a non-specific sign which is likely to be present in any unwell neonate, independent of the presence or absence of respiratory pathology. Immaturity within neural pathways and vagal predominance result in any systemic stress, triggering apnoeas. Also, the respiratory reserve is severely limited in neonates, and an increase in the metabolic oxygen demand will be met initially by tachypnoea, which can only be sustained in the short to medium term and will subsequently progress to hypopnoea and apnoeas, due to respiratory muscle fatigue

◆ Peripheral hypoperfusion: similarly, this is a non-specific sign which is likely to be present in patients with respiratory, cardiovascular, septic, and metabolic pathologies. An early presenting feature of neonatal illness reported by parents is an inability to feed which often precedes hospital presentation by several days. In patients with respiratory pathology, this inability to feed results from the fact that they cannot sustain an adequate respiratory function via nasal breathing during feeding. With cardiac or septic pathologies, the infant cannot meet the metabolic demand during feeding, as this is an energy-demanding process in itself. The net result is that poor feeding for several days results in hypovolaemia and a calorie deficit, often manifest as failure to regain birthweight or further weight loss.

The differential diagnosis in this patient would be:

◆ Congenital cardiac anomaly: duct-dependent lesions will present at 1–2 weeks of life with peripheral hypoperfusion and cyanosis. Signs of heart failure may be present

- Sepsis: group B streptococcal infection from perinatal materno-fetal transmission. This may present as generalized septic shock or meningitis. A history of group B streptococcal status is usually available from the mother if she has undergone routine antenatal care
- Metabolic disorder: the potential specific diagnosis within this broad category is beyond the scope of this text, lying firmly in the remit of neonatal specialists. However, these disorders will generally present with a non-specific collapse, resembling neonatal sepsis and universal hypoglycaemia, and may be accompanied by seizures.

Case update: resuscitation and treatments

The patient's ventilation is immediately supported with manual ventilation via an appropriate bag and mask, and monitoring is applied. Initial observations demonstrate a HR of 180, NIBP of 45/25 mmHg, and peripheral capillary refill of >5 s. A capillary blood sample reveals a blood glucose of 1.2 mmol/L, pH of 7.10, $PaCO_2$ of 9 kPa, PaO_2 of 5 kPa, a base deficit of –6 mol/L, and lactate of 4 mmol/L.

Comment on these findings, and discuss the interventions required

These results indicate tachycardia, hypotension, and a mixed metabolic and respiratory acidosis, all of which are compatible with a cardiac, septic, or metabolic pathology so, at this stage, do not aid with specifying the diagnosis. However, the initial resuscitation principles are the same, irrespective of the diagnosis:

- Physiological parameters: the normal range for the HR in a newborn is 140–160 bpm, but rates of 180–190 are commonly observed when the child is upset. Rather than noting the systolic and diastolic BPs, it is often more helpful to consider the MAP in neonates. This should equate to the gestational age in weeks for the first few months of life; for example, this patient with a gestational age of 41 weeks should have an MAP of 41 mmHg, so he is hypotensive with her current MAP of 32 mmHg
- Blood gas results: whilst most anaesthetists are familiar with the interpretation of arterial samples, a re-adjustment of normal values is required for capillary samples. A mild respiratory acidosis is expected with elevated $PaCO_2$ and decreased PaO_2 values, compared to arterial sampling. However, the base deficit and lactate should be within normal limits, with values outwith suggesting a metabolic component to the blood gas disturbance.

Interventions required include the provision of respiratory and cardiovascular support, the treatment of acidosis and hypoglycaemia, specific therapies to cover potential diagnoses, and referral for definitive care.

◆ Respiratory support: this patient's airway may be threatened by virtue of an impaired consciousness, but she is likely to require urgent intubation and ventilation for respiratory support. In the short term, ventilation may be augmented with either a T-piece during periods of spontaneous effort or a neonatal self-inflating bag during apnoea. The application of positive pressure through both of these devices will lead to gastric insufflation, and early NG or orogastric tube insertion should be performed to minimize abdominal distension and diaphragmatic splinting

◆ Cardiovascular support:

• Access: securing IV access in neonates often presents considerable challenges to the anaesthetist. Veins are often easily visible through the relatively transparent skin but are typically difficult to cannulate, due to their small bore, tortuous pathway, and fragility. The dorsum of the hand or foot are reasonable sites for first attempts, and the long saphenous vein often affords a relatively consistent position, anterior to the medial malleolus, even when it cannot be seen. Scalp veins are often cannulated by neonatologists but can be difficult to secure, rendering them liable to displacement during resuscitation and transport. In the collapsed neonate, due consideration to intraosseous cannulation should be given early in the resuscitation phase, both with manual and automated systems, minimizing the risks of multiple access attempts and hence prolonging the periods of hypotension and hypoglycaemia whilst exacerbating hypothermia. Note the umbilical venous approach for central cannulation is only available to neonatologists in the immediate post-natal period and is not an option for anaesthetists, even if the umbilical cord clamp is still on when the patient presents

• Fluids: the presence of tachycardia, hypotension, and peripheral capillary shutdown necessitates fluid therapy; however, whilst administering fluid boluses, it should be borne in mind the potential for congenital cardiac pathology with the risk of excessive fluid replacement precipitating acute heart failure. In initial stages, a bolus of 20 mL/kg of normal saline is appropriate, with further boluses of 10 mL/kg titrated, depending on the trends of the cardiovascular parameters over at least 15 min following a fluid bolus. Glucose-containing fluids should never be administered as a volume bolus; however, this patient does require a loading dose of glucose as therapy for hypoglycaemia, and 2 mL/kg of 10% glucose, as per advanced paediatric life support (APLS) guidelines, with subsequent treatments, as necessary, following a recheck of blood sugar levels

- Inotropes: a broad-spectrum sympathomimetic agent is indicated in the collapsed neonate. Dopamine is often used in paediatric and neonatal units, in dose ranges of 5–20 micrograms/kg/min. Many anaesthetists are more familiar with the use of adrenaline infusions in the resuscitation phase of adults and children, and this is equally appropriate in the management of a collapsed neonate. The dose range is 0.1–1 micrograms/kg/min. Agents, such as noradrenline or dobutamine, are rarely indicated as first-line therapies and should only be considered on the advice of a neonatologist. As with all drugs, but particularly drug infusions, great care must be exercised when preparing these agents, as the dilutions and concentrations will be unfamiliar to many staff, and cross-checking of the prescription and preparation of these infusions is advised

- Anaesthesia: the collapsed neonate is likely to require anaesthesia during the resuscitation phase to facilitate ongoing interventions, controlled ventilation, and transport to definitive care. This should not be performed until volume resuscitation is well under way, multiple ports of venous access have been secured, and the appropriate staff, equipment, and drugs have been prepared, in anticipation of further deterioration

  - Equipment: the equipment required to anaesthetize a 3 kg neonate is no different to that required for a 100 kg adult, and all national guidelines on skilled assistance, pre-use checks, and monitoring standards are equally applicable. Either cuffed or uncuffed tracheal tubes are suitable, with no evidence to suggest a higher complication rate from microcuffed tubes, which are sized from 3.0 mm upwards. The laryngoscope blade is the choice of the individual anaesthetist, but straight blades, e.g. a Robertshaw blade, are often favoured, although MacIntosh zero blades are effective for neonatal intubation. Ventilators, often stocked in EDs, are generally unsuitable for neonatal ventilation, due to excessive deadspace in the circuits and the inability to deliver small tidal volumes

  - Drugs: commonly used induction agents, such as propofol and thiopentone, will be likely to cause significant hypotension, even in reduced dosing, if administered to the collapsed neonate. Etomidate is not used in neonatal or paediatric practice. The ideal induction agent in this clinical situation is ketamine, administered IV, at a dose of 1–2 mg/kg. This will provide an acceptable plane of anaesthesia, without compromising the BP. Midazolam and fentanyl may also be used as adjuncts, but caution should be applied, unless familiar with the use of these agents in sick children. Suxamethonium is still the recommended muscle relaxant, in doses of 1–2 mg/kg, to provide muscle relaxation for intubation, being mindful that fasciculations are usually not observed in small children. Bolus doses of adrenaline (1 microgram/kg) and atropine (20 micrograms/kg) and saline fluid boluses should be prepared and be immediately ready prior to induction. Where there has been an unsatisfactory response to 40–60 mL/kg of fluid boluses, commencing an adrenaline infusion prior to induction is recommended.

Case update: stabilization

The patient fails to respond adequately to 40 mL/kg of saline boluses and is still requiring intermittent manual ventilation for progressive apnoeas. One IV line and one intraosseous line have been sited, and an adrenaline infusion has been commenced at 0.2 micrograms/kg/min. Benzylpenicillin and gentamicin have been administered. Anaesthesia has been induced with 2 mg/kg of ketamine and 2 mg/kg of suxamethonium, and a size 3.5 tracheal tube has been inserted without difficulty. The paediatric intensive care retrieval team have been called to transport this patient to the paediatric ICU (PICU); their arrival time is estimated at 2 hours.

What measures should be instituted whilst awaiting the retrieval team's arrival?

The referring team is required to deliver paediatric intensive care until the arrival of the retrieval team. This is a standard of care, as outlined by the Royal College of Anaesthetists, and there should be appropriate staffing, equipment, training, and governance systems established to ensure that an appropriate standard of care can be delivered. The key principles of paediatric critical care delivery are best outlined on a systems basis:

◆ A—airway: the tracheal tube position must be securely fixed, ideally with zinc oxide tapes, over the maxillary regions, rather than tube ties which often let smaller tubes slip. The tube should be suctioned with a soft suction catheter; the appropriate size is double that of the internal diameter of the tracheal tube, e.g. a 7F catheter for a 3.5 mm or a 10F catheter for a 5 mm tube

◆ B—breathing: unless a paediatric-specific ventilator is available, it is likely that manual ventilation will be required. A problem with adult ventilators is that they are unable to deliver appropriately small tidal volumes without excessive pressures and that the volume of the pressure-monitoring apparatus prevents an adequate tidal volume. As such, hand ventilation may be the optimal strategy, either with a T-piece or a self-inflating bag. Capillary or venous blood gases should be checked at the commencement of ventilation and at around 30-min intervals, and ventilation rates titrated accordingly. Whilst neonatal practice is to avoid delivering 100% oxygen, this is acceptable in the short-term situation, and the use of oxygen–air blenders, or other similar devices, should only be undertaken where appropriate expertise is available. A CXR should be performed after intubation to confirm the tracheal tube position. A gastric tube should be inserted in all patients for drainage of any gastric insufflation that may impede an efficient ventilation

+ C—circulation: additional 20 mL/kg boluses of saline may be administered, as required, for hypotension, although, if >80–100 mL/kg are required, the haematology profile should be checked, as haemodilution is likely and blood or platelet transfusions may be indicated. In all patients, maintenance fluids should be administered, using the 4–2–1 mL/kg/hour formula where 4 mL/kg/hour is administered for the first 10 kg of body weight, plus 2 mL/kg/hour for a body weight of 10–20 kg, and an additional 1 mL/kg/hour for any body weight over 20 kg, if necessary. In this 3.5 kg patient, the maintenance infusion rate would be 14 mL/hour. The exact composition of the fluid may be dependent on local or regional guidance, but an isotonic mix of saline and glucose is recommended. It is important that dextrose is a component of maintenance fluids; otherwise, hypoglycaemia is a likely consequence. The adrenaline infusion should be titrated to a rate achieving an MAP comparable to the patient's post-conceptual age in weeks. Any points of venous or osseous access should be well secured. Central venous or arterial access is not normally indicated in this stabilization phase, unless staff with the appropriate skills are present

+ D—disability/neurology: it is vital that the patient remains adequately sedated and relaxed during the stabilization and transport phase. Inadequate sedation may trigger tachycardia and hypertension that may be misinterpreted as cardiovascular instability. Inadequate relaxation will allow coughing which may displace the tracheal tube, trigger profound vagal reflexes, and will certainly impede effective ventilation. The standard infusions used are morphine, midazolam, and a relaxant such as vecuronium or rocuronium. These should all be prepared, according to local monographs, and be double-checked before administration to the patient. The standard infusion rates are morphine 20 micrograms/kg/hour, midazolam 0.1 micrograms/kg/hour, and vecuronium 0.1 mg/kg/hour, though these should always be discussed with the PICU team before commencing, and the infusion rates titrated to response. Pupillary responses should be checked at regular intervals

◆ Environment: attention should be paid at all times to maintaining the environmental temperature to mitigate hypothermia in the neonate. Ideally, the ambient air temperature should be turned up to 26–28°C, though this may prove uncomfortable for staff. Forced air warming devices should be used, wherever possible, and prolonged periods with the skin exposed, e.g. for a central line insertion, should be avoided. Preparation for the retrieval team arriving includes ensuring all notes and prescriptions are documented and copies are made of the relevant paperwork.

Summary

The management of a collapsed neonate is a challenging situation that may present at any acute-receiving facility, including those without inpatient neonatal and paediatric services. It is the responsibility of the ED and anaesthesia team to resuscitate and stabilize these patients prior to the arrival of the retrieval team. Neonatal collapse may be due to complex cardiac, septic, and metabolic pathologies; however, the core treatment principles should be initiated which will optimize the condition of the neonate prior to transfer, including:

◆ Early recognition of the acutely unwell neonate: detection of apnoeas, poor peripheral perfusion, drowsiness

◆ Prompt intervention to stabilize cardiorespiratory decompensation: manual respiratory support; early IV or intraosseous access with fluid boluses; inotropic infusion; anaesthesia and intubation, if failing to respond to initial therapies

◆ Stabilization and preparation for retrieval team transport: securing tubes and lines; assessing the adequacy of ventilation; maintaining the fluid balance and glycaemic status; preventing hypothermia.

Further reading

Kattwinkel J, Perlman JM, Aziz K, *et al*.; American Heart Association (2010). Neonatal resuscitation: 2010 American Heart Association Guidelines for Cardiopulmonary Resuscitation and Emergency Cardiovascular Care. *Pediatrics*, **126**, e1400–13.

Paediatric Intensive Care Society (2010). *Standards for the care of critically ill children*, 4th edn. Available at: <http://www.ukpics.org.uk/documents/PICS_standards.pdf>.

Case 14.3

Time-critical transfers by referring clinicians

Background

The development of stand-alone retrieval services across the globe has enhanced the quality of care on transport for critically ill and injured patients. These retrieval teams cover neonatal, paediatric, obstetric and adult patients and may utilize tertiary level intensive therapies such as inhaled nitric oxide, IABPs, active cooling and extracorporeal life support. However, the capacity for retrieval team support may be overwhelmed due to multiple demands for transport or transport logistics, for example adverse weather. In specific clinical situations there may be an urgency to transport the patient to the site of definitive care where a delay waiting on a retrieval team necessitates transport by the referring hospital team. This discussion outlines the key decision making issues when considering referring vs retrieval team transport.

Learning outcomes

1 Identify advantages and disadvantages of retrieval team transport

2 Outline the principles of equipment for referring team transport

3 Outline the process for referring team transport.

CPD matrix matches

2A11; 2D07; 2F01

Case history: identifying the advantages and disadvantages of retrieval team transport

An 11-year-old boy has fallen off his bicycle and crashed into a tree at high speed, striking his head on the main trunk. He was reported to be GCS 10 at the scene but has become increasingly drowsy en route into hospital, and he was GCS 6 on arrival in your ED, 20 min after the incident. He has been anaesthetized and ventilated, and a CT of the head demonstrates a large bifrontal extradural haematomas (see Figure 14.5). You work in a large district general hospital

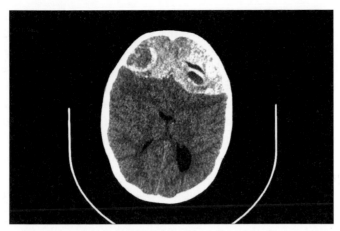

Fig. 14.5 Large bifrontal extradural haematomas.

which has general and trauma surgeons, paediatricians, and anaesthetists, but no neurosurgery or paediatric intensive care facilities. Your nearest neurosurgical unit is 100 miles away.

What are the options for the emergency management of this child's life-threatening injury?

This child needs an emergency evacuation of his intracranial haematoma. There are essentially three options to facilitate this procedure: perform the surgery in the referring hospital, referring team transport, or retrieval team transport to the neurosurgical centre.

- Local surgery: a discussion on the surgical options is outwith the scope of this anaesthetic text; however, cases have been reported where lifesaving haematoma decompression, by way of burr holes, has been performed by remote and rural practitioners, with limited experience, under the telephone guidance of neurosurgeons. There is no doubt that many of these procedures have been successful in the past, but great concern has been expressed regarding this practice from neurosurgeons. Whilst the emergency burr hole may relieve critical intracranial hypertension, the referring practitioner may have very limited ability or equipment to deal with persistent arterial or venous bleeding and may, in fact, release a relative tamponade that leads to major haemorrhage. The risk of this is such that the standard neurosurgical approach to these cases is typically by craniotomy, so that bleeding vessels may be identified and ligated in the primary procedure, a procedure such as this being beyond the scope of a referring unit

- Referring team transport: transfer of this ventilated patient by one of the local anaesthetists may appear, on the face of it, to be the most rapid method of achieving definitive care, but there are many facets to review. The Royal College of Anaesthetists mandates that any unit which receives critically ill patients must have the capacity to transfer them to definitive care, which includes the consideration of staff, equipment, protocols, and a governance system relating to transport episodes. Any ventilated patient must be accompanied by an anaesthetist on transport. Guidelines, produced by the AAGBI, state that any anaesthetist transferring a patient, such as this child with a traumatic brain injury, must be trained in paediatric anaesthesia, neurocritical care, and transport medicine. There should be nominated senior staff responsible in each referring unit for producing transport protocols, delivering a programme of ongoing education, liaising with receiving centres, and ensuring equipment is maintained serviceable

- Medical escort: the accompanying anaesthetist must be familiar with delivering critical care in a transport environment, with respect to the hazards of equipment failure, tube and line disconnections, acceleration and deceleration forces, and movement artefact on monitors. This is often the senior anaesthetist present in the referring unit; however, the team often faces difficult decisions, as there may be patients requiring ongoing clinical care requiring the senior anaesthetist. It is important that a junior member of the anaesthetic team, with limited transport experience, is not selected to transfer these critically injured patients

- Medical assistant: similarly, experience in functioning in the transport environment is more important than the exact grade or specific profession of the accompanying assistant. It may be that an intensive care or ED nurse, an operating department practitioner, or a critical care paramedic has the most experience with transport processes and equipment, and hence is the most suited team member to accompany the physician

- Retrieval team transport: transfer by a specialized retrieval team is associated with improved outcomes for critically injured patients. The rate of adverse clinical incidents on transport, including airway complications, cardiopulmonary arrest, and loss of vascular access, is significantly less (1.5% vs 61%) with a retrieval team vs a non-specialized team transport. Also, illness severity-adjusted mortality is over 50% greater in patients transported by referring hospital teams. Transports by referring hospital teams take around 25% longer, and more critical care interventions are typically required on admission to the receiving unit. Evidence therefore strongly favours the transport of all critically ill patients by retrieval teams; however, within the realm of time-critical neurosurgical transfers, a great deal of contention remains. The Society of British Neurosurgeons suggest that more patients may come to harm waiting on retrieval team transports, although the evidence supporting this statement relates to practice from 20 to 30 years ago. Hence, there is the need for a three-way conversation between the referring unit, the retrieval team, and the neurosurgeon to determine the appropriate transport pathway for the patient, with the ultimate goal being to achieve intracranial decompression as soon as possible, and certainly within 4 hours of injury.

Case update: outlining the principles of equipment for referring team transport

It has been decided that the most time-efficient transport option is for the anaesthetic registrar and an intensive care nurse from the referring unit, both of whom have experience in the transport environment. The patient is presently ventilated in the ED and is clinically stable.

What equipment is required for the safe transport of this patient?

The transport team requires equipment that is able to deliver a mobile intensive care service. This equipment should be pre-identified, specifically detailed for transport, and be regularly checked and maintained. There is no place for assembling transport equipment in an ad hoc fashion, whilst concurrently trying to clinically manage a critically ill patient. There should be a senior clinician nominated in each referring unit who has the responsibility for equipment procurement and maintenance, and liaising with receiving units to ensure collaborative working from transport protocols. The equipment required includes:

- Trolley: a unit which has to perform a number of intensive care transports should ideally have a dedicated transport trolley, e.g. the Ferno® CCT6. This allows intensive care equipment, such as pumps, ventilators, and monitors, to be securely mounted, enhancing staff and patient safety and minimizing the risk of damage to this equipment. The critical care trolleys will have a locking mechanism to dock securely to the ambulance chassis, further enhancing patient and staff safety

- Monitor: the generic specifications of the monitor require it to be self-powered, with a battery life of several hours, and ideally with spare battery capacity. In addition to meeting all minimal monitoring standards, the monitor must be able to continuously monitor the $ETCO_2$ and at least one invasive pressure, typically arterial. Using invasive, rather than non-invasive, BP monitoring considerably reduces battery power drain and should be utilized on any transfers of critically ill children. Continuous arterial pressure monitoring also allows the immediate detection of a physiological instability that may be invoked, due to acceleration or turning G-forces whilst in motion. The monitor should be mounted on the transport trolley by a secured bracket

◆ Ventilator: transport ventilators are usually relatively simple devices, compared to modern intensive care ventilators; however, they have proven to be robust, waterproof, windproof, and shockproof, and they have the capacity to run for prolonged periods of time without mains power. Options from the Pac and Oxylog series are used widely throughout the UK. The patient should be stabilized on the transport ventilator for some time prior to departure, and ABGs checked to confirm adequate ventilation before moving. Again, there are mounts for both of these types of ventilator for transport trolleys

◆ Oxygen: oxygen supplies should be calculated for the journey, based on current minute ventilation, oxygen requirements, and the anticipated duration of the journey. It is then reasonable to double this calculation to ensure a safety margin. Running out of oxygen during an intensive care transport may lead to patient death and is indefensible. Oxygen will be carried in the ambulance, and it is the transfer team's responsibility to ensure supplies are adequate before leaving the referring unit. They can be changed easily prior to departure. Oxygen requirements can be estimated by the following formula:

$$O_2 \text{ requirement} = (FiO_2 \times \text{minute ventilation}) \times 2$$

Note that many transport platforms are moving to the newer lightweight style of the oxygen cylinder; for example, the BOC ZF, an F sized cylinder which would normally contain 1300 L of oxygen, but this is compressed to around 250 atm (i.e. around double that of a normal cylinder), so it contains around 2500 L of oxygen, enough for approximately 4 hours of ventilation at an FiO_2 of 1.0 in an adult ventilated at 12 x 750 mL.

◆ Pumps: anywhere from three to six infusion pumps will be required for an emergency intensive care transport to infuse sedative and analgesic agents, fluids, vasoactive drugs, and muscle relaxants. Ideally, all of these drugs should be delivered by infusion, rather than boluses, to maintain stability on transfer. The pumps should have a battery life that exceeds the duration of transport, and spare batteries carried where possible. Many modern frontline ambulances have a 12–240 V inverter system where the mains AC power can be delivered from the vehicle's electrical system when the engine is on, which should be used, wherever possible

◆ Additional equipment and drugs: additional and emergency equipment for airway management, vascular access, and intercostal chest drainage should be carried on all retrievals. Drug bags should include several hours' supplies of sedation, muscle relaxation, analgesia, and adequate emergency drugs to support arrhythmias or hypotension. These should all be checked as within expiry dates and that all stock is present as part of the transfer equipment routine daily checks.

Case update: outlining the logistical processes for referring team transport

The anaesthetic registrar and the ICU nurse have assembled and checked the transport equipment. The patient has been packaged on a critical care transport trolley, and full invasive monitoring established. He is settled on the transport ventilator, with ABGs confirming satisfactory oxygen and carbon dioxide tensions. Infusions of propofol, alfentanil, and rocuronium are running, and good venous access is secured.

What are the necessary logistical processes to be implemented in order to effectively transfer this patient?

Discussion

◆ Communication:

- Ambulance service: it is vital that all communications with the ambulance service clearly outline that this is a long-distance intensive care transport with a ventilated patient and an accompanying medical team. This may influence the tasking, depending on crew availability and experience and vehicle availability. Some provision for repatriating the transport team to the base hospital should be outlined, particularly where a considerable amount of equipment has been transported, though this should not delay the departure of the team

- Receiving unit: the receiving unit should be called immediately prior to departure to update on the patient's clinical status and estimated arrival time. The arrival destination should be reconfirmed, e.g. ED, intensive care, or theatre, and, if the team is unfamiliar with the location request, someone from the referring unit should meet the ambulance on arrival. Any specific therapies should be requested, so that they can be made ready in advance at the receiving unit, e.g. drug infusions, blood availability, specific ventilator settings, cooling or warming devices, in order to enhance the efficiency of handover. The transfer team should pass a contact mobile telephone number to the receiving unit

• Relatives: contact details should be taken from the relatives by the transfer team and passed on to the receiving unit. The relatives should be updated on the patient's clinical condition and the anticipated outline of events and interventions over the subsequent hours. They should be given directions as to where to go and a contact point in the receiving unit, and they must have a clear explanation that they must not attempt to follow the ambulance, as this will risk their own and the patient's safety

◆ Patient transfers: even for a relatively straightforward road transport, such as this case, there will be a considerable number of intermediate patient moves, each of which poses a risk to the patient's safety. During loading and unloading of the trolley to and from the ambulance, close attention must be paid by the transport team to the ventilator tubing, drug infusion lines, and monitoring lines, as there is a high chance they might get snagged on various components of the ambulance. Ideally, all tubing and lines should be packaged within the patient's securing harness, or vacuum mattress if used, to minimize the risk. Outwith specialist transport teams, ambulance service colleagues may not be familiar with moving ventilated patients around; hence, it is vital that the team is vigilant during these periods. As soon as the patient is loaded into the ambulance, the ventilator should be transferred to the ambulance oxygen supply, and, if available, the pumps and monitors powered by the vehicle's mains AC supply. After every change in oxygen supply, adequate ventilation should be confirmed by patient examination

◆ Handover: copies of all notes and documentation will be provided for the receiving team, and they will have been briefed by the referring unit, but a concise verbal 'hands-off' handover should be given by the transport team to everyone in the receiving unit on arrival. Ideally, this should follow an SBAR format and be delivered in 1 minute or less. Assuming the patient is stable, this should be delivered prior to any change of equipment or patient moves. Further detailed questions should be addressed after the handover. An example of an SBAR handover for this patient would be:

• Situation:
'This is an 11-year-old 40 kg male with an extradural haematoma.'
• Background:
'He fell off his bike and struck a tree at high speed. Initial GCS was 10 at the scene, deteriorating to 6 by arrival in the ED. He was anaesthetized and transferred for a CT scan. No other injuries or relevant past medical history have been identified.'

- Assessment:

  'He has a 6.5 ETT taped at 17 cm. He is ventilated at a rate of 14 by 400 mL, with an FiO$_2$ of 0.45. The ETCO$_2$ has been between 4 and 4.5 kPa which correlates closely with the arterial PaCO$_2$. The HR has been 80–90, and the MAP at least 80 mmHg. He has two peripheral IVs and a left radial arterial line. Therapies include infusions of propofol at 10 mL/hour and alfentanil at 3 mL/hour. He last had a bolus of rocuronium 20 min ago. There were no major abnormalities on FBC or U&E.'

- Recommendations:

  'He has been stable on transport and is ready for transfer to your operating theatre for haematoma evacuation. He will need a blood cross-match performed urgently. Does anyone have any immediate questions?'

Summary

Evidence indicates that the transfer of critically ill patients is more effectively performed by specialized retrieval teams. However, transport service capacity, logistical issues, or clinical urgency may necessitate transfer by referring unit teams. The complexity of this should not be underestimated, and all units should have dedicated transport equipment that is comprehensively checked on a regular basis, transport protocols, and support from senior staff in the transport process. Clear and concise communication regarding transport planning and handover of patient details will minimize the potential for misunderstanding and errors.

Further reading

Association of Anaesthetists of Great Britain and Ireland (2006). *Recommendations for the safe transfer of patients with brain injury.* Available at: <http://www.aagbi.org/sites/default/files/braininjury.pdf>.

Royal College of Anaesthetists (2014). *Guidelines on the provision of anaesthetic services.* Available at: <http://www.rcoa.ac.uk/system/files/GPAS-FULL-2014_3.pdf>.

The stridulous infant

Background

Respiratory distress in infants and small children is very common, particularly over the winter months, and is typically mild and self-limiting. A very small minority will need escalation to critical care support, however, when respiratory decompensation occurs and may be alarmingly rapid, needing urgent institution of ventilatory therapy. Many of these children will present to GPs or EDs with what appears to be non-specific malaise or upper respiratory tract symptoms, and identifying those with clinical features which may suggest significant pathology is often challenging.

Learning outcomes

1 Identify the signs and symptoms suggestive of impending respiratory failure

2 Have an awareness of the underlying pathologies

3 Outline a management plan for the stridulous infant

4 Prepare for emergency anaesthesia of the stridulous infant.

CPD matrix matches

1C01; 2D01

Case history: identifying the signs and symptoms suggestive of impending respiratory failure

An 18-month-old female infant presents to the ED in your district general hospital. She has a 2-day history of general non-specific malaise, has been pyrexial, and has not been feeding well. Her mother has brought her into the ED, as her breathing has become noisy, and she appears to be coughing and struggling for breath at times. She is previously well. You have been called down to review her from an airway and breathing perspective, as the ED doctor is concerned she may need anaesthetic support.

What clinical features are suggestive of severe respiratory compromise?

Severe airway or respiratory pathologies can often be detected on a focussed primary ABC survey, without going into detailed examination and investigation. This will allow prompt escalation and activation of senior and theatre support where necessary.

- A—airway: before starting to examine the patient, you may be struck by the noisy breathing from the end of the bed. Key elements to elicit are the respiratory phase, i.e. inspiratory or expiratory. Inspiratory noises can either be stertor or stridor; expiratory noises may be grunting or wheeze

  - Stertor: is generated due to turbulent airflow through the supraglottic airway, typically due to partial obstruction from a hypotonic oropharynx, generally sounding like snoring. This is generally exclusively an inspiratory noise seen during sleep, which may be resolved by simple manoeuvres, like head and neck positioning, or, in extreme cases, with oropharyngeal or nasopharyngeal airways. Stertor in the awake patient is suggestive of significant upper airway obstruction

  - Stridor: this should be considered an airway 'red flag' until proven otherwise. All practising anaesthetists will be most familiar with the high-pitched inspiratory noise of laryngospasm triggered due to an inadequate depth of anaesthesia. This inspiratory sound is triggered by high-velocity airflow through an airway narrowing between the glottis and the carina. There may be some expiratory component to the noise if the obstruction is severe. Irrespective of the aetiology, any infant with stridor requires an immediate anaesthetic assessment, with consideration for escalation to critical care

  - Grunting: this end-expiratory noise is a compensatory mechanism for respiratory compromise, in which the patient partially closes their glottis during inspiration, effectively generating resistance to expiration and hence an intrinsic PEEP (sometimes referred to as auto-PEEP). This is a feature of failure of gas exchange, where either hypoxia or hypercarbia are stimulating the ventilatory drive, and can often be overcome by providing a small amount of external CPAP

  - Wheeze: is not usually audible without a stethoscope but, if so, suggests a severe lower airway obstruction, with marked restriction to expiration. Patients have supranormal levels of intrinsic PEEP, and the RR will have a prolonged expiratory phase in order to facilitate an adequate carbon dioxide clearance.

Other assessment points in the airway examination include excluding the presence of foreign bodies, secretions, or blood, and identifying congenital abnormalities which may impact the airway patency, e.g. Pierre–Robin sequence, mucopolysaccharidoses, or cleft palate. Whilst these disorders may not immediately compromise the airway in isolation, in combination with any additional insult, e.g. a mild viral URTI, they may result in airway obstruction.

- ◆ B—breathing: similarly, a focussed primary breathing assessment may be performed from the end of the bed, prior to direct auscultation with a stethoscope. Key points to identify include:

  - Rate: the RR varies with age and the concurrent state of the child. The RR in a newborn is around 40–60/min but may be 70–80/min when the child is upset. At 12–18 months, the normal RR will be 25–30/min, decreasing to 15–20/min for primary school-aged children and to adult values by teenage years. More important than the absolute rate itself is the trend over time, and many units use early warning charts to document the trends which give vital information on the progression. In response to an inadequate gas exchange, the RR will steadily increase, up to rates of 60–70 breaths/min which can only be sustained for a relatively short period of time, and will subsequently rapidly fall to hypopnoea, promptly followed by apnoea. Always determine that any fall in the RR is accompanied by a clinical improvement, as, if not, external ventilatory support is likely to be required urgently

  - Work of breathing: an all-encompassing term that includes the presence of any, or all, of tracheal tug, intercostal indrawing, asymmetrical chest movement, subcostal recession, and abdominal paradoxical (see-saw) respiration. The presence of any of these clinical features is a compensatory mechanism to increase the negative intrathoracic pressure and increase the minute ventilation, as a result of an airway obstruction or an inadequate gas exchange due to pulmonary pathology. There is no single feature that is of more concern than the others, but rather the increasing magnitude of each and the presence of multiple signs point towards a marked increase in the work of breathing, which will often be accompanied by an increased RR, this situation being unsustainable in the longer term without external support.

    Chest palpation and auscultation and pulse oximetry are obviously part of the respiratory assessment but may yield little additional information, particularly if the child is crying or moving around, where oximetry also often fails to provide accurate data.

- ◆ C—circulation: a full examination of the cardiovascular system is essential in the management of any unwell infant, but, for the purposes of a rapid assessment of the child with a compromised respiratory function, it is unlikely to add further to the diagnostic process or planning management. Key points to detect on the primary survey are peripheral perfusion, usually measured by the CRT, with a refill time >2 s indicating an inadequate perfusion and >5 s indicating severe hypoperfusion. Similarly, the patient's colour will gave a rapid indication of the general physiological state, with a pink child indicating an adequate perfusion and oxygenation, cyanosis indicating hypoxia, but usually in the presence of an adequate cardiac output (mostly related to congenital cyanotic heart disease), and a pale or mottled child indicating a critical problem with oxygenation and perfusion

- D—disability/neurology: assessing a formal GCS in an unwell infant is challenging and often inaccurate. Most reliable is to perform a neurological assessment on an AVPU scale:
  - A: **a**lert approximates to GCS 14–15
  - V: response to a **v**erbal stimulus is GCS 12–13
  - P: response to a **p**ainful stimulus is GCS 9–11
  - U: **u**nconscious is GCS 8 or less.

Case update: having an awareness of the underlying pathologies

You assess your patient in the ED. Your primary ABCD survey demonstrates that she has a loud inspiratory stridor and is drooling at the mouth. Her RR is 40–50 breaths/min, and she has a markedly increased work of breathing, signified by tracheal tug, intercostal indrawing, and abdominal paradoxical respiration. She appears peripherally warm and is flushed. She is slightly drowsy at times but is quite miserable and gets upset when you try to approach her and examine her. The nurses cannot get any monitoring on her and do not want to upset her with further attempts.

What is the differential diagnosis for this patient's underlying pathology?

This patient has stridor with severe respiratory distress. Irrespective of the aetiology, this is a potentially life-threatening situation which requires a consultant review and may require high-risk emergency anaesthesia. The differential diagnosis for an upper airway obstruction includes:

- Foreign body: this should be a differential for any child (or adult) presenting with an acute airway obstruction. Often the history of foreign body ingestion will be absent in children, as it often occurs when they are unsupervised or playing with siblings. Features which suggest this diagnosis include an abrupt onset in an otherwise well child with no other symptoms. Any form of a viral prodrome is usually absent, although it cannot be excluded in the child who may have ingested a foreign body whilst having a concurrent URTI

- Croup: this is the commonest cause of an upper airway obstruction in children aged between 1 and 2 years. Also known as laryngotracheobronchitis, it is a viral infection causing inflammation of the upper airways, most often caused by parainfluenza viruses but may also be caused by other respiratory viruses such as adenovirus, respiratory syncytial virus (RSV), and influenza A. Key features in the presentation include a viral prodrome for 24–48 hours and the classical 'barking cough', though the patients are usually not systemically unwell otherwise

- Epiglottitis: this is the classical red alert condition which presents with an acute airway obstruction in stridulous infants which are systemically toxic. Patients are often drooling at the mouth, due to odynophagia. These patients are often quiet and prefer to be in the sitting position. Any attempt to lie the patient down for examination usually exacerbates the airway obstruction. The incidence of epiglottitis has significantly decreased over the last 10 years, as children are now routinely vaccinated against the causative agent *Haemophilus influenzae*. However, due to adverse publicity related to other vaccination schedules, some parents choose to withhold all vaccines from their children, and, as such, bacterial epiglottitis must remain on a differential diagnosis list

- Tracheitis: bacterial tracheitis can be considered the intermediate pathology between croup and epiglottitis. Patients usually present with the systemic features of bacterial infection, including pyrexia, tachycardia, and hypotension, and with the airway manifestations of croup such as the barking cough and stridor. Drooling may, or may not, be present. These patients can deteriorate rapidly if the airway obstruction reaches a critical stage

- Lower respiratory pathology: any severe lower respiratory pathology in an infant may compromise gas exchange, such that an increased work of breathing is present, which, on occasion, may be associated with a mild inspiratory stridor, due to high-velocity airflow through a relatively narrow airway. In this age group, common pathologies include viral pneumonias, which may be particularly severe, requiring prolonged ventilation, and caused by adenovirus, influenza (including H1N1), parainfluenza, and RSV. Bacterial pneumonia or congenital abnormalities, such as cysts, may also present in this age group.

Case update: outlining a management plan for the stridulous infant

After examination, you suspect your patient has croup, bacterial tracheitis, or epiglottitis. The patient's increased work of breathing and stridor persist. You are concerned that she looks like she is becoming exhausted and may need invasive respiratory support. Your consultant will attend shortly, and, in the interim, you need to outline a management plan.

What investigations, staff, and equipment will be required to manage this patient?

This patient will be managed based on the progress of the clinical condition and response to interventions. It is unlikely that any specific investigation will influence management in the acute situation; however, they may direct subsequent intensive care management.

Investigations

- Blood tests: FBC or biochemistry will not affect how the patient's airway is managed. They will likely be required once the acute situation has been stabilized, but it would be generally inadvisable to embark upon blood sampling at this stage. Blood gases may inform the stage of respiratory decompensation, but careful consideration must be given to this. Arterial sampling is not likely to be possible, and, whilst venous or capillary sampling is used routinely in paediatric and neonatal care, the sampling procedure is likely to cause great distress which may also exacerbate airway compromise. If these samples are taken, they provide no information on the oxygenation state of the patient but give a reasonable indication of the carbon dioxide retention and acid–base status

- Radiology: similarly, the acute airway management is unlikely to be immediately influenced by chest radiograph imaging; however, it may be useful to detect a severe pneumonia or pneumothorax (which may result from a ruptured congenital cyst), prior to intubation. Plain film imaging purely for airway assessment is unhelpful, though, if performed for other reasons, it may be possible to denote the 'steeple sign' of a narrowed upper airway in croup or a swollen epiglottis on a lateral neck film

- Microbiology: samples from nasal swabs, respiratory secretions, and blood cultures will inform on appropriate antimicrobial therapies and the duration of treatment. Taking any of these samples in the awake child with a compromised airway will exacerbate the problem and should be deferred until the airway is secured.

Staff

This patient needs to be managed in an operating theatre by a consultant anaesthetist, ideally one with recent paediatric experience, if available. Where resources allow, this patient's anaesthesia would ideally be performed by at least two anaesthetists. The full theatre team, including the operating department practitioner and theatre nurses, must be present. Due consideration to alerting an ENT surgeon should be given, and, where a local service exists for an ENT surgeon with paediatric experience, they should be requested to be present for the induction of anaesthesia in severe cases. Anecdotes exist of ENT surgeons from tertiary paediatric units attending a district general hospital in an emergency manner for airway support, though this is very dependent on local resources. The receiving PICU should be notified as early as possible, as the patient will need retrieval to the ICU, once the airway has been secured.

Equipment

The full range of anaesthetic equipment for anaesthetizing an 18-month-old child must be present, as per AAGBI recommendations. Emergency drugs should be prepared in advance, including atropine and adrenaline; boluses of fluid and agents to maintain anaesthesia and muscle relaxation, once the airway has been secured, must be immediately to hand. A selection of laryngoscope blades and tracheal tubes should be selected by the operator. It is inappropriate to suggest that one profile of laryngoscope blade is superior to another for this situation, but the most important factor is that the intubating anaesthetist has familiarity with the blade selected. A MacIntosh blade may be perfectly suitable, there being no obligation to use a straight blade in this or any other paediatric patient. If an ENT surgeon is available, a paediatric tracheostomy tray will be required in theatre. The utility of fibreoptic scopes is likely to be limited in a small airway with inflammation, secretions, or other abnormality, but more anaesthetists would be comfortable using this in a difficult airway situation as a rescue device, so it is reasonable to have one on standby. The external diameter of a paediatric bronchoscope limits the tracheal tube size that can be used, with the following approximate guidelines:

- A 2.2 mm scope: no suction channel, minimum tracheal tube internal diameter (ID) 3.0 mm
- A 2.8 mm scope: no suction channel, minimum tracheal tube ID 4.0 mm
- A 4 mm scope: usually with suction ports, minimum tracheal tube ID 5.0 mm.

Case update: prepare for emergency anaesthesia of the stridulous infant

This infant's respiratory function has deteriorated, with impending respiratory exhaustion, intermittent apnoeas, decreasing stridor (a sign of reduced air-flow), and drowsiness. You have transferred the patient to theatre, still sitting on her mother's lap, and a full theatre team and an adult ENT surgeon have been requested and will attend urgently. The PICU retrieval team are mobilizing but will take 90 min till arrival in your unit.

You are likely to need to anaesthetize this patient to secure their airway and support the respiratory function. Outline the ongoing management of this child

Whilst awaiting the arrival of the full theatre team and senior anaesthetic and ENT support, you may consider some non-invasive therapies before progressing to anaesthesia and intubation.

Inhaled therapies

- Oxygen: at all times, there should be attempts to provide supplemental oxygen to this patient. This should be delivered at high flow, without fear of respiratory depression from carbon dioxide retention. A careful balance must be achieved between attempting to deliver oxygen and upsetting the patient further, and hence increasing their oxygen demand. Ideally, a reservoir bag–mask, held in the vicinity of the patient's mouth and nose, often by the mother, will provide some oxygen supplementation. If the patient is sleeping or drowsy, it may be possible to apply the mask and/or nasal cannulae without disturbing the patient. Wherever possible, avoid manually ventilating the patient with a bag–valve–mask, as, in the situation of a partially occluded airway, most of this ventilated gas is likely to enter the stomach and subsequently impede diaphragmatic excursion

- Adrenaline: adrenaline nebulizers are a very effective treatment for croup, typically delivered as 5 mg of adrenaline in 5 mL of saline via standard nebulizers. This often results in a prompt resolution of croup-related stridor; however, the effect is often short-lived, and this may need repeating. More than 3–4 nebulizers over 1–2 hours suggest progressive disease that may require invasive support

- Bronchodilators: agents, such as salbutamol or ipratropium, are likely to have little effect on upper airway obstruction.

Systemic treatments

◆ Steroids: this is the mainstay of management in croup and usually results in the resolution of symptoms within 6 hours, which may avoid the need for intubation if adrenaline nebulizers are delivered in the interim period. The specific agent and route is unimportant, as long as a corticosteroid is administered early in the patient's admission. This may be oral prednisolone, IV or oral dexamethasone, or IV hydrocortisone. The combination of early steroids and adrenaline nebulizers mitigates the need for intubation in around 98% of patients with croup

◆ Antibiotics: often at this stage in the management, the differentiation between a bacterial or viral aetiology has not been completed, and it is appropriate to cover all patients who show signs of sepsis with airway obstruction with antibiotics. These are best delivered intravenously; however, the same caveats apply in that the airway should not be risked purely for the purposes of IV cannulation for the administration of antibiotics. A third-generation cephalosporin, usually ceftriaxone, will provide adequate cover for *Haemophilus influenzae* and for the common pathogens for bacterial tracheitis, typically Gram-positive cocci.

Anaesthestic management

An infant with a compromised stridulous airway will typically receive an inhalational induction of anaesthesia. There is growing experience using propofol TIVA for small children with airway obstructions, the benefits including a sustained delivery of anaesthetic and a rapid titratability and reversibility, even when the airway is compromised; however, this technique should be reserved for experts practising regularly with TIVA in children. Inhalational induction will be performed in the operating theatre, with the surgical team scrubbed in the event that an emergency surgical airway is required—there are few anaesthetists who possess up-to-date skills in performing surgical airways in children. Questions that are often raised include the following.

When to get IV access?

IV access should be established at a time when this will cause minimal upset to the child. It may be that, early in the admission, a topical local anaesthetic, such as Emla®, can be applied, and cannulation can be performed in the awake patient by a skilled operator. Often concerns that this will cause undue upset defers cannulation attempts, till the patient is anaesthetized, but this should be a priority once the induction has started, and attempts to secure the airway must not be performed without IV access. In the event of a severe deterioration on induction in a patient with poor venous access, an immediate deferral to intra-osseus access should occur.

In what position should the child be induced?

If the patient is maintaining an airway, whilst sitting on the mother's lap or similar, one should consider commencing the inhalational induction in this position. Attempts to separate the child from her mother or position on an operating table are likely to cause upset and exacerbate the airway occlusion. Oxygen and sevoflurane can be gently introduced into the atmosphere around the patient's face, by a cupped hand or breathing circuit without a face mask, progressing to the application of the mask, and taking the child from the mother as the induction progresses. A full explanation of details to the parent and a briefing of the primary plan and backup plan to the theatre team must be explicit before commencing induction.

Once an adequate depth of anaesthesia has been achieved, IV access obtained, and full monitoring established, laryngoscopy should proceed by the most experienced anaesthetist present. Adjuncts, such as a bougie, may be required, and significant downsizing of the tracheal tube should be anticipated, even when the larynx appears normal, in the case of bacterial tracheitis or tracheal stenosis. Once the airway is secured, the patient should have anaesthesia maintained, muscle relaxation, and preparation for transfer to the regional PICU.

Summary

Management of the stridulous infant is challenging for any anaesthetic team, and a high risk of patient harm exists if these cases are managed without meticulous preparation. Early recognition of a significant respiratory compromise and an impending ventilatory failure is vital, triggering a team response to prepare the necessary anaesthetic equipment and requesting support from additional staff from surgery and anaesthetics. Any interventions must be carefully balanced against worsening the airway compromise, with the ultimate aim of securing a safe airway prior to patient transfer.

Further reading

Bjornson CL and Johnson DW (2008). Croup. *Lancet*, **371**, 329–39.

Aeromedical transport considerations in acute lung injury

Background

Aeromedical critical care transport is a highly specialized field of transport medicine. Many factors may prove to compromise the patient's safety, including the hazards of loading and unloading, the physiological effects of acceleration and altitude, and equipment failure or malfunction in a restricted environment. On rare occasions, a non-transport anaesthetist may be asked to transfer a patient in an emergency from a referring unit to a regional centre by air. This case will outline some of the key considerations for aeromedical transport.

Learning outcomes

1 Understand the indications for aeromedical transport
2 Understand the physiological effects of altitude
3 Logistical considerations of aeromedical transfer.

CPD matrix matching

2A02; 2A11

Case history: understanding the indications for aeromedical transport

You are working in a remote, but large, district general hospital which has 24/7 anaesthetic, surgery, and ED cover, which is 120 miles from the regional network's major trauma centre. You are called to be on standby in the ED one evening for a young male that has come off his motorbike at high speed and hit a small group of trees. Your primary survey reveals he has a compromised airway by way of blood and dental fractures; his respiration is laboured with a flail chest and reduced air entry on the left; his abdomen is soft, and he has a suspected left femoral fracture. His GCS on arrival was E2 M5 V2, and you proceed to perform an uneventful RSI for stabilization of his airway, respiratory support, and anticipating a neurological deterioration. He is taken for a whole body CT which shows he has small intraparenchymal haemorrhages with mild cerebral oedema, fractures of the left ribs 1 to 4, and a small haemopneumothorax. He appears to have a small dissection of his aortic arch, but there is no active bleeding at the moment. He is cardiovascularly stable after a small bolus of volume resuscitation, and his femur has been stabilized with a Kendrick splint. He requires emergency transfer to the regional cardiothoracic unit in the event that thoracic surgery is needed.

What are the advantages and disadvantages of aeromedical vs road transport for this patient?

This is a complex and critically ill patient with a life-threatening injury. Transfer will be challenging, and a progression of his aortic injury may be terminal, irrespective of any interventions. Once cardiorespiratory stability has been achieved, he should be transferred in a time-sensitive manner, but at all time bearing in mind that any severe physiological disturbance may rupture any formed aortic clot and precipitate a catastrophic haemorrhage. There are many factors which must be taken into account to determine the optimal transport modality for this patient:

- Road transport: a local road ambulance is usually the most readily available option, though, in remote areas, front-line ambulance resources are often limited to 1–2 crews, serving a large geographical area. Advantages of road transport include a degree of familiarity with the layout for most anaesthetists, reasonable access to the patient, the ability to stop the vehicle if complex interventions need to be performed, and the ability to divert to a hospital en route if there are any equipment or vehicle malfunctions. Disadvantages mainly relate to the speed and smoothness of transfer. As an approximation, 120 miles would take 2.5–3 hours, depending on the road, weather, and traffic conditions. Driving at speeds in excess of the national speed limit is possible in modern vehicles and can be supported with a police escort to enhance safety, but this becomes challenging for staff in the back to manage the patient effectively, due to noise, vibration, and G-forces

- Rotary wing: helicopter transport is often perceived as the most rapid form of emergency patient transport, with evidence supporting that emergency patient transport at distances over 45 miles is optimally performed by rotary wing over road ambulance transport. Advantages may include the ability to travel from a referring hospital helicopter landing site (HLS) to a receiving unit HLS, thereby negating the need for any secondary road transfers. Transport is also relatively smooth in the cruise, depending on the weather. A standard civilian air ambulance will cruise at around 120 knots, meaning

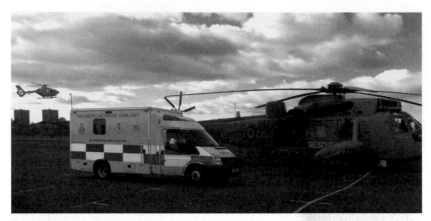

Fig. 14.6 Most helicopter retrievals currently require a secondary road transport at the receiving unit.

that a helicopter flight for this patient will take around an hour or so, plus loading and unloading times. Apart from the speed of transfer, there are many disadvantages to helicopter transport; the aircraft is unlikely to be at the referring unit at the time dispatch is required, unless based there, so an additional time delay may be factored in. If neither the referring nor the receiving units have an HLS on site, a secondary road transport will be required (see Figure 14.6), and, even if an HLS is present, there may be weather or lighting limitations to its use, necessitating a diversion to an alternative HLS at short notice. Weather conditions, such as cloud base and temperature, in conjunction with the terrain to be traversed, may limit the aircraft's capabilities. Notwithstanding the logistical difficulties, many anaesthetists are not familiar with the operating environment in an air ambulance, with respect to the restricted space and limited access to the patient, the negligible scope for performing patient interventions, and the impact of noise and vibration on patient monitoring

- Fixed wing: this is unequivocally the fastest and smoothest way to transport patients over longer distances, with a recommendation that distances over 150 miles be performed preferentially by fixed wing. Purpose-built air ambulance aeroplanes, such as the Beechcraft King Air (see Figure 14.7), which is in use globally for this purpose, have large cargo doors, with mechanical stretcher lifts, 240 V AC power, extensive oxygen supplies, and a cruising speed of around 240 knots. This would give a flying time of around 30 min for this patient's journey. However, every fixed wing journey will require a secondary road transfer before and after each flight, and, as well as adding considerable delay to mobilization, this increases the risk of tube,

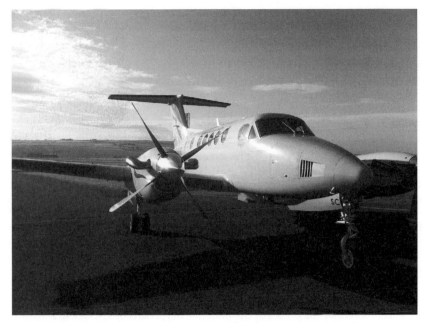

Fig. 14.7 The Scottish Ambulance Service Beechcraft KingAir 200 aircraft.

line, or monitor displacement every time the patient is transferred in and out of a vehicle. Fixed wing aircraft are much less subject to weather limitations than helicopters, but nonetheless extremely cold temperatures or fog may prevent landing at the desired destination airport. As with helicopters, the aircraft will often have to attend from a base airport which may add further delay into the process.

For this patient, arguments could be made for and against each of the three transport platforms. Road ambulances will be the most readily available and present the fewest challenges for the non-transport specialist, but they will be the slowest option. If a helicopter is available and the weather is favourable, this may be the quickest option but is the most difficult working environment for the anaesthetist. Fixed wing transfer has the drawbacks of secondary road transport but is likely to be faster and smoother, and it may be the preferred option for this patient.

Case update: understanding the physiological effects of altitude and forces of flight

There is a helicopter presently on your hospital HLS which is available for immediate dispatch, and the receiving cardiothoracic unit also has an HLS on site. You choose to perform this transport by helicopter. The weather is favourable, and your route on a direct track will take you to 5000 ft (1500 m) to clear the nearest mountains. Your estimated total transfer time will be 80 min, including loading and unloading at either end.

What physical factors during the flight may influence the patient's physiology, and what can be done to minimize disturbances to the patient?

There are many issues relating to the working environment within an air ambulance helicopter, but external forces may have a severe impact on the patient's cardiorespiratory status and must be anticipated in advance of a flight.

Barometric pressure

• Oxygenation: as a general rule, the barometric pressure decreases by 10% per 1000 m ascent from sea level, this being subject to local weather conditions, and reducing less so at altitudes >5000 m. For a proposed flight at 1500 m, one would anticipate a 15% fall in the barometric pressure from around 101 kPa at sea level to 85 kPa, with a subsequent reduction in the atmospheric oxygen pressure from around 21 kPa to 18 kPa. This will have negligible effects on either the crew's or the patient's oxygenation. The key implication for this fall in oxygen pressure would be, if a patient was spontaneously ventilating on high-flow oxygen by a trauma mask at sea level and only just maintaining an adequate oxygenation, the 15% reduction in partial pressure will worsen hypoxia. Managing this situation would include requesting a low-level flight or using a pressurized aircraft

• Pressure: the patient in this case has a pneumothorax, the gas volume of which will expand in direct proportion with the fall in atmospheric pressure at altitude. If the pneumothorax is of considerable size, this may cause tension effects, and an elective intercostal drainage should be performed prior to air transport in any patient with a pneumothorax. Other air spaces which may distend include the middle ear, sinuses, and bowel, or any pathological air, e.g. a pneumocranium or pneumoperitoneum. Unlike commercial aircrafts which have a 'cabin altitude' of 1800–2000 m, air ambulance aeroplanes can pressurize the cabin to sea level, i.e. 101 kPa, negating the effects of oxygen reduction and gas space expansion; however, a rapid decompression may occur at any stage, and an intrathoracic drainage should be performed prior to any flight. Also, sea level cabin pressurization considerably increases fuel consumption and causes repeated stresses on the air frame, so it should only be requested when clinically necessary

• G-forces and positioning: the acceleration and deceleration forces in a helicopter are typically gentle and should not cause excessive redistribution of venous blood. Some manoeuvres after take-off and on approaching landing require sharp turns, and the pilot should be briefed to avoid such manoeuvres wherever possible. Low-level flying will result in an unsatisfactory transport experience for the patient, due to the multiple severe directional changes. A helicopter flies with a typical 'nose-down' pitch which, over the period of the hour or so of the flight, may be undesired in view of the intracranial injury this patient has sustained. This is unavoidable, due to the physics of a helicopter flight, but it may be possible to package the patient in the transport vacuum mattress with a slightly head-up attitude to counter the effects during flight. This is in contrast to a fixed wing aircraft which flies with a 'nose-up' pitch and tends to manoeuvre less aggressively than a helicopter. However, the linear G-forces on take-off and landing are considerable and unavoidable. These should be anticipated at these stages of flight, with extreme attention to detail to the BP and treatment, as necessary

Case update: logistical considerations of aeromedical transfer

You have prepared the patient for helicopter transport. He is intubated and ventilated on a transport ventilator, with standard and invasive pressure monitoring on a transport monitor. He is sedated with a low-dose propofol infusion and has had opioid analgesia and a bolus of muscle relaxant. He has been packaged on a vacuum mattress and has a cervical collar applied. A left intercostal chest drainage has drained around 100 mL of blood and is swinging with ventilation. The aircraft is ready on the helipad outside your ED.

What are the logistical considerations to transferring this patient by helicopter?

This critically ill patient will be challenging to manage in a well-staffed operating theatre or ICU, so this will be a considerable order of magnitude more difficult to manage in a helicopter.

Clinical environment

Once loaded into an air ambulance helicopter, access to the patient is usually very limited. Access to an injection port should be readily available, without having to unstrap either the patient or staff member from their safety harnesses. The aim during preparation for transfer should be to have the patient as stable as possible and packaged in such a manner that minimal interventions are anticipated in flight. Any major interventions that require the team to come out of their harnesses must involve the pilot, who may elect instead to divert to the nearest safe landing site. Defibrillation can be safely performed in flight, but only after approval from the pilot, as there may be transient interference on the aircraft's electrical systems. The monitor and ventilator should be secured to aviation-approved air frame mounting brackets, and all carry-on items must be stowed securely in the appropriate cargo area. Adequate oxygen supplies within the aircraft must be ensured prior to departure.

Communication

As with road transfer, the receiving unit must be briefed of the patient's condition and an estimated arrival time prior to departure. Once in flight, all communications out of the aircraft are limited to being relayed via the pilot and air traffic control or via the flight paramedic's VHF radio through ambulance control. Direct communication with a receiving unit would only be possible via satellite phones which are not regularly carried on most UK air ambulance helicopters. Standard mobile phones do interfere significantly with the VHF radio system in the aircraft, and they lose signal once over 500–1000 m altitude, so they cannot be used.

Weather

The route may have to be diverted or the destination altered, depending on the weather. In general, helicopters can fly through cloud on instrument flight rules (IFR), provided the temperature is above 5°C. At temperatures lower than this, a helicopter cannot fly through cloud, as there is a risk of icing on the rotor blades which significantly compromises performance and may necessitate an emergency landing.

Summary

Aeromedical transfer of critically ill patients requires careful consideration of the risk–benefit ratio. Advantages, including speed and a relatively smooth transport platform, may be offset against drawbacks, including a restricted clinical environment, limited communications, and the effects of a fall in the barometric pressure on both internal air-filled spaces and on oxygenation.

Further reading

Martin T (2001). *Handbook of patient transportation*. Greenwich Medical Media Ltd, London.

Martin T (2006). *Aeromedical transportation: a clinical guide*, 2nd edn. Ashgate Publishing Ltd, Aldershot.

Chapter 15

Pain medicine

Dr Prit Singh
Dr Joanna Renée

Complex regional pain syndrome

Background

Complex regional pain syndrome (CRPS) is a severe, chronic pain condition that can be triggered by a minor injury (or can even occur spontaneously), which leads to distal regional symptoms and signs. It has a long protracted course and is associated with significant disability and a reduced quality of life. The incidence from various studies is quoted between 5 and 26/100 000. Females are more affected than males (3–4:1). The incidence peaks in the 6th decade. Upper limbs are generally more affected than lower limbs (3:2). Nine out of ten cases do not have a predisposing nerve injury. It can affect more than one limb and, in certain cases, the opposite limb too. It has also been associated with asthma, migraine, MI, traumatic brain injury, osteoporosis, and ACE inhibitor intake.

Learning outcomes

1 Recognize the clinical features of CRPS
2 Outline potential management strategies for CRPS.

CPD matrix matches

2E02; 2E03

Case history

A young, motivated athlete suffered a soft tissue injury of his left ankle, whilst training. Initially, he was seen by the trauma doctors in the A&E department and was discharged home with adequate advice and analgesia. It is almost 6 months since his injury now, and he has visited various physicians, with not much relief of his pain. He has come to see you now with a sharp, burning pain in his left leg, with associated changes to the colour of the skin, decreased hair growth, and abnormal nail changes.

What are the key points you would assess from this patient's history?

A comprehensive history should be elicited from the patient. The history should include details of the pain condition, including the onset, severity, radiation,

Table 15.1 CRPS diagnosis: the Budapest criteria

Category	Sign (you can see or feel a problem)	Symptom (the patient reports a problem)
1. Sensory	**Allodynia** (to light touch and/or temperature sensation and/or deep somatic pressure and/or joint movement) and/or **hyperalgesia** (to pinprick)	**Hyperaesthesia** does also qualify as a symptom
2. Vasomotor	Temperature asymmetry and/or skin colour changes and/or skin colour asymmetry	If you notice temperature asymmetry, it must be >1°C
3. Sudomotor/oedema	Oedema and/or sweating changes and/or sweating asymmetry	
4. Motor/trophic	Decreased range of motion and/or motor function (weakness, tremor, dystonia) and/or trophic changes (hair/nail/skin)	

(A) The patient has continuing pain which is disproportionate to the inciting event.

(B) The patient has at least one sign in two or more of the categories.

(C) The patient reports at least one symptom from three or more of the categories.

(D) No other diagnosis can better explain the signs and symptoms.

Data from Harden RN et al., 'Proposed new diagnostic criteria for complex regional pain syndrome', *Pain Medicine*, 2007, 8, 4, pp. 326–331.

character, alleviating and exacerbating factors, effects on sleep, social interactions, mood, and the various treatment modalities utilized and their effect on the pain problem. A requisite number of symptoms are required to diagnose CRPS in an individual, as shown in Table 15.1.

A detailed examination of the area will reveal various signs associated with CRPS in this patient. A full systemic examination should also be carried out for completeness.

What clinical features may you elicit on examination?

The characteristic clinical features of CRPS involve a combination of negative (sensory loss) and positive symptoms (hyperalgesia and allodynia), similar to neuropathic pain. However, according to the new definition, they cannot be classified as neuropathic pain as described in Table 15.1. In severe cases, the limb may be distorted, and the patient may display features of neglect.

How is the diagnosis confirmed?

The physician diagnosing the case should be aware of the Budapest criteria, which have a sensitivity of 0.85 and specificity of 0.69, compared to the previous International Association for the Study of Pain (IASP) criteria which had high sensitivity, but a very low specificity, for diagnosing CRPS. The new criteria rely on history and clinical examination and any additional tests are not recommended. Other tests may be done to exclude differential diagnoses, e.g. nerve conduction studies and electromyography (EMG).

Discuss the pathophysiology of complex regional pain syndrome

There are multiple pathophysiological mechanisms involved in the progression of CRPS, and it can change with time. The following have been implicated in CRPS: inflammation, sympathetic nervous dysfunction (coupling with the sensory system and catecholamine dysfunction), genetic and psychological factors, autoimmune dysfunction, peripheral and central sensitization, and cortical plasticity and reorganization. There is a complex interplay between most of these factors, resulting in the symptoms and signs.

Outline a management strategy for this patient

There is no definitive treatment for CRPS. Patients who are diagnosed with CRPS should be managed by a multidisciplinary approach, and the following four areas should be considered, with each patient requiring individualized care. The evidence base for these strategies are elucidated in the following paragraphs:

- Pharmacological management (including medicines and interventions)
- Rehabilitation: physical and vocational
- Psychological therapies
- Self-management skills with adequate patient information and education.

Although medications are often used to manage cases of CRPS, there is either no or insufficient evidence for the use of conventional analgesics, local anaesthetics, or first- and second-line anti-neuropathic agents.

There is limited evidence for ketamine and gabapentin for short-term use. Certain free radical scavengers, like dimethyl sulfoxide (DMSO) and N-acetylcysteine (NAC), have been used with moderate evidence. DMSO is used for 'warm'-type CRPS, and NAC for 'cold'-type CRPS. There is insufficient evidence for the use of botulinum toxin, capsaicin cream, muscle relaxants, or benzodiazepines. Calcitonin has been used, but the evidence is not clear. There may be some benefit for the use of bisphosphonates and calcium channel blockers.

Various interventions, like percutaneous and IV sympathetic blocks, have been used; however, there is no evidence for the effectiveness of these blocks. Surgical sympathectomy has been shown to have limited evidence for pain relief. Spinal cord stimulation, when used in carefully selected patients, results in better pain scores and an improved quality of life.

Physiotherapy and occupational therapy have been shown to have a beneficial effect in the management of CRPS and have been recommended as part of multidisciplinary care. There is minimal evidence for transcutaneous electrical nerve stimulation (TENS) or rehabilitation medicine. There is a paucity of evidence for the role of psychological management. Self-management has been shown to improve confidence in patients.

Summary

CRPS has been known in the past by various names and is a debilitating chronic condition, characterized by extreme pain in the affected limb. It is associated with sensory, motor, vasomotor, and sudomotor changes and may or may not be associated with nerve injury. Patients complain of limb dysfunction and psychosocial distress. Different diagnostic criteria have been used in the past, the most recent being the Budapest criteria, which are divided into four components and have improved the management of patients suffering from CRPS.

Further reading

Body in Mind. Available at: <http://www.bodyinmind.org>.

Butler D and Moseley L (2003). *Explain pain*. NOI Group Publications, Adelaide.

Goebel A, Barker CH, Turner-Stokes L, *et al.* (2012). *Complex regional pain syndrome in adults: UK guidelines for diagnosis, referral and management in primary and secondary care*. Royal College of Physicians, London.

Harden RN, Bruehl S, Stanton-Hicks M, and Wilson PR (2007). Proposed new diagnostic criteria for complex regional pain syndrome. *Pain Medicine*, **8**, 326–31.

The Knowledge Network. *Chronic pain*. Available at: <http://www.knowledge.scot.nhs.uk/pain.aspx>.

Phantom limb pain

Background

Phantom limb pain (PLP) is frequently described by post-amputation patients as sharp, shooting, stabbing, burning, or cramp-like. Patients may also experience residual limb or 'stump' pain which too can become chronic. Stump pain is strongly associated with PLP, and, although treatment for each pain may overlap, it is important to differentiate between the two.

Learning outcomes

1 Recognize the risk factors for the development of PLP

2 Identify both pharmacological and non-pharmacological strategies for the long-term management of PLP.

CPD matrix matches

2E01; 2E03

Case history

A 58-year-old gentleman with type II diabetes is listed for theatre for a below-knee amputation. He has diabetic nephropathy, background retinopathy, and peripheral neuropathy with reduced sensation of both feet. He has had rest pain at night for 9 months, secondary to his peripheral vascular disease. He describes a constant burning pain of the soles of his feet, despite them being cold to touch, and a throbbing ache in his calves worsened by walking.

He also has a non-healing ulcer on his right heel for 3 months which has been treated with antibiotics in the community. In this area, he experiences intermittent throbbing and a sharp, shooting pain radiating from his heel to mid calf. The area of the ulcer itself is numb, and he has reduced sensation to touch, distal to his ankle.

Other significant past medical history includes hypertension, hypercholesterolaemia, and mild COPD. He is a current smoker, with minimal alcohol intake. He had an uneventful general anaesthetic 13 years ago after injuring his arm in a DIY-related incident. He is overweight with a BMI of 32. His airway assessment is unremarkable, and he has a full top denture. His current medications include ramipril, simvastatin, insulin, aspirin, inhalers, and co-codamol 30/500 (two tablets four times daily), and tramadol 50 mg (as required).

Blood results show an Hb of 15.2 g/dL, WCC 6.9×10^9/L, Plt 353×10^9/L, Na$^+$ 139 mmol/L, K$^+$ 4.8 mmol/L, urea 8.1 mmol/L, Cr 140 micromoles/L, and an eGFR of 54. Coagulation and LFTs are normal. ECG shows a sinus rhythm, with borderline left ventricular hypertrophy.

He is concerned about PLP and would like to know more about it.

What is phantom limb pain? What is the incidence? What are the risk factors for developing phantom limb pain?

Phantom sensations are feelings perceived to be coming from the missing body part, such as itching, tingling, or movement, and can often be painful. Phantom pain has been reported in many different amputated body parts as well as limbs, such as breast, penis, rectum, bladder, eyes, and teeth. Up to 80% of amputee patients experience PLP, usually occurring shortly after the operation. Some patients have resolution of symptoms after a few months, but, in many, the symptoms persist. Occasionally, patients have no phantom symptoms, until many years later when it may spontaneously arise or be triggered by an event such as trauma (physical or emotional) or even a spinal anaesthetic.

PLP appears to be more prevalent in patients who had pain in the limb prior to amputation. Indeed, the pain is often similar in nature. It is also more common in lower limb and bilateral amputees.

Your patient asks why phantom limb pain happens and if there is anything that can be done to prevent it

The exact cause of PLP has been deliberated and investigated for many years, and unsurprisingly, like most pain states, it appears to be multifactorial.

The brain and nervous system display neuroplasticity and are constantly processing information, adapting, and restructuring as a consequence. This shapes our individual pain experience and is influenced by many factors such as past experience of pain, genetics, the environment, social and cultural background, and personality. This is known as 'the biopsychosocial model of pain'.

In patients with PLP, structural changes have been shown in the somatosensory cortex, dorsal horn of the spinal cord (central sensitization), thalamus, brainstem, and the peripheral nerves. These changes are usually characterized by an increased excitability of neurones, combined with a reduction of inhibitory pathways.

PLP (again, like many pain states) can also be mediated by the sympathetic nervous system, causing an exacerbation of pain in response to emotion and stress. Furthermore, in the residual limb, neuromas develop, secondary to nerve trauma (surgery), and can also be triggered spontaneously by an increase in circulating catecholamines.

Another common finding is changes in the somatosensory cortex where the area representing the missing limb is 'remapped' and receives sensory messages from other areas. This can result in patients feeling phantom sensation and phantom pain when a different area of the body is stimulated.

A lot of focus on preventing PLP has been around the perioperative period and whether we can prevent or modify the changes that take place at the time of amputation. Several strategies have been studied and mainly involve minimizing perioperative pain signalling. High levels of acute pain have been associated with the development of chronic post-surgical pain, as have nerve damage and pre-existing pain—all factors common to many amputees.

The evidence is often conflicting, as frequently the studies have been of relatively small patient numbers or suffer from inadequate randomization. Follow-up data are often difficult to interpret, due to the patient population characteristics. Patients who commonly present for limb amputation have significant comorbidities, and, in many studies, the patients do not survive to the endpoints.

What is the role for central neuraxial blockade in the development of phantom limb pain?

Epidurals and spinals undoubtedly provide superior acute pain control for amputation, but it is unclear whether they can influence the development of PLP. An ongoing epidural local anaesthetic (up to 3 days) may have a beneficial effect on long-term outcomes, as may a combination of epidural clonidine and diamorphine. Epidural ketamine does not appear to have an effect on PLP.

Is peripheral neural blockade beneficial?

Most studies looking at this strategy were examining a catheter placed perineurally, with an infusion for up to 72 hours post-operatively. Unfortunately, no studies have shown a long-term reduction in PLP with this method. In addition, analgesia for acute stump pain was found to be inferior to an epidural local anaesthetic. This would be a useful adjunct to systemic analgesia for those patients unsuitable for central neural blockade.

Are there any adjunctive medications that might impact on phantom limb pain?

IV ketamine and oral gabapentin have also been tried for the prevention of PLP, with disappointing results. Most patients in this group have pre-existing pain, and it is likely that blocking pain signalling at the stage of surgery does not reverse the existing central changes. It may be possible to prevent further changes secondary to nerve damage, but evidence for perioperative prevention is limited.

Case update

Your patient underwent his amputation under spinal anaesthesia with diamorphine plus a femoral nerve block with a catheter, followed by a local anaesthetic infusion for 2 days. He was very comfortable throughout and was able to participate with physiotherapy the next day.

Nine months later, you meet this patient again at his first appointment at the chronic pain clinic. He has adapted well to life with an amputated limb and is mobilizing with a prosthesis for short periods. His post-operative course was uneventful, and he is considering returning to work soon. However, he has troubling pain where his right leg used to be, particularly at night. His sleep quality is poor, and he finds himself getting up to sleep in a chair on most nights. He feels exhausted and unable to concentrate. He sometimes gets the pain during the day, particularly at times when he 'really does not need it', often at times of stress. His daytime pain is distracting, although this is less severe than at night. He describes the feeling as tense or gripping. His GP started amitriptyline at night which was titrated to 30 mg, but he was intolerant of the side effects such as dry mouth, urinary retention, and excessive sleepiness. He has started gabapentin, now at a dose of 300 mg three times day. Initially, he slept better at night but is unsure if it is having any real effect on his pain.

What more do you want to know about the history?

He has already described the characteristics of his pain, its variation during the day, the effect on his sleep, and the effects of analgesic medications. To complete a pain history, you ask him more about his pain. Is there anything he can do to make it better or worse? Does he have any other sensations? Does he have stump pain? Is his pain similar to his preoperative pain?

He reports that his leg feels better when he takes his prosthesis off and especially when he is relaxing in the evening. He does not think anything else changes his pain. His stump is tender after wearing the prosthesis, and occasionally he feels a tight sensation when at rest. He does admit that sometimes his pain feels like his preoperative burning pain but thinks this must be foolish, as the ulcerated foot has now gone.

It is important to elicit a detailed medication history. What other medication does he take and at what dose? Ask about each analgesic he takes, if it helps, if he has side effects. Are there any other medications he has tried? Has he tried other treatments like physiotherapy or acupuncture? His current medications are ramipril, simvastatin, insulin, aspirin, inhalers, and co-codamol 30/500 as before. He no longer takes tramadol, as it was ineffective, and he started gabapentin 2 months ago. His physiotherapy has formally finished, but he continues to follow their advice.

What other factors in the history may influence your management plan?

How does he manage with his daily activities? Find out what he can and cannot do. Who lives at home with him? Does he require any help or social support? What does his work involve, and how does he think he will manage?

Your patient is able to do most things around the house. He manages all personal care and is happy with transfers. He has a wheelchair for mobilizing and rarely uses it indoors now. He uses a stick for walking. He is at home with his wife who is relatively fit, and she does the housework and shopping. They also have a son and a daughter who are nearby and regularly visit. He owns a hardware store which he runs with his son who has been looking after the business since his father's operation. He is keen to return to work and has been recently involved with the accounts side of the business. He does worry about lifting and moving stock and also about what he would do if he had a lot of pain when he was on his own in the shop.

Does his pain affect his mood or his outlook on life?
What concerns does he have about his pain?
What does he hope to gain from the pain clinic?

This patient appears to be a stoic gentleman and initially denies any low mood. He states that 'anyone in this situation would get a bit down', but he tries to keep a positive outlook and wants to find a way to 'deal with it'. After speaking to you at the pre-assessment visit, he expected he would have some phantom pain and has since read about it on the internet. He is concerned that it will not get any better and that he will continue to be too exhausted to go back to work. He wants to have good-quality sleep.

Many health professionals who deal with patients and their pain utilize validated questionnaires. These can provide useful information and can be a guide to success of treatment. Many of these tools exist; some examples are the Brief Pain Inventory, the McGill Pain Questionnaire, the Hospital Anxiety and Depression Scale, the Pain Catastrophising Scale, and the self-report version of the Leeds Assessment of Neuropathic Symptoms and Signs.

Examination is also important, and, for most pain patients, it will focus on the appearance and temperature of the skin, the sensation to light touch and pin prick, and, if applicable, the range of movement. Often a neurological examination and/or palpation of the painful area are performed.

What is the prognosis of phantom limb pain?

Several studies have looked at the persistence of PLP and found that symptoms reduce in most patients. Around 60% of patients with PLP symptoms will have their symptoms remaining after 2 years, but the severity and frequency of the attacks will usually decrease. The pain is usually intermittent and is often similar in nature to the pre-amputation pain. Over time, the limb may feel shortened, a phenomenon known as 'telescoping'.

What therapies are available for phantom limb pain?

Pharmacology

There is little evidence for the effectiveness of simple analgesics, such as paracetamol and NSAIDs, in PLP. Antidepressants and anticonvulsants are effective for neuropathic pain, and gabapentin has some evidence of short-term benefit in PLP, but there is inadequate evidence for other medications in this class. Opioids have some effect on neuropathic pain, and studies have shown possible benefit for PLP. Short-term effects have also been shown in controlled studies of ketamine and calcitonin, although the numbers of patients were small.

Physical therapies

Whilst there is little evidence for an effective pharmacology treatment, physical treatments have been shown to make significant improvements to a patient's pain and quality of life. Many types of physical treatment, such as TENS, sensory discrimination, acupuncture, massage, mirror therapy, and graded motor imagery, have been utilized, with good effects, although evidence is limited. These methods often target the changes within the nervous system, attempting to manipulate the neuroplasticity of the brain and alter the cortical reorganization that has occurred in these patients. It is also important to establish any problems with the residual limb and prosthesis fitting which can aggravate the phantom limb.

Surgery

Repeated surgery is not of benefit, unless there is an obvious pathology of the residual stump. Attempts in the past to remove neuromas have unfortunately worsened symptoms. Spinal cord stimulation has been used for refractory pain, with some success, but further studies are needed.

Other pain management strategies

As for all patients living with chronic pain, learning new ways of managing life and coping with chronic pain can make significant differences to their quality of life. There are many resources available to provide an understanding of pain and ways of dealing with it. The biopsychosocial approach involves physiotherapy, psychology, and medicine which can be accessed individually or as part of the chronic pain service.

Pain specialist physiotherapy is about learning movements and techniques that increase function and ability such as pacing and goal setting.

Pain specialist psychology addresses stress, mood, thoughts, and feelings and teaches relaxation and techniques such as mindfulness.

Social support is also important, and there are many useful organizations and resources. There are local (e.g. the Pain Association Scotland), national (e.g. Pain Concern), international (e.g. IASP), and condition-specific groups (e.g. the Limbless Association).

You discuss with your patient the options for treatment for PLP, and he is keen to avoid multiple medications and side effects. You advise him to gradually titrate the gabapentin up to 900 mg three times a day, with advice to regularly consider its effectiveness and side effects. You reassure him that there are other medications that he can try if he feels gabapentin is not for him. You also suggest that, when he is on a stable dose, he tries gradually reducing his co-codamol, as this may be an unnecessary medication for pain relief, now his stump has healed.

You discuss other therapies, and he is not keen for treatments that involve touching his residual limb and so decides not to try the TENS machine you have suggested.

He has insight into his condition and appears motivated, so you refer him to a pain management programme for physiotherapy and possibly psychology. You give him advice about local organizations and some web-based resources, along with a leaflet about Airing Pain, the online radio station broadcasted by Pain Concern. He appears pleased and relieved that there are several helpful options and thanks you for your time.

Summary

PLP is pain perceived to be from the amputated body part. It is experienced in up to 80% of amputee patients and is often persistent. It is more common in patients with pre-existing pain and is thought to be due to several mechanisms, including nervous system changes such as central sensitization, remapping of the homunculus, and neuroma formation. Many strategies have been used for the prevention of PLP, although there is little evidence of effectiveness, except possibly for epidural anaesthesia. For longer-term management, there is more evidence for non-pharmacological treatments than for medication, and, in general, as for most pain patients, a biopsychosocial approach should be taken.

Further reading

Alviar MJ, Hale T, and Dungca M (2011). Pharmacologic interventions for treating phantom limb pain. *Cochrane Database of Systematic Reviews*, **12**, CD006380.

Flor H (2002). Phantom limb pain: characteristics, causes, and treatment. *Lancet Neurology*, **1**, 182–9.

Jackson M and Simpson K (2004). Pain after amputation. *Continuing Education in Anaesthesia, Critical Care & Pain*, **4**, 20–3.

Nikolajsen L and Jensen TS (2001). Phantom limb pain. *British Journal of Anaesthesia*, **87**, 107–16.

Ypsilantis E and Tang TY (2010). Pre-emptive analgesia for chronic limb pain after amputation for peripheral vascular disease: a systematic review. *Annals of Vascular Surgery*, **24**, 1139–46.

Chronic post-surgical pain

Background

Chronic post-surgical pain (CPSP) is one of the most common complications after surgery or trauma, occurring in up to 40% of patients. It causes significant morbidity to patients and accounts for a considerable proportion of activity in chronic pain clinics in the UK.

Learning outcomes

1 Define the incidence of CPSP between various surgical specialties
2 Recognize the complex interactions between biophysical, social, and pathological factors.

CPD matrix matches

2E1

Case history

An anxious 32-year-old female has presented to the chronic pain clinic with constant, severe pain of her anterior chest wall and axilla. She underwent a mastectomy and an axillary node clearance 4 years ago, followed by a course of radiotherapy. The pain is shooting and burning in nature, and she reports her skin is 'sensitive', resulting in difficulty wearing tight clothing. Her sleep is disturbed, and the pain greatly limits the use of her arm. She reports having had some pain post-operatively, but the shooting and burning she describes started gradually during her radiotherapy and has worsened over time.

How is chronic post-surgical pain defined?

So far, there is no universal definition of CPSP. A working definition which is endorsed by IASP, has the following features:

♦ Pain after a surgical procedure
♦ Pain present for >2 months

- Other causes of pain excluded (infection/malignancy)
- Pain other than that existing pre-surgery.

Outline the risk factors for patients having major procedures developing chronic post-surgical pain and how these can be predicted

Certain major procedures have prolonged healing times, and pain can be an issue for >8 weeks but may eventually settle down with no residual effects. This is one of the reasons that different incidences have been quoted in various papers, ranging between a fifth and up to half of all surgical patients. It has been suggested that 2–10% of people suffering from CPSP have severe disabling pain. Table 15.2 is representative of the incidence of CPSP from specific surgeries.

CPSP has a complex biopsychosocial interaction. It is associated with an increased use of analgesics and a decrease in the activities of daily living, which consequently affect the quality of life of patients and have significant economic costs to the health care and social support system.

What are the risk factors for chronic post-surgical pain?

A number of risk factors have been identified for the development of chronic or persistent post-surgical pain. These factors can be divided into preoperative, intraoperative, or post-operative factors and are illustrated in Table 15.3.

These factors can also be broadly divided into patient factors and medical or surgical factors. The patient factors, in turn, have various forces acting upon

Table 15.2 Incidence of CPSP

Type of operation	Incidence of chronic pain (%)	Estimated incidence of severe chronic pain (VAS >5/10) (%)
Amputation	30–85	5–10
Thoracotomy	5–65	10
Mastectomy	11–57	5–10
Inguinal hernia	5–63	5–10
Coronary bypass	30–50	5–10
Caesarean section	6–55	4
Cholecystectomy	3–50	Not estimated
Vasectomy	0–37	Not estimated
Dental surgery	5–13	Not estimated

Adapted from *The Lancet*, 367, 9522, Kehlet H et al., 'Persistent postsurgical pain: risk factors and prevention', pp. 1618–1625, Copyright 2006, with permission from Elsevier; and Adapted from Macrae WA, 'Chronic post-surgical pain: 10 years on', *British Journal of Anaesthesia*, 2008, 101, 1, pp. 77–86, by permission of Oxford University Press.

Table 15.3 Risk factors for CPSP

Preoperative factors	Pre-existing pain, moderate to severe, lasting >1 month
	Repeat surgery
	Psychological vulnerability (e.g. catastrophizing)
	Preoperative anxiety
	Female gender
	Younger age (adults)
	Workers' compensation
	Genetic predisposition
	Inefficient DNIC
Intraoperative factors	Surgical approach with risk of nerve damage
Post-operative factors	Pain (acute, moderate to severe)
	Radiotherapy
	Chemotherapy
	Depression
	Psychological vulnerability
	Neuroticism and anxiety

them, e.g. the effects of genotype, the medical history, or psychosocial factors. The medical and surgical factors would include the type of surgery, anaesthesia, and analgesics.

What are the patient factors that may influence the development of chronic post-surgical pain?

Demographic factors

Age seems to be inversely related to the incidence of CPSP in certain surgeries and associated medical conditions. In various studies looking at hernia and breast surgery, it was found that an increasing age is associated with a lower incidence of CPSP. This could be attributed to other factors e.g. within each age group there may have been differences in the pathology, recurrence of tumour, extensive or aggressive radio- or chemotherapy. After various adjustments of the factors already mentioned, it has been suggested that there is approximately a 5% reduction in persistent pain per year in breast and hernia surgery.

A very young age may be a protective factor, especially in children <3 months. Children undergoing a thoracotomy have also been found to have a lower incidence of chronic pain than in adults. In contrast, it is found that elderly patients suffering from shingles have a much higher risk of developing post-herpetic neuralgia. The female gender has been found to have a higher incidence of persistent surgical pain, especially if they suffer from premorbid generalized body pains, e.g. fibromyalgia.

Psychosocial factors

Biopsychosocial factors play a major role in chronic pain and more recently, have been recognized to also play a significant role in acute post operative pain. Other factors identified as predictors for chronic post surgical pain include depression, psychological vulnerability, stress, and late return to work. Hypervigilance, a factor associated with fibromyalgia, may also play a role in CPSP.

Genetic factors

This area has been of interest recently. Genetic polymorphism of COMT enzyme and its relation to heightened pain to experimental stimuli, as well as to the development of temporomandibular joint pain, have been acknowledged by various authors. Another enzyme GCH1, a haplotype of this enzyme type, has effects on decreasing the sensitivity to pain in cancerous and other surgical interventions. Despite these genetic polymorphisms, the exact markers which can predict CPSP have not yet been found.

Many clinicians also have found that certain chronic pain conditions, like fibromyalgia, migraine, irritable bowel syndrome (IBS), and irritable bladder, could be associated with CPSP. The exact genetic mechanisms are still not known. It has been found that such individuals are more prone to having higher post-operative pain scores, which may or may not, however, be related to a higher incidence of CPSP.

Preoperative pain

Preoperative pain is consistently found to be a predictor for persistent post-surgical pain in certain surgeries such as amputation and mastectomy (mainly phantom pain), herniorrhaphy, and cholecystectomy. However, studies of preoperative pain in patients who undergo total hip arthroplasty do not correlate with the development of chronic pain at a later time. Despite various studies, preoperative pain is still not proven to be an independent risk factor for CPSP. Perhaps it is a combination of this with the neuroplastic changes at the time of surgery and the lack of adequate analgesia post-operatively which leads to the development of chronic pain.

Acute post-operative pain

The severity of acute post-operative pain has been consistently found to have a strong correlation with CPSP. This was first seen in patients who underwent thoracic surgery. Multiple studies have since had similar findings across a whole range of surgeries, including inguinal hernia surgery, breast cancer surgery, Caesarean sections, and hip arthroplasty. These findings support the hypothesis that repetitive nociceptive stimulation during the perioperative period results in permanent changes in the CNS in the form of central sensitization, which results in persistent pain. In patients undergoing cholecystectomy, it was found that the overall severity of pain was a better predictor for the development of persistent pain, rather than the maximum pain scores; thus, the duration of post-operative pain may also play a role.

Surgical factors

The size of the operation does not have a simple correlation with chronic pain. The duration of the surgery, however, has been found by a few investigators to be of significance in the development CPSP. This could be attributed to more serious pathology or complications, or perhaps other health issues which may affect the complexity of the surgery and the eventual outcome. Patients undergoing surgeries longer than 3 hours in duration have a higher incidence of CPSP and a generally poorer outcome. Similarly, more complex breast surgeries also have a higher incidence of chronic pain.

The surgical approach also plays a part in the development of chronic pain. Laparoscopic or minimally invasive approaches result in less chronic pain after hernia and cholecystectomy surgeries. Patients who have repeat hernia repair surgery were found to have higher moderate to severe pain scores, up to a year after the surgery. Complications, including re-operation, infection, and rebleeding, were also factors associated with persistent post-operative pain.

Other co-existing factors, such as the expertise of the surgeon, ambulatory or inpatient surgery, and the reason for surgery, are still areas of controversy for the development of CPSP. Patients undergoing radiotherapy have a higher incidence of CPSP, independently of other variables.

Do different anaesthetic and analgesic strategies minimize the risk of chronic post-surgical pain?

Pain at the time of surgery and in the immediate perioperative period is thought to sensitize the CNS and eventually to be a forerunner to persistent pain. Approaches to limit this are often used in day-to-day practice. However, to date, there have been conflicting results. There have been some positive studies for various surgeries like hernia repair, Caesarean section, hysterectomy, and thoracotomy. Despite the current lack of consensus, it is still reasonable to continue to deliver a multimodal, individualized approach for analgesia for all surgeries, in an attempt to reduce the incidence of CPSP.

Can you predict patients at risk of chronic post-surgical pain preoperatively?

A combined scoring system to predict acute post-operative pain has been proposed, consisting of variables, including age, gender, and preoperative pain. This has not yet been validated, due to the lack of large numbers of population required for individual procedure risk stratification. There have been other tests that are used to predict acute post-operative pain, using heat packs or ice water. Unfortunately, these tests have failed to be predictive of CPSP.

Recent research has concentrated on neurophysiological assessment, in the form of the quality of the endogenous inhibitory system by diffuse noxious inhibitory control (DNIC) testing, and seems promising as a predictor of CPSP.

Summary

Chronic pain after surgery is common. In recent years, there have been advances in the understanding of the pathophysiological processes, but its management and prevention still remain inadequate. Although much work still needs to be done to address the issues mentioned earlier, it is thought that improving acute post-operative pain management is one of the key strategies to prevent CPSP. There may be certain barriers to overcome (organizational, technical, and cultural) to achieve improvement.

Education of medical professionals and the general public will play an important role in the extent and disability of this problem, and it may deter some patients from undergoing inappropriate and unnecessary procedures.

The identification of high-risk patients is a major goal for the future. This may help to develop preventative strategies and avoid treatments with side effects for patients who are not at risk of developing chronic pain after surgery. Due to a lack of appropriate data for such strategies, an effective perioperative pain management and nerve-sparing surgical techniques are the major focus at the present time for the prevention of CPSP.

Further reading

Macrae WA (2008). Chronic post-surgical pain: 10 years on. *British Journal of Anaesthesia*, **101**, 77–86.

Macrae WA and Davies HTO (1999). Chronic post-surgical pain. In: Crombie IK, Linton S, Croft P, Von Korff M, and LeResche L, eds. *Epidemiology of pain*, pp. 125–42. IASP Press, Seattle.

Nikolajsen L, Brandsborg B, Lucht U, Jensen TS, and Kehlet H (2006). Chronic pain following total hip arthroplasty: a nationwide questionnaire study. *Acta Anaesthesiologica Scandinavica*, **50**, 495–500.

Peters ML, Sommer M, de Rijke JM, et al. (2007). Somatic and psychologic predictors of long-term unfavorable outcome after surgical intervention. *Annals of Surgery*, **245**, 487–94.

Poleshuck EL, Katz J, Andrus CH, et al. (2006). Risk factors for chronic pain following breast cancer surgery: a prospective study. *Journal of Pain*, **7**, 626–34.

Poobalan AS, Bruce J, Smith WC, King PM, Krukowski ZH, and Chambers WA (2003). A review of chronic pain after inguinal herniorrhaphy. *Clinical Journal of Pain*, **19**, 48–54.

Schnabel A and Pogatzki-Zahn E (2010). Predictors of chronic pain following surgery. What do we know? *Schmerz* **24**, 517–31; 532–3.

Schug SA and Pogatzki-Zahn EM (2011).Chronic pain after surgery or injury. *IASP Pain: Clinical Updates*, **19**, Issue 1.

Searle RD and Simpson KH (2010). Chronic post-surgical pain. *Continuing Education in Anaesthesia, Critical Care & Pain*, **10**, 12–14.

Visser EJ (2006). Chronic post-surgical pain: epidemiology and clinical implications for acute pain management. *Acute Pain*, **8**, 73–81.

Yarnitsky D, Crispel Y, Eisenberg E, *et al.* (2008). Prediction of chronic post-operative pain: pre-operative DNIC testing identifies patients at risk. *Pain*, **138**, 22–8.

Regional vs systemic analgesia

Background

Epidural nerve block has become a significant advance in neuraxial anaesthesia and analgesia. The procedure is commonly performed as a sole anaesthetic or in combination with spinal or general anaesthetic. The duration of anaesthesia or analgesia is prolonged when epidural catheters are used. Patients are able to control their pain with patient-controlled epidural analgesia (PCEA), in a manner similar to that of IV PCA. Epidural analgesia is a widely used technique for the management of acute pain in adults and children, particularly after surgery and occasionally in trauma situations, and in parturients.

PCA refers to a method of pain relief that allows a patient to self-administer small doses of an analgesic agent, as required. Most often, the term PCA is associated with programmable infusion pumps that deliver opioid medications intravenously. However, these opioids can be delivered in other ways, regionally (central neuraxial or peripheral) or systemically.

Learning outcomes

1 Discuss the risks and benefits of regional anaesthesia in elective and emergency surgical situations
2 Have an awareness of the impact of different perioperative regimens on long-term post-operative outcomes.

CPD matrix matches

2E01

Case history

You are the registrar in anaesthesia and have been asked by your educational supervisor to deliver a talk to junior surgical trainees regarding the efficacy of epidural vs IV PCA for various kinds of major surgeries.

Outline the evidence regarding those mentioned techniques

Epidural catheters can be inserted at different levels, according to the proposed surgery or, in rare occasions, the type of trauma. Upper thoracic levels are used for cardiothoracic surgeries. Lower thoracic levels are used for GI and vascular surgery and, in certain instances, for urological or gynaecological surgery. For lower limb surgeries, most urology, gynaecological, and major plastic surgery, and obstetric anaesthesia or analgesia, epidurals are normally sited in the lumbar region.

Due to the variety of levels used for different surgeries, the different modes of administration (continuous vs PCEA), and the number drugs used for epidural analgesia, it is very difficult to interpret the data. In summary, regional anaesthesia has been shown to be more efficacious than systemic opioid-based PCA, regardless of these variables. A meta-analysis assessing the efficacy of opioid-based PCA vs epidural analgesia for various surgeries concluded that epidural analgesia provided better analgesia at rest and in movement (dynamic pain scores) for the first 72 hours after surgery. The epidural group also had a lower incidence of sedation and PONV. However, patients with epidurals had a higher incidence of pruritus, urinary retention, and motor block.

These results were seen in groups which had either a local anaesthetic, or a local anaesthetic and an opioid mixture, or an opioid only (lipophilic drugs), but not in groups which only used hydrophilic opioids.

Comment on the epidural use in elective and emergency abdominal surgery

An assessment of post-operative pain control after intra-abdominal surgery confirmed that patients who had epidural analgesia (continuous, thoracic) had lower pain scores at rest and in movement, compared to patients using IV PCA, as well as the duration of ileus. There was not any difference in the length of stay.

The benefits of post-operative epidural analgesia in patients for abdominal procedures include a reduction in a range of adverse outcomes. Pain scores (at rest and in movement), arrhythmias, the duration of post-operative invasive ventilation, the length of ICU stay, stress hormone concentrations (adrenaline, noradrenaline, cortisol, and glucose), and the duration of ileus are all lower in groups treated with regional, rather than systemic, analgesia. The rate of renal failure is reduced in patients treated with local anaesthetic-only thoracic epidurals.

Do epidurals influence post-operative pulmonary morbidity?

It has been shown that patients treated with epidurals have a reduction in 24-hour consumption of morphine and improved lung volumes on spirometry testing. They also had higher PaO_2 levels, reduced pulmonary infections, and an overall reduction in pulmonary complications, compared to patients treated with systemic opioids. The observed incidence of chest infections in patients on systemic opioids is 12%, compared to an incidence for patients receiving epidurals of 8%.

How does epidural use influence post-operative pain?

Patients undergoing elective abdominal aortic surgery have lower pain scores (up to 72 hours) when using thoracic epidural catheters for post-operative pain relief, compared to a systemic opioid administration. In colorectal surgical patients, pain scores and the duration of ileus were reduced in patients with epidurals.

Discuss the implications of regional analgesia techniques in cardiothoracic surgery

The insertion of high thoracic epidurals results in reduced pain scores and a lesser incidence of dysrhythmias and pulmonary complications, and a decreased time to extubation, compared to systemic opioid analgesia. However, there is widespread concern of epidural haematomas, due to the fact that high-dose anticoagulation is typically used during cardiac surgery, and therefore the use of regional anaesthesia during cardiac procedures must involve a risk–benefit assessment on an individual patient basis.

Discuss the benefits of epidurals in major lower limb orthopaedic surgery

Comparing lumbar epidural blockade to systemic opioid analgesia for major lower limb joint replacement surgeries reported better dynamic pain scores in the epidural group and no difference in adverse effects between the two groups. Immediate and long-term post-operative knee movement was significantly better with epidural nerve block, compared to the systemic analgesia group.

Can epidurals be used in trauma patients?

The insertion of epidural analgesia in patients with rib fractures provides superior analgesia, compared to IV PCA. Patients with severe chest injury who have epidural also have improved pulmonary function and a favourable immune response, with a reduced rate of nosocomial pneumonia, compared to systemic opioid therapy.

Outline the differences between continuous epidural analgesia and patient-controlled epidural analgesia

It has been suggested that continuous epidural analgesia (CEA) provides superior analgesia, compared to PCEA, with regard to overall pain (static and dynamic) measurement. However, patients treated with CEA have a higher incidence of nausea and vomiting and motor block. It is probable that CEA results in a relative excess of local anaesthetic delivery, beyond that of the patient's requirement for analgesia, and some side effects may be offset if using PCEA. As the literature currently stands, there is little evidence to advocate one strategy over the other for epidural drug delivery.

Summary

Most of the evidence cited previously has come from various systematic reviews and meta-analyses and would be categorized as level 1 evidence. It favours the use of epidural analgesia, compared to IV PCA, for a variety of surgeries. It has been clearly shown that they provide better post-operative pain control, have lesser associated morbidity and a favourable stress response, and provide better immune function. The data at present do not equate to better outcomes or lesser mortality. Overall, epidurals should be considered in major high-risk colorectal, vascular, lower limb, and cardiothoracic surgery, after an adequate individual risk–benefit stratification.

Further reading

Ballantyne JC, Carr DB, deFerranti S, *et al.* (1998). The comparative effects of postoperative analgesic therapies on pulmonary outcome: cumulative meta-analyses of randomized, controlled trials. *Anesthesia & Analgesia*, **86**, 598–612.

Bauer C, Hentz JG, Ducrocq X, *et al.* (2007). Lung function after lobectomy: a randomized, double-blinded trial comparing thoracic epidural ropivacaine/sufentanil and intravenous morphine for patient-controlled analgesia. *Anesthesia & Analgesia*, **105**, 238–44.

Bulger EM, Edwards T, Klotz P, and Jurkovich GJ (2004). Epidural analgesia improves outcome after multiple rib fractures. *Surgery*, **136**, 426–30.

Capdevila X, Barthelet Y, Biboulet P, Ryckwaert Y, Rubenovitch J, and d'Athis F (1999). Effects of perioperative analgesic technique on the surgical outcome and duration of rehabilitation after major knee surgery. *Anesthesiology*, **91**, 8–15.

Carrier FM, Turgeon AF, Nicole PC, *et al.* (2009). Effect of epidural analgesia in patients with traumatic rib fractures: a systematic review and meta-analysis of randomized controlled trials. *Canadian Journal of Anaesthesia*, **56**, 230–42.

Choi PT, Bhandari M, Scott J, and Douketis J (2003). Epidural analgesia for pain relief following hip and knee replacement. *Cochrane Database of Systematic Reviews*, **3**, CD003071.

Corning JL(1885). Spinal anaesthesia and local medication of the cord. *New York Medical Journal*, **42**, 483–5.

Curbelo MM (1949). Continuous peridural segmental anesthesia by means of a ureteral catheter. *Current Researches in Anesthesia & Analgesia*, **28**, 13–23.

Fowler SJ, Symons J, Sabato S, and Myles PS (2008). Epidural analgesia compared with peripheral nerve blockade after major knee surgery: a systematic review and meta-analysis of randomized trials. *British Journal of Anaesthesia*, **100**, 154–64.

Guay J (2006). The benefits of adding epidural analgesia to general anesthesia: a metaanalysis. *Journal of Anesthesia*, **20**, 335–40.

Liu SS, Block BM, and Wu CL (2004). Effects of perioperative central neuraxial analgesia on outcome after coronary artery bypass surgery: a meta-analysis. *Anesthesiology*, **101**, 153–61.

Liu SS and Wu CL (2007). Effect of postoperative analgesia on major postoperative complications: a systematic update of the evidence. *Anesthesia & Analgesia*, **104**, 689–702.

Liu SS and Wu CL (2007). The effect of analgesic technique on postoperative patient-reported outcomes including analgesia: a systematic review. *Anesthesia & Analgesia*, **105**, 789–808.

Macintyre PE, Schug SA, Scott DA, Visser EJ, and Walker SM; APM:SE Working Group of the Australian and New Zealand College of Anaesthetists and Faculty of Pain Medicine (2010). *Acute pain management: scientific evidence*, 3rd edn. Australian and New Zealand College of Anaesthetists and Faculty of Pain Medicine, Melbourne.

Marret E, Remy C, and Bonnet F (2007). Meta-analysis of epidural analgesia versus parenteral opioid analgesia after colorectal surgery. *British Journal of Surgery*, **94**, 665–73.

Moon MR, Luchette FA, Gibson SW, *et al.* (1999). Prospective, randomized comparison of epidural versus parenteral opioid analgesia in thoracic trauma. *Annals of Surgery*, **229**, 684–91; discussion 691–2.

National Health and Medical Research Council (1999). *A guide to the development, implementation and evaluation of clinical practice guidelines*. Available at: <http://www.nhmrc.gov.au/_files_nhmrc/publications/attachments/cp30.pdf>.

Nishimori M, Ballantyne JC, and Low JH (2006). Epidural pain relief versus systemic opioid-based pain relief for abdominal aortic surgery. *Cochrane Database of Systematic Reviews*, **3**, CD005059.

Popping DM, Elia N, Marret E, et al. (2008). Protective effects of epidural analgesia on pulmonary complications after abdominal and thoracic surgery: a meta-analysis. *Archives of Surgery*, **143**, 990–9.

Tenenbein PK, Debrouwere R, Maguire D, et al. (2008). Thoracic epidural analgesia improves pulmonary function in patients undergoing cardiac surgery. *Canadian Journal of Anesthesia*, **55**, 344–50.

Werawatganon T and Charuluxanun S (2005). Patient controlled intravenous opioid analgesia versus continuous epidural analgesia for pain after intra-abdominal surgery. *Cochrane Database of Systematic Reviews*, **1**, CD004088.

Wu CL, Cohen SR, Richman JM, et al. (2005). Efficacy of postoperative patient-controlled and continuous infusion epidural analgesia versus intravenous patient-controlled analgesia with opioids: a meta-analysis. *Anesthesiology*, **103**, 1079–88.

Wu CL, Jani ND, Perkins FM, and Barquist E (1999). Thoracic epidural analgesia versus intravenous patient-controlled analgesia for the treatment of rib fracture pain after motor vehicle crash. *Journal of Trauma*, **47**, 564–7.

Managing chronic pain patients for elective surgery

Background

With every patient, there are different issues surrounding pain management, and the patient with chronic pain presenting acutely can be a particular challenge.

Recent data suggest that chronic pain is as prevalent as one in six of the population. Only a small proportion of those are referred to specialist pain services, and yet many are seen by virtually all other medical specialties and allied professions. Chronic pain results in changes to the nervous system, producing hyperaesthesia, allodynia, and central sensitization. Unfortunately, due to these factors, the chronic pain patient's acute pain experience is usually worse than that of the rest of the surgical population. Chronic pain patients often have a fear of increased pain and worry their pain will be severe and uncontrolled. They may display hypervigilance, fear, and anxiety.

Learning outcomes

1 Recognize the difficulties in managing patients with chronic pain through the perioperative period
2 Understand the need for additional analgesia whilst still meeting background analgesic requirements
3 Have a familiarity with dose conversions between differing routes of administration and opioid agents.

CPD matrix matches

2E01; 2E02

Case history

You have been referred an anxious 46-year-old female who is scheduled for major lower bowel resection for surgical management of inflammatory bowel disease. She has had several procedures before and suffers from chronic abdominal pain. She has attended the chronic pain clinic in the past and is on several analgesic medications. She has been in hospital for a few weeks, with an inadequate response to medical management, and has become increasingly more frail and in more pain. It is anticipated that she will be undergoing a prolonged open procedure.

What needs to be considered when managing this patient's pain?

Pain is an unpleasant sensory and emotional experience, and pain perception is affected by biological, psychological, and social influences—the biopsychosocial model of pain. How a person experiences pain is modified not only by specific receptors in the body (the usual target for pharmacological treatment), but also by many processes within the brain and nervous system which, in turn, are affected by emotions, beliefs, and circumstances. These powerful influences are more challenging to treat and, in chronic pain, often require time and perseverance.

Chronic pain patients are likely to have consulted a number of health professionals, seeking either relief of their pain or investigation into its cause. They may be on a number of analgesic medications, and some patients will be on strong opioids.

Pre-assessment

As with any surgical patient, a thorough history and assessment is required. In addition to your pre-assessment questions, ask about the patient's pain. Where is it? How often do they have it? What does it feel like? Does it affect sleep, mood, working life, daily activities? What makes it worse or better? Any information about their pain can be valuable.

Information should be obtained about previous pain management, acute and chronic. Ask about treatments tried, including medications, how effective they were, and why they were stopped or changed. A lot of people with problematic pain have tried several strategies before, and the treatment was either ineffective or intolerable. Look through medical notes—anaesthetic charts, medicine prescription charts, and clinic letters—and establish how post-operative pain was managed previously. Ask how the patient felt about these past experiences. You may find she had a wonderful experience with one operation, but a dreadful time with another which will help you plan your own management.

Case update

Your patient describes her abdominal pain as a deep, almost constant, ache with intermittent episodes of sharp, stabbing pain in her lower abdomen. She also complains of sharp, burning pain across her abdomen, worse around previous surgical scars. The pain can wake her at night, is often related to food, but it can come on at any time. Before this episode, her pain, although present, was controlled. It interfered less with her day-to-day life than previously, and she had recently returned to studying for her university degree. She scores her usual pain level as 4/10 on a verbal rating scale (VRS).

Since her admission, her pain has been much worse and more continuous. Her usual medications include paracetamol, slow-release morphine 50 mg, short-acting oral morphine 15 mg, as required (taken twice on normal days, sometimes more, up to six times per day), gabapentin 600 mg three times daily, sulfasalazine, and lactulose. During this admission, she has had IV antibiotics and steroids. She has been intermittently nil by mouth and has been mainly receiving subcutaneous morphine 10 mg for analgesia.

In the past, she has tried amitriptyline which did not help her pain significantly but did leave her feeling drowsy and with a terribly dry mouth. Prior to starting morphine, she took tramadol and codeine which did not work well for her pain and worsened her inflammatory bowel symptoms. She completed a pain management programme a year ago where she learned relaxation skills to help her cope with her pain symptoms. She practises this 2–3 times a week.

She had a laparotomy with bowel resection 3 years ago, following a severe flare-up, requiring high dependency care. Her anaesthetic management at that time was general anaesthesia with opiates and a ketamine bolus, followed by morphine PCA. She had a lot of pain post-operatively, and the acute pain team were involved. She is currently 62 kg.

A letter from the chronic pain clinic suggests, in addition to the pain from her inflammatory bowel disease, she suffers from CPSP with hyperalgesia and allodynia around the area of her abdominal scars.

Who may be able to assist you with planning this patient's analgesia?

It is important to make the acute pain team aware of any patients with potentially complicated analgesia and to discuss your plan with them. It may also be useful to inform the chronic pain consultant involved with the patient, particularly if they are still seeing the patient regularly or if you have any questions about their treatment.

How would you manage this patient's opioid therapy through the perioperative period?

Patients on chronic opioid therapy may include chronic pain patients, cancer patients, and patients with substance misuse disorders. For many of these patients, a dose reduction is part of their long-term treatment plan. Patients can be anxious about increasing their opioid, which may be perceived as a failure or setback, and also fearful of anticipated pain. The acute situation is not the time to be focussed on reducing the background opioid dosage, and the patient, and staff involved in their care, should be aware of this. A more realistic aim would be to discharge the patient with a regime similar to what they were prescribed prior to admission, or a clear plan with that goal in mind. Occasionally, an operation does reduce, or remove, the cause of pain, such as in some cases of cancer surgery or neurosurgery, and the dosage of opioid should be decreased cautiously, bearing in mind that an abrupt cessation may result in withdrawal symptoms.

The selection of opioid and the route of administration depends on the individual patient's situation. The aim is to administer a suitable dose that provides satisfactory pain relief and to avoid detrimental effects, including opioid toxicity. Ideally, the background opioid dose should be maintained, and the acute pain treated in addition.

In this patient's circumstance, where she has been acutely unwell and has not been able to take oral medications, opioids must be provided by another route. An appropriate solution would be a background IV morphine infusion, combined with PCA. This approach would usually require high dependency care to ensure appropriate monitoring is provided.

Discuss the oral to intravenous opioid conversion equivalences

Your patient takes morphine sulphate, slow-release tablets, totalling 100 mg/24 hours and equalling 33 mg/24 hours intravenously. This dose would be provided by an infusion with concentrations of morphine sulphate of 2 mg/mL at 0.5–1 mL/hour. Her daily requirements in hospital are likely to be higher and should be calculated from her medicine chart. It is likely the 10 mg morphine subcutaneous injections she has been receiving are inadequate, and she may require an initial loading dose of morphine to control her pain. Once the morphine PCA is in place, the patient should be reviewed after a few hours to ensure optimal pain control. Direct comparison of opioids and consequent equianalgesic doses can be difficult to ascertain. Local guidance should be consulted. Table 15.4 provides a guide with information drawn from personal knowledge and corroborated by several sources such as the *British National Formulary*'s Prescribing in Palliative Care, MIMS online, and the Scottish Intercollegiate Guidelines Network guideline (see Further reading at the end of this case).

If opioid switching is necessary, an opioid conversion tool should be consulted to calculate equivalent doses (see also Table 15.5). Some physicians, when

Table 15.4 Opioid equivalence table

	Dose equivalent
Morphine PO	10 mg
Morphine IM/SC	5 mg
Morphine IV	3.3 mg
Morphine epidural	1 mg
Diamorphine SC/IV	3 mg
Tramadol PO	50–100 mg
Dihydrocodeine PO	100 mg
Codeine PO	80–100 mg
Oxycodone PO	5—6.6 mg
Oxycodone IV	3—5 mg
Fentanyl IV	100 micrograms

PO, oral; IM, intramuscular; SC, subcutaneous; IV, intravenous.

Note: this is a guide only. Any change in opioids should be done with caution, due to interindividual variations of cross-tolerance and metabolism.

Table 15.5 Transdermal opioid conversion tables

Transdermal fentanyl (micrograms/hour)	Fentanyl dose in 24 hours (micrograms)	Oral morphine equivalent (mg/24 hours)	Immediate-release oral morphine dose, 4-hourly (mg)
25	600	60–120	<20
50	1200	120–200	20–30
75	1800	180–300	40–50
100	2400	240–400	40–60

Transdermal buprenorphine (micrograms/hour)	Buprenorphine dose in 24 hours (micrograms)	Oral morphine equivalent (mg/24 hours)	Immediate-release oral morphine dose, 4-hourly (mg)
BuTrans® 5	120	10–15	2.5–5
BuTrans® 10	240	15–25	5
BuTrans® 20	480	25–80	5–15
Transtec® 35	840	85–120	20
Transtec® 52.5	1260	125–150	25
Transtec® 70	1680	160–200	30

Based on recommendations by the manufacturers and *British National Formulary*.

switching opioids, e.g. from fentanyl to morphine, advocate reducing the 24-hour dose by up to 50%, as patients genetically differ in cross-tolerance to opioids, and there is a risk of inducing opiate toxicity. This is less of an issue in the hospital setting where the patient can be monitored closely, and, during a dose reduction, the patient can be given additional opioid at any time, if required. Close monitoring is particularly desirable for the patient on high-dose opioids (>200mg of oral morphine equivalent/24hours).

What are the general guidelines for dealing with any patient requiring opioids?

◆ Minimize the number of routes of administration and of the different types of opioids. For example, if a patient's background opioid is a fentanyl patch and this is to continue, a fentanyl PCA would be an appropriate option. The more complicated things are, the higher the risk of drug error and opioid toxicity

◆ Write clear prescriptions, and document your plan in the medical notes. You may have formulated a perfect strategy, but unless it is communicated effectively, it will be lost when the out-of-hours team are dealing with the patient.

What non-opiate analgesia may be of use for this patient?

◆ Paracetamol reduces opioid requirements significantly. Some patients do not perceive it has benefits, but an explanation of its usefulness in increasing the efficacy of opiate medications usually helps with compliance

◆ NSAIDs are very effective analgesics. Of course, there are important contraindications (renal impairment, coagulopathy, and atopic asthma, to name a few), but ask at the pre-assessment visit if the patient is able to take them without side effects. Check with the surgeon if there are concerns about perioperative effects, e.g. in some orthopaedic surgery. Surgeons may be happy for NSAIDs to be prescribed as required or as a once-only medication. If the oral route is unavailable, IV and PR formulations can be used. Consider prescribing a PPI if concerned about gastric irritation (and continue for 2–3 days post-treatment)

◆ Local anaesthetics are used extensively to treat pain in the hospital setting. Where possible, use it. Consider it for every procedure—local infiltration, peripheral nerve blocks and catheters, neuraxial blockade, wound catheters or intravenous infusion. Local anaesthetics are particularly useful for wound pain and can be given in the recovery area, if necessary; ask the surgeon to do this if any concerns about injecting the wound area

- Ketamine, an NMDA antagonist, is a useful opioid-sparing analgesic, particularly for neuropathic pain (and it is increasingly recognized that acute surgical pain will often have a neuropathic element). Advise patients about side effects, as they are likely to be better tolerated if forewarned, e.g. hallucinations and dark dreams. It can be given as a bolus intraoperatively and/or a subcutaneous or IV infusion perioperatively. Many hospital wards are now comfortable managing subcutaneous ketamine infusions, alleviating the need for HDU care

- Clonidine, a centrally acting α2-agonist, is also a good opioid-sparing analgesic. Most often used perioperatively via the IV or epidural route, it can also come in immediate and slow-release tablets and patches. It is used in many conditions such as hypertension, restless legs, and opioid withdrawal. If administered intravenously, it can be given as a titrated bolus, with close monitoring for hypotension and bradycardia, or by infusion. As this is not used routinely for many cases, a patient on a clonidine infusion will require care in a high dependency area, with instructions clearly documented, including common adverse effects—as mentioned previously, plus drowsiness, dry mouth, headache, postural hypotension, and anxiety.

Is intravenous or oral opioid analgesia optimal?

- Oral opioids should be used whenever enteral fluids are well tolerated. This general principle applies to many medications. It removes the need for repeated IV or subcutaneous cannula insertions; it saves on resources and time for staff and is one move closer to the patient getting back to normal.

Whatever treatment you administer, it will be more effective if it is discussed beforehand with the patient. Explain how it will work, and reassure them that there is something that can be done for their pain. Remember that pain perception, and therefore pain relief, is about much more than just a few receptors in the CNS. The brain is a powerful tool; it can create pain when there is no physical stimulus and hide it where there is obvious tissue damage. Be empathetic, and your treatment will be more successful.

Case update

Your patient has her operation under general anaesthesia with a thoracic epidural. Post-operatively, she returns to the HDU where her background morphine infusion and PCA are continued, with a plain local anaesthetic epidural infusion. She is also prescribed regular paracetamol. On day 2, she is allowed sips of water; her oral morphine and gabapentin are restarted, and her background morphine infusion discontinued. You go to see her on day 3 when her epidural has been removed, and she is comfortable with her PCA and oral medication. She is hoping to be discharged to the ward today and expects her PCA to stop soon. Overall, she is pleased with the analgesia she received and thanks you for taking care of her.

Summary

Patients with chronic pain can be challenging to manage in the acute setting. The mainstay of acute perioperative analgesia is opioid medications, and there are many useful adjuncts such as local anaesthesia. Patients who are already established on opioid therapy need careful management at this time to avoid withdrawal syndrome, opioid toxicity, and uncontrolled pain. As with all pain management, communication is the key—including with the patient.

Further reading

British National Formulary. *Prescribing in palliative care*, March 2013.

British Pain Society (2010). *Opioids for persistent pain: good practice*. Available at: <http://www.britishpainsociety.org/book_opioid_main.pdf>.

Chou R, Fanciullo GJ, Fine PG, *et al.* (2009). Clinical guidelines for the use of chronic opioid therapy in chronic noncancer pain. *Journal of Pain*, **10**, 113–230.

Kehlet H, Jensen TS, and Woolf CJ (2006). Persistent postsurgical pain: risk factors and prevention. *Lancet*, **367**, 1618–25.

Lewis N and Williams J (2005). Acute pain management in patients receiving opioids for chronic and cancer pain. *Continuing Education in Anaesthesia, Critical Care & Pain*, **5**, 127–9.

Macintyre PE, Schug SA, Scott DA, Visser EJ, and Walker SM; APM:SE Working Group of the Australian and New Zealand College of Anaesthetists and Faculty of Pain Medicine (2010). *Acute pain management: scientific evidence*, 3rd edn. Australian and New Zealand College of Anaesthetists and Faculty of Pain Medicine, Melbourne.

Macrae WA (2008). Chronic post-surgical pain: 10 years on. *British Journal of Anaesthesia*, **101**, 77–86.

MIMS Online. *Opioid analgesics: approximate potency equivalence with oral morphine.* Available at:<http://www.mims.co.uk/Guidelines/1146201/Opioid-Analgesics-Approximate-Potency-Equivalence-Oral-Morphine/>.

Scottish Intercollegiate Guidelines Network (2008). *Control of pain in adults with cancer*, SIGN guideline 106. Available at: <http://www.sign.ac.uk/pdf/qrg106.pdf>.

Appendix 1

Royal College of Anaesthetists CPD matrix: level 2

See Figure A1.1 for the Royal College of Anaesthetists CPD matrix: level 1;
Figure A1.2 for the Royal College of Anaesthetists CPD matrix: level 2;
Figure A1.3 for the Royal College of Anaesthetists CPD matrix: level 3.

1	Scientific Principles*	Emergency Management and Resuscitation	Airway Management	Pain Medicine	Patient Safety	Legal Aspects of Practice	IT Skills	Education and Training	Healthcare Management
	Physiology and biochemistry (1AA01)	Anaphylaxis (1BA01)	Airway assessment (1CA01)	Assessment of acute pain (1DA01)	Infection control (1EA01)	Consent (1FA01)	Use of patient record systems (1GA01)	Roles and responsibilities of clinical supervisors (1HA01)	Critical incident reporting (1IA01)
	Pharmacology and therapeutics (1AA02)	Can't intubate, can't ventilate (1BA02)	Basic airway management (1CA02)	Management of acute pain (1DA02)	Level 2 and Level 3 child protection training (see recommendations and competencies) (1EA02)	Mental capacity and deprivation of liberty safeguards (1FA02)	Basic search methodology (1GA02)	Personal education and learning (1HA02)	Team leadership and resource management (1IA02)
	Physics and clinical measurement (1AA03)	Basic life support (all age groups and special situations) (1BA03)			Protection of vulnerable adults (1EA03)	Data protection (1FA03)			Human factors in anaesthetic practice (1IA03)
		Advanced life support (relevant to practice) (1BA04)			Blood product checking protocols (to comply with local requirements) (1EA04)	Equality and diversity (1FA04)			Understanding of complaints process (1IA04)
					Venous thromboembolism prophylaxis (1EA05)	Ethics (1FA05)			Quality improvement (1IA05)

*At least one lecture/e-Learning session/CEACCP article to be completed relevant to your clinical practice for each of the three aspects of Scientific principles detailed in one revalidation cycle.

Fig. A1.1 Royal College of Anaesthetists CPD matrix: level 1. Reproduced with permission of the Royal College of Anaesthetists.

General	Obstetrics	ICM	Paediatrics	Pain Medicine	Neuro	Regional Anaesthesia	Education and Training
Advanced airway management (1A01)	Analgesia for labour (1B01)	Assessment of the critically ill patient (1C01)	Assessment and initial management of the critically ill child (1D01)	Advanced management of perioperative pain (1E01)	Initial management: of brain injury (traumatic or spontaneous intracranial haemorrhage) (1F01)	Indications, benefits and risks of RA (1G01)	Work-place based assessment (1H01)
Principles of assessment and management of major trauma (including burns) (1A02)	General anaesthesia for elective and emergency LSCS (1B02)	Initiation and management of ventilatory support (1C02)	Perioperative care of children (1D02)	Management of acute non-surgical pain (1E02)	Initial management of spinal injured patients (1F02)	Principles of performing local, regional and neuraxial techniques (1G02)	Educational supervisor training (1H02)
Preoperative assessment and preparation for surgery (1A03)	Regional anaesthesia for elective and emergency LSCS (1B03)	Diagnosis and management of shock, infection and sepsis (1C03)	Vascular access techniques (1D03)	Basic assessment and management of chronic pain (1E03)	Management of patients with neuro trauma for imaging (1F03)	Use of nerve/plexus location techniques (1G03)	
Advanced patient monitoring techniques (1A04)	Regional anaesthesia complications in the pregnant patient (1B04)	Support of threatened and failing organ systems (1C04)	Fluid management for children (1D04)			Recognition and management of side effects and complications of regional anaesthesia (1G04)	
Fluid management and blood product usage (1A05)	Management of obstetric emergencies (1B05)	Sedation techniques for ICU patients (1C05)	Analgesia for children (1D05)				
Perioperative emergencies (1A06)	Assessment of the critically ill parturient (1B06)	End of life issues and organ donation (1C06)	Sedation techniques for children (1D06)				
Perioperative management for surgical specialties not listed elsewhere (1A07)	Principles of newborn resuscitation (1B07)	Management of the ICU (1C07)	Team working between DGHs and PIC retrieval teams (1D07)				
Anaesthetic management for non-operative procedures (1A08)							
Anaesthesia for non-obstetric procedures in the pregnant patient (1A09)							
Sedation techniques for adults (1A10)							
Patient transfer skills (1A11)							
Developments in allied clinical specialties (relevant to practice) (1A12)							

Fig. A1.2 Royal College of Anaesthetists CPD matrix: level 2. Reproduced with permission of the Royal College of Anaesthetists.

3	Faculty/specialist society (where there is no website shown there are currently no specific recommendations for Level 3 CPD in this special interest area)
Airway management	(3A01)
ENT, maxillo-facial and dental surgery	(3A02)
General, urological and gynaecological surgery	(3A03)
Hepatobiliary surgery	(3A04)
Vascular surgery	(3A05) www.vasgbi.com/CPD.php
Day surgery	(3A06) www.daysurgeryuk.net/bads
Sedation practice	(3A07)
Orthopaedic surgery	(3A08)
Regional anaesthesia	(3A09)
Trauma management (including pre-hospital care)	(3A10)
Transfer medicine	(3A11)
Ophthalmic	(3A12) www.boas.org/cpd.html
Bariatric	(3A13) www.sobauk.com/index.php?option=com_phocadownload&view=file&id=17:royal-college-of-anaesthetists-cpd-programme-skills&itemid=61
Military anaesthesia	(3A14) www.rcoa.ac.uk/sites/default/files/CPD-MILITARY-2013.pdf
Obstetrics	(3B00) www.oaa-anaes.ac.uk/content.asp?ContentID=328
Adult ICM	(3C00) www.ficm.ac.uk/cpdandrevalidation.ashx
Paediatrics and paediatric ICM	(3D00) www.apagbi.org.uk/professionals/professional-standards/safeguarding
Pain medicine	(3E00) www.rcoa.ac.uk/faculty-of-pain-medicine/cpd
Neuro (including neuro critical care)	(3F00) www.nasgbi.org.uk/pages/neuroanaesthesia-cpd
Cardiothoracic	(3G00) www.acta.org.uk/ACTAS3CurrentTraining.asp
Plastic/burns	(3H00)
Other clinical	(3J00)
Other non-clinical	(3J00)
IT skills	(3J01) www.scata.org.uk/mediawiki/images/8/8c/CPD_1-3list_SCATAFeb2011.pdf
Education and training	(3J02) www.seauk.org/?q=node/57
Research	(3J03)

Fig. A1.3 Royal College of Anaesthetists CPD matrix: level 3. Reproduced with permission of the Royal College of Anaesthetists.

Appendix 2

List of cross-references between chapters

Chapter	Cross referenced with
Chapter 1—General anaesthesia	
1.1 Waiting times: improving theatre productivity and minimizing expenditure	
1.2 Assessing and explaining risk and predicting outcome	4.3 Regional anaesthesia in the elderly patient 8.2 Acute epiglottitis 9.3 Elective aorto-femoral arterial revascularization 10.1 Lung isolation techniques 12.1 Laparoscopic radical prostatectomy
1.3 'Did I really do that?' Managing the aftermath of a serious adverse event	
1.4 Current approaches to complex colorectal surgery	
Chapter 2—Trauma and resuscitation	
2.1 Major haemorrhage	2.4 General anaesthesia for major trauma 5.1 Major obstetric haemorrhage 11.1 Anaesthesia for major liver resection
2.2 Burns	8.4 Airway obstruction
2.3 Sepsis	5.5 Severe sepsis in pregnancy 12.3 Percutaneous nephrolithotomy
2.4 General anaesthesia for major trauma	2.1 Major haemorrhage 7.1 Principles of neuroanaesthesia 13.1 Cervical spinal injury 14.1 Pre-hospital management of a multiple injured trauma patient
Chapter 3—Day case anaesthesia	
3.1 Post-operative nausea and vomiting	
3.2 Day case dental anaesthesia	

(*continued*)

Chapter	Cross referenced with
Chapter 4—Regional anaesthesia	
4.1 Lower limb anaesthesia	
4.2 Upper limb regional anaesthesia	
4.3 Regional anaesthesia in the elderly patient	1.2 Assessing and explaining risk and predicting outcome
Chapter 5—Obstetric anaesthesia	
5.1 Major obstetric haemorrhage	2.1 Major haemorrhage
5.2 Pre-eclampsia	
5.3 Morbidly obese in obstetrics	
5.4 Peripartum cardiomyopathy	
5.5 Severe sepsis in pregnancy	2.3 Sepsis
Chapter 6—Paediatric anaesthesia	
6.1 Prematurity	
6.2 Intravenous fluids for children	8.1 Bleeding tonsils 13.4 Morquio's syndrome 14.2 The collapsed neonate
6.3 The uncooperative child	
6.4 Pyloric stenosis	
Chapter 7—Neuroanaesthesia	
7.1 Principes of neuroanaesthesia	2.4 General anaesthesia for major trauma
7.2 Acute subdural haematoma	
7.3 Endovascular treatment of subarachnoid haemorrhage due to ruptured berry aneurysm	7.4 Clipping of aneurysm
7.4 Clipping of aneurysm	7.3 Endovascular treatment of subarachnoid haemorrhage due to ruptured berry aneurysm
7.5 Posterior fossa craniectomy	
7.6 Awake craniotomy	
Chapter 8—Ear, nose, and throat anaesthesia	
8.1 Bleeding tonsils	6.2 Intravenous fluids for children
8.2 Acute epiglottitis	1.2 Assessing and explaining risk and predicting outcome 14.4 The stridulous infant
8.3 Inhaled foreign body	
8.4 Airway obstruction	2.2 Burns Chapter 13 Introduction 13.2 Acromegaly 13.3 Thyroid tumour

Chapter	Cross referenced with
Chapter 9—Vascular anaesthesia	
9.1 Ruptured abdominal aorticx aneurysm	9.1 Ruptured abdominal aortic aneurysm
9.2 Carotid endarterectomy	
9.3 Elective aorto-femoral arterial revascularization	1.2 Assessing and explaining risk and predicting outcome
Chapter 10—Cardiothoracic anaesthesia	
10.1 Lung isolation techniques	1.2 Assessing and explaining risk and predicting outcome
10.2 Off-pump cardiopulmonary bypass	
10.3 Valve replacement surgery	
10.4 Transcatheter cardiac valve surgery	
Chapter 11—Hepatobiliary and transplant anaesthesia	
11.1 Anaesthesia for major liver resection	2.1 Major haemorrhage
11.2 Acute liver failure	
11.3 Anaesthesia following renal transplantation	
11.4 Management of the brainstem-dead organ donor	
Chapter 12—Urology	
12.1 Laparoscopic radical prostatectomy	1.2 Assessing and explaining risk and predicting outcome
12.2 Total cystectomy with ileal conduit formation	
12.3 Percutaneous nephrolithotomy	2.3 Sepsis
12.4 Transurethral resection of the prostate	
Chapter 13—The difficult airway	
Introduction	8.4 Airway obstruction
13.1 Cervical spine injury	2.4 General anaesthesia for major trauma 14.1 Pre-hospital management of a multiple injured trauma patient
13.2 Acromegaly	8.4 Airway obstruction 13.3 Thyroid tumour
13.3 Thyroid tumour	8.4 Airway obstruction 13.2 Acromegaly
13.4 Morquio's syndrome	6.2 Intravenous fluid for children

(continued)

Chapter	Cross referenced with
Chapter 14—Transport and retrieval medicine	
14.1 Pre-hospital management of a multiple injured trauma victim	2.4 General anaesthesia for major trauma 13.1 Cervical spine injury
14.2 The collapsed neonate	6.2 Intravenous fluid for children
14.3 Time critical transfers by referring clinicians	
14.4 The stridulous infant	8.2 Acute epiglottitis
14.5 Aeromedical transport considerations in acute lung injury	
Chapter 15—Pain medicine	
15.1 Chronic regional pain syndrome	
15.2 Phantom limb pain	
15.3 Chronic post-surgical pain	
15.4 Regional vs systemic analgesia	15.5 Managing chronic pain patients for elective surgery
15.5 Managing chronic pain patients for elective surgery	15.4 Regional vs systemic analgesia

Index

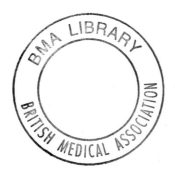